COMMUNITY RESOURCES
FOR OLDER ADULTS

EDITION

I am dedicating this book to Jani Malkiewicz who, after 20 years, continues to encourage and offer her unconditional support for all of my travels and endeavors.

—RRW

I am dedicating this book to my husband, Steven Sheetz, for his support, thoughtful words, understanding when I needed time to write, and much-needed hugs during the entire process.

—KAR

COMMUNITY RESOURCES FOR OLDER ADULTS
Programs and Services in an Era of Change

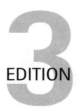

EDITION

Robbyn R. Wacker
University of Northern Colorado
Karen A. Roberto
Virginia Polytechnic Institute and State University

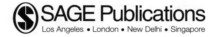
SAGE Publications
Los Angeles • London • New Delhi • Singapore

For information:

Sage Publications, Inc.
2455 Teller Road
Thousand Oaks, California 91320
E-mail: order@sagepub.com

Sage Publications Ltd.
1 Oliver's Yard
55 City Road
London EC1Y 1SP
United Kingdom

Sage Publications India Pvt. Ltd.
B 1/I 1 Mohan Cooperative Industrial Area
Mathura Road, New Delhi 110 044
India

Sage Publications Asia-Pacific Pte. Ltd.
33 Pekin Street #02-01
Far East Square
Singapore 048763

Printed in the United States of America.

Library of Congress Cataloging-in-Publication Data

Wacker, Robbyn R. Community resources for older adults : programs and services in an era of change / Robbyn R. Wacker, Karen A. Roberto.—3rd ed.
      p. cm.
Includes bibliographical references and index.
ISBN 978-1-4129-5129-6 (cloth : alk. paper)

    1. Older people—Services for—United States. 2. Community health services for older people—United States. 3. Old age assistance—United States. 4. Older volunteers in social service—United States. I. Roberto, Karen A. II. Title.

HV1461.W32 2008
362.6'30973—dc22   2007031735

This book is printed on acid-free paper.

07   08   09   10   11   10   9   8   7   6   5   4   3   2   1

Acquisitions Editor:	Kassie Graves
Editorial Assistant:	Veronica Novak
Production Editor:	Karen Wiley
Copy Editor:	Susan Jarvis
Typesetter:	C&M Digitals (P) Ltd.
Proofreader:	Tracy Marcynzsyn
Indexer:	Kay Dusheck
Cover Designer:	Gail Buschman
Marketing Manager:	Carmel Withers

Brief Contents

Detailed Contents

PART II THE CONTINUUM OF SERVICES

4 Information and Assistance   53

5 Volunteer and Intergenerational Programs   73

6 Education Programs   93

7 Senior Centers and Recreation   115

8 Employment Programs   137

9 Income Programs   151

10 Nutrition and Meal Programs   167

11 Health Care and Wellness   189

12 Mental Health Services   219

13 Legal Services   239

14 Transportation   261

15 Housing   283

16 Care Management   311

17 Home Care Services   331

PART III   PREPARING FOR THE FUTURE

20 Programs and Services in an Era of Change   393

The Authors' Purpose

Students preparing for careers in gerontology and related areas need more than a description of existing community resources available for older adults. They need to understand how programs come to exist through federal legislation, who uses these resources, how they are delivered, and the challenges service providers face in meeting the needs of the aging baby boom cohort.

We have developed a text that gives students a basic understanding of aging policy that created the "aging network" and of theories that can be used to explain help-seeking behavior. Each chapter provides the reader with an in-depth review of the programs and services provided by the "aging network" and the private sector, current scholarship in each topic area, and national and internet resources. Students will learn to identify the challenges inherent in providing services to older adults through case studies, learning activities, and best-practice models. Instructors can use these learning activities to stimulate critical thinking about service delivery and to explore what changes might be needed in the future. We hope that *Community Resources for Older Adults* is a text that both you and your students enjoy.

Robbyn R. Wacker
University of Northern Colorado

Karen A. Roberto
Virginia Polytechnic Institute and State University

Acknowledgments

As is typical of a project of this magnitude, many people have helped us along the way. Some did so willingly, others by default because they were in the right (or maybe wrong) place at a time that we needed help. We would like to take this opportunity to acknowledge those persons who made undertaking the revisions for this edition a pleasant and manageable experience. First, we thank former and current graduate students at the University of Northern Colorado (UNC) and at Virginia Polytechnic Institute and State University (Virginia Tech) for all their help in collecting articles, tracking down references, and offering feedback. They include Sonja Rizzolo-Letzen from UNC and Nancy Brossoie, Erica Husser, Marya McPherson, and Pamela Murphy from Virginia Tech. Our secretarial staff Carlene Arthur and Frances Braafhart supported us in many ways. We appreciate the assistance of Sharon Larson, Region VIII Administration on Aging, for providing so much information on the Older Americans Act and its history. Thanks to Linda Piper, former director of the Weld County Area Agency on Aging, who was our co-author for the first two editions of the text. We are also indebted to the reviewers who offered their insights for the third edition:

Varsha Pandya, Ohio University

Denise Gammonley, University of Central Florida

Joaquin Anguera, San Diego State University

M. C. "Terry" Hokenstad, Case Western University

Shanta Sharma, Henderson State University

Patricia K. Cianciolo, Northern Michigan University

Sandy Cook-Fong, University of Nebraska, Kearney

Louise Murray, UNC Charlotte

Daphne Joslin, William Paterson University

Rochelle Elaine Rottenberg, St. Catherine/St. Thomas

A big thank you goes to Kassie Graves and her staff at Sage, who aptly guided us through the revision of the second edition.

Robbyn R. Wacker
Karen A. Roberto

PART I

The Social Context of Community Resource Delivery

1

On the Threshold of a New Era

What will society in the United States be like in the year 2030? It is hard to know exactly how different our daily lives will be, but we do know that by the year 2030 our society will be experiencing something that none other has experienced. As we move through the twenty-first century, more Americans than ever before will be in their seventh, eighth, and ninth decades of life. By the year 2030, the first members of the baby boom generation, born in 1946, will be 84 years of age, and the youngest members, born in 1964, will be 65. By the year 2030, there will be about 71.5 million people aged 65 and older—more than twice the number in 2000 (Federal Interagency Forum on Aging-Related Statistics, 2004). Demographically, the baby boom cohort is sandwiched between two smaller cohorts. As a result of its enormous size and vast racial and ethnic diversity, it has commanded attention at every stage of its life course. In the 1960s, school systems were forced to react to the soaring enrollments of the baby boom cohort; soon social institutions that serve the older population will be challenged to respond to the baby boomers as well.

Will this graying of our population dramatically change our society? As demographers, economists, gerontologists, and sociologists debate this question, we can be relatively safe in predicting that, because of their unique characteristics, the aging baby boomers will cause a reexamination of current aging policies and services. Unlike the generations before them, collectively they will be better educated, better off financially, living in the suburbs, and beneficiaries of the programs that were put in place for their grandparents. On the other hand, this giant cohort is tremendously diverse. About 89% of boomers have completed high school and 29% have a bachelor's degree or more (MetLife, 2005a). Although boomers' earnings are comparable with their parents' at a similar stage in life, the distribution of wealth in the United States has become more unequal in the past two decades; it is projected that 2% of boomers will live in poverty and 5% will live in near-poverty (up to 125% of the poverty line) in 2030 (Smith, 2003). Race and ethnicity are related to poverty in late life. About 7.5% of White elders lived below the poverty level in 2004, compared with 23.9% of Black elders, 13.6% of Asian elders, and 18.7% of Hispanic elders (Administration on Aging [AoA], 2005a). The high rates of poverty will no doubt have implications for the financial wellbeing and quality of life of persons of all races and ethnicities in later life.

Another unique characteristic of the boomer cohort is their marriage and family patterns as compared with those of their parents and grandparents. Boomers tended to marry later, and have smaller families and higher rates of divorce than their parents. Approximately 14% of boomers are divorced, compared with 7% of people age 65 and older (MetLife, 2005a). In addition, the percentage of boomers who never married (12.6%) is significantly higher than for prior generations (4–5%). As a result, boomers are redefining the traditional definition of "family" and thereby increasing the complexity of kin networks. Boomer families take many forms, including single-parent families, step-families, cohabiting heterosexual and same-gender couples, childless families, and intergenerational families. Because families play a key role in providing instrumental and emotional support, as well as long-term care, to their older members, it is uncertain how these changes will influence family support patterns. For example, will adult children feel an obligation to care for both biological and step-parents? Will families who choose not to have children be at risk of having fewer informal resources? Will friends and families of choice be acknowledged and accepted as important sources of support and caregivers for lesbian, gay, bisexual, and transgender elders? Although the exact influence of family composition changes on the use of formal services is not known, we can anticipate that community programs and services will play a significant role in the lives of *all* older adults.

Collectively, these demographic characteristics will shape the type, amount, and nature of community resources in the future. They will increase the demand for home health care and retirement housing options. Many baby boomers will move into third, fourth, and even fifth careers and seek educational opportunities and greater flexibility in work and retirement options. The social safety net may need to be expanded for the underclass and lower class. The sheer numbers of aged boomers will challenge policy makers to rethink health care, retirement programs, and pension plans. Even now, projections—both dire and not so dire—are being made about Social Security and Medicare. Thus demographic characteristics of the next generation of older adults will have direct implications on social policies that, in turn, support programs and services for older adults. In this next section, we discuss a few more of the salient demographic characteristics of the boomer cohort.

GROWTH OF THE OLDER POPULATION

The projected growth in the older population is shown in Exhibit 1.1. In 1950, 12.3 million persons (8.2% of the population) were aged 65 and older. By 2004, that number increased to 36.3 million (12.4% of the population; AoA, 2005a), and it is expected to grow to 71.5 million (19.6% of the population) by 2030 (Federal Interagency Forum on Aging-Related Statistics, 2004). Members of the older population are also aging. In 2004, 18.5 million persons were between the ages of 65 and 74, 13.0 million persons constituted the 75–84 age group, and 4.9 million people were 85 years of age and older (AoA, 2005a). Moreover, persons 85 years of age and older represent the fastest-growing part of the older adult population. The population aged 85 and older will more than double from approximately 4.2 million in 2000 to 9.6 million in 2030 and will increase to 20.9 million by 2050 (Federal Interagency Forum on Aging-Related Statistics, 2004).

What are the social implications of such an increase in the older adult population? Many writers in the popular press suggest that the increase in the number of older adults signals an impending social and fiscal crisis and that aged persons will become a financial burden to society (e.g., Bryant, 2001; Samuelson, 2005). Others (Dychtwald, 2000; Friedan, 1995; Gambone, 2001) argue that a "crisis mentality" overlooks other important demographic factors. Although it is true that the United States, along with other developed nations, will experience an increase in the older adult population, the number of older adults has steadily increased during the past 130 years. This steady increase has allowed society to adapt to the changes of an aging population. Many scholars believe society will be able to adapt to this new cohort of older adults as well (Schulz & Binstock, 2006).

The assumption that older adults will place a burden on society is often based on the economic dependency ratio. The economic dependency ratio is the ratio of persons in the total population (including Armed Forces overseas and children) who are not in the labor force per 100 of those who are in the labor force. For every 100 persons in the 2004 labor force, about 65 persons were not. Of this group, about 44 were under the age of 16, and 21 were 16 to 64 years of age. The part of the dependency ratio that has been steadily increasing is the portion attributable to older persons. It is projected to rise to 22.6 older retired persons per 100 workers by 2014 (U.S. Bureau of Labor Statistics, 2005) and, on the basis of current projections of the composition of the population, will continue to rise with the aging of the baby boomers.

The increase in the number of older adults, however, does not automatically result in a greater social burden. The aging population presents serious challenges that face all sectors of society. Meeting these challenges will require a new vision of American life that reaches beyond the immediate challenge of the aging of the boomers and promotes active engagement and a high quality of life throughout the lifespan (AARP, 2005a).

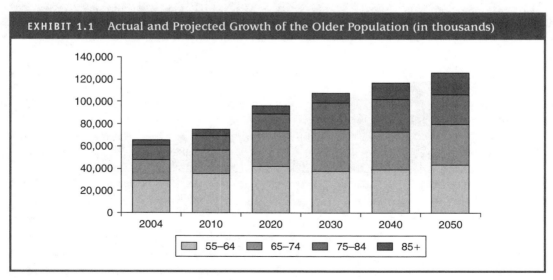

EXHIBIT 1.1   Actual and Projected Growth of the Older Population (in thousands)

Source: Data from U.S. Bureau of the Census (2000a, 2004a).

GROWTH OF THE OLDER POPULATION OF RACIAL AND ETHNIC MINORITIES

With the aging of the baby boomers, the older population is growing more diverse. Approximately 17% of baby boomers are from racial and ethnic minority groups: 8% are Black, 4% are Asian/Pacific Islander, and less than 1% (0.8%) are American Indian or Alaskan Native (U.S. Bureau of the Census, 2000a, 2004b). Fewer than 10% of boomers are of Hispanic origin. Although non-Hispanic White older adults will still represent a greater percentage of those over age 65 in the year 2050, the percentages of Hispanics and of non-Hispanic Blacks, American Indians, and Asian Americans will increase dramatically. Exhibit 1.2 illustrates the percentage of older adults by race for the years 2004 and 2050 (U.S. Bureau of the Census, 2000a, 2004a). This growing minority of the elder population brings new challenges and opportunities for providers of community programs and services (Goins, Mitchell, & Wu, 2006; Olson, 2001).

GROWTH IN THE NUMBER OF OLDER ADULTS LIVING ALONE

A final demographic characteristic with social service implications is the increase in the number of older adults who will be living alone. In 2004, 38% of all noninstitutionalized persons aged 65 years and older lived alone, representing 39.7% of older women and 18.8% of older men (AoA, 2005a). Living arrangements also varied by racial and ethnic status.

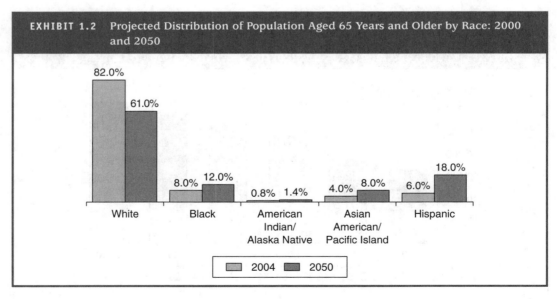

EXHIBIT 1.2   Projected Distribution of Population Aged 65 Years and Older by Race: 2000 and 2050

Source: Data from U.S. Bureau of the Census (2000a, 2004a).

Among both non-Hispanic White and Black women aged 65 and older, approximately 41% lived alone compared with 26.7% of Asian and 24.8% of Hispanic older women. In contrast, 18.7% of non-Hispanic older White men lived alone compared with 26.6% of Black, 9.9% of Asian and Pacific Islander, and 15.7% of Hispanic older men (Federal Interagency Forum on Aging-Related Statistics, 2006). Moreover, the percentage of older men and women living alone increased with age. Among women aged 75 and over, for example, approximately 50% live alone compared with about 30% of women aged 65–74 (AoA, 2005a). Differences in living arrangements of adults aged 65+ by sex, race, and Hispanic origin can be seen in Exhibit 1.3. Most notable is the generally high percentage of men who live with their spouses compared with women and the large percentage of women living alone, across all groups. Living with relatives occurs more than twice as often with Black and Hispanic women than with non-Hispanic women.

Older adults who live alone are more likely to live in poverty. In 2002, approximately 19.2% of persons aged 65 and older living alone were living in poverty compared with 5.1% of older married couples (U.S. Bureau of the Census, 2003). Sex, race, and ethnicity further differentiate the percentage of older adults living in poverty. For example, 40.6% of older Black women living alone were in poverty compared with 12.3% of older Black women living with their spouses. Similarly, 47.1% of older Hispanic women living alone lived in poverty compared with 14.9% of their married counterparts.

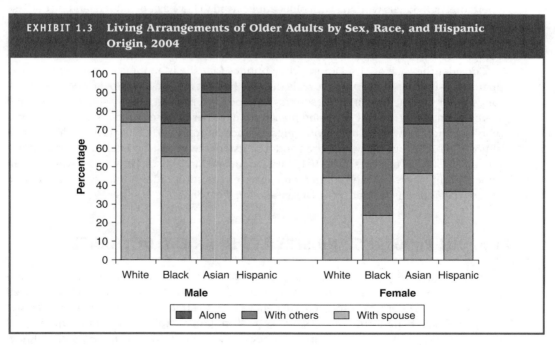

EXHIBIT 1.3   **Living Arrangements of Older Adults by Sex, Race, and Hispanic Origin, 2004**

Source: Federal Interagency Forum (2006).

IMPLICATIONS OF DEMOGRAPHIC CHARACTERISTICS FOR COMMUNITY RESOURCES

These selected demographic projections and unique characteristics have a number of implications for the delivery of community resources to older adults. The growth in the older adult population will increase the demand for all types of services. Professionals working to deliver the programs and services designed to improve the quality of life of older adults will thus be challenged to do even more with less. Because of the diverse nature of the boomer population with regard to ethnicity, income, family history, and life experience, professionals will be expected to be knowledgeable about a wide range of services and programs that serve both mainstream and disenfranchised individuals. Community programmers also must recognize and accommodate cultural diversity and remove the social and cultural barriers to service accessibility. A concerted effort needs to be made to design culturally appropriate programs and interventions that are responsive to the needs of minority communities (AoA, 2001a; Center on an Aging Society, 2004). Professionals must be visionaries in planning and developing services and programs to meet the needs of this new cohort with its diverse characteristics.

Now that we have had a chance to consider the challenges that lie ahead for services and programs that assist older adults, let's return to the present and consider more immediate issues. In every community, resources are designed to assist older adults in a variety of ways. Therefore, individuals working with older adults need to have a good understanding of these resources as well as the patterns of service use by older adults and their families. Anyone who has ever worked with older adults knows that the problems they confront tend to be complex and multifaceted.

Consider the case of Mrs. Duran, who confides that she is about to be evicted from her apartment. Further questioning reveals that she has not received her Social Security check for two months. She has limited resources for food, has received a utility shutoff notice, and has been unable to renew her insulin prescription for her diabetes. Or consider Mr. Jackson, who does not know what to do with himself since he retired. He has played golf or fished almost every day but is getting bored and disillusioned with retirement life. What community resources can be accessed to help Mrs. Duran and Mr. Jackson? Advocates who have an understanding of various programs and services assisting older adults can recommend appropriate options for both Mrs. Duran and Mr. Jackson.

A TEXT ABOUT PROGRAMS AND SERVICES IN AN ERA OF CHANGE

Because of the multiple challenges that older adults can experience and the changing demographics of the older adult population, we have created a text that provides a broad-based discussion of community resources. We believe that, to effectively meet the needs of older adults who can benefit from using services and programs, professionals must understand the social and psychological dynamics of help-seeking behavior. It is not enough to know what services are available and appropriate; practitioners must also be armed with theoretical knowledge to understand *why* a daughter, despite her exhaustion, refuses to bring her father to the local adult day program and *why* an older adult, who barely survives on a small pension, refuses to apply for additional income support that would make life a bit more bearable. In addition, we believe that practitioners must understand service use patterns and how families interact with the formal network when they need assistance in caring for their older family members. Greater understanding of these patterns can better prepare students and practitioners for understanding the dynamics of when and how families choose to use the formal network.

We also believe that simple descriptions of existing programs and services that assist older adults would provide an incomplete picture. Practitioners and students should benefit from the interplay that exists between research and practice because research results have practical applications for the delivery of services and programs. In each chapter, we draw from empirical research to describe who uses and provides such programs. We also include information about program outcomes when available.

Next, professionals need to be alerted to the infinite number of programs and services in communities that exist outside those funded through the Older Americans Act (OAA) of 1965 and subsequent amendments. Thus we attempt to introduce readers to many programs that are both publicly and privately funded. Moreover, we discuss the different ways in which aging programs have successfully networked with one another to develop public and private partnerships in an attempt to reach more older adults.

In preparing the third edition of this book, we maintained the organizational structure of previous editions while updating and expanding the content to address the changes in community programs and services available to older adults throughout the United States. In addition to including the most up-to-date statistical data available, we have described important updates and additions to federal policies that provide the underlying framework for aging services and resolutions from the 2005 White House Conference on Aging for meeting the needs of the current and future generations of aging adults. Each chapter includes reference to the latest research and highlights new programs and services that serve as examples of innovative ways in which communities are meeting the needs of older adults and their families. We acknowledge the increasing diversity among members of the aging population by addressing the need for cultural competency in service delivery and including new research findings (when available) and illustrative examples of resources and programs for older adults from different racial, ethnic, cultural, and faith groups as well as older persons living in rural areas, and for older adults who are gay, lesbian, bisexual, or transgender. The increasing availability of information online has allowed us to add many new web-based resources for students to access further information about a particular issue, policy, program, or service.

ORGANIZATION OF THE BOOK

This book consists of three parts. In addition to this chapter, Part I has two other chapters. Chapter 2 presents a brief review of major aging policies, including Social Security, Medicare, and the OAA, the basis for the existence of many older adult programs. Chapter 3 explains the patterns of service use by older adults and the theories that can predict help-seeking behavior.

Part II of the book is based on the concept of the *continuum of care*. Conceptually, the continuum of care is a system of social, personal, financial, and medical services that supports the wellbeing of any older adult, regardless of the person's level of functioning. The goal, of course, is to have the appropriate services available to match the presenting needs. The continuum is often conceptualized in a linear way—older adults move from one end of the continuum (independence) to the other (dependence), and services exist at every point along the continuum to meet their social, medical, and personal needs. In addition, services impinge differently on the personal autonomy of their participants. For example, those who attend senior centers come and go as they please and make choices about their level of participation. In contrast, a nursing home is the most restrictive environment and impinges a great deal on personal autonomy and choice.

We have opted to depict the continuum of care as a more dynamic and interactive system (see Exhibit 1.4). Rather than moving in a linear fashion from independence to dependence, older adults move in and out of areas of service need as they experience changing levels of independence and dependence, health and illness, and financial stability and instability. For example, older adults just discharged from the hospital may need in-home services as well as home-delivered meals. Yet, as they become less dependent, they may access services offered at the senior center. Those who are striving to maintain their independence can access services along the continuum.

Therefore, Part II presents the variety of community resources available for older adults and is divided into three sections, based on our depiction of the continuum of care. The first section presents information about *community services*. These are services that benefit older adults with low levels of dependency and impinge little on their personal autonomy. These services offer participants opportunities to enhance personal and social wellbeing. Specifically, we address information and referral services (Chapter 4), volunteer and intergenerational programs (Chapter 5), education (Chapter 6), senior centers (Chapter 7), employment programs (Chapter 8), and income assistance programs (Chapter 9).

Support services are discussed in the second section of Part II. These services help older adults who need assistance in maintaining their level of functioning. Support services include nutrition programs (Chapter 10), health and wellness programs (Chapter 11), mental health services (Chapter 12), legal services (Chapter 13), transportation (Chapter 14), and housing (Chapter 15).

The final chapters in Part II provide information about community-based and institutional long-term care services. These are services to assist individuals who have greater dependency needs. Chapters included in this section are on care management (Chapter 16), home care (Chapter 17), respite care (Chapter 18), and nursing homes (Chapter 19).

We have organized each chapter in Part II to include policy background, a description of users and programs, and future concerns. Each chapter includes case studies to help readers think critically about the service delivery issues. These cases were developed on the basis of actual experiences we have encountered (names and situations were altered to protect individuals' identity). In addition, best-practice models that highlight creative and unique programs and sources for additional information are presented. The best-practice models

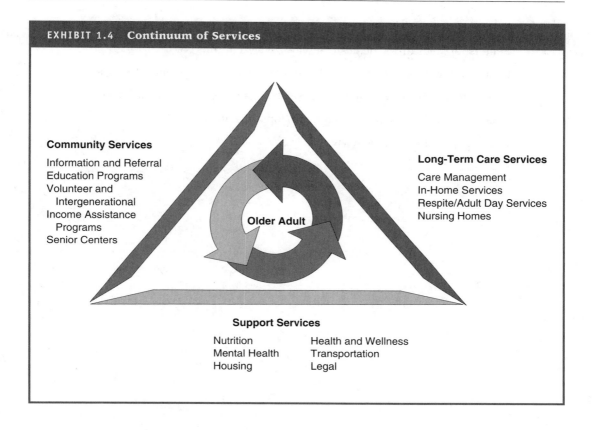

EXHIBIT 1.4   Continuum of Services

Community Services

Information and Referral
Education Programs
Volunteer and
    Intergenerational
Income Assistance
    Programs
Senior Centers

Older Adult

Long-Term Care Services

Care Management
In-Home Services
Respite/Adult Day Services
Nursing Homes

Support Services

Nutrition   Health and Wellness
Mental Health   Transportation
Housing   Legal

are representative of the programs and services that exist in various communities. Learning activities designed to expand understanding of the issues are also included. Additional resources, including the names and addresses of professional organizations and internet resources, are located at the end of each chapter.

Part III contains the final chapter on programs and services for the future (Chapter 20). This chapter presents an in-depth look at the challenges that lie ahead for the aging network.

Accessing Updated Information

Because statistical profiles of older adults are constantly being updated and because Congress frequently enacts legislation that affects the existence of community resources and programs, information presented in texts such as this can become quickly outdated. To keep up with these changes, we recommend regular visits to the following websites and others suggested throughout this book:

Administration on Aging: www.aoa.gov

Centers for Medicare & Medicaid Services: www.cms.hhs.gov

Data Warehouse on Trends in Health and Aging: www.cdc.gov/nchs/agingact.htm

Federal Interagency Forum on Aging-Related Statistics: www.agingstats.gov

FIRSTGOV for Seniors: www.firstgov.gov/Topics/Seniors.shtml

U.S. Bureau of the Census: www.census.gov

2

Legislative Foundations for Programs, Services, and Benefits Supporting Older Adults

It had been a busy week at the Area Agency on Aging office. Dorothy, the administrative assistant, was tidying up her desk on Friday afternoon and thinking about all the people the office had helped that week. Mrs. Wright, in her early 80s, came first to her mind. Mrs. Wright's husband had just undergone surgery for throat cancer. For the next couple of months, he would be restricted to a liquid diet for most of his meals. A low-income couple, but at not poverty level, the Wrights could not afford the full cost of a nutritional food supplement at their local grocery store. The Wrights found out about the Area Agency on Aging's food supplement program from their doctor. It had saved them nearly half the cost of the two cases a week required for Mr. Wright while he was recovering. With her many years' experience working at the agency's front desk, Dorothy knew that this couple would not have qualified for welfare assistance. She realized, yet again, how important the Older Americans Act (OAA) programs were to many people.

In countless communities across the country, local Area Agencies on Aging (AAAs) work to help older adults such as the Wrights. All Americans aged 60 and older can benefit from services provided by the "aging network" because of legislation enacted more than 30 years ago. On July 14, 1965, President Lyndon B. Johnson signed into law the OAA, thus launching milestone legislation in the evolution of the nation's public policy for older adults. The OAA is one of many laws that have been enacted to assist older adults in maintaining their physical, social, psychological, and financial wellbeing. This chapter will discuss some of the important laws that laid the foundation for the creation of programs, services, and benefits for older adults. We begin with a review of some of the more notable aging legislation enacted.

LEGISLATIVE FOUNDATIONS OF SOCIAL PROGRAMS AND SERVICES

Long before the enactment of the OAA, policies designed to protect older adults from the vicissitudes of old age were slowly put into place (see Exhibit 2.1). For example, in 1920 the Civil

EXHIBIT 2.1   A National Policy on Aging: Selected Historical Highlights

1920   The **Civil Service Retirement Act** was enacted to provide a retirement system for many government employees. including Members of the U.S. Congress and those in the uniformed aid civil services.

1927   The **American Association for Old Age Security** organized to further national interest in old age legislation.

1935   The **Social Security Act** was passed and signed into law by President Roosevelt "to provide protection as a matter of right for the American worker in retirement."

1937   The **Railroad Retirement Act** was enacted to provide annuity pensions for retired railroad employees and their families

1937   The **U.S. Housing Act** stimulated passage of enabling legislation in a majority of states, to provide low-rent public housing.

1950   The first **National Conference on Aging** conference was held in Washington, D.C., sponsored by the Federal Security Agency.

1950   The **Social Security Act** was amended to establish a program of aid to the permanently and totally disabled and to broaden aid to dependent children to include relatives with whom the child was living.

1956   Special **staff on aging** were assigned coordinating responsibilities for aging within the Office of the Secretary of Health, Education, and Welfare.

1959   The **Housing Act** was amended, authorizing a direct loan program of nonprofit rental projects for the elderly at low interest rates. Provisions also reduced the eligible age for public low-rent housing for low-income older persons to age 62 for women and age 50 for disabled individuals.

1961   The first **White House Conference on Aging** convened in Washington. D.C.

1961   Social Security amendments lowered the retirement age for men from age 65 to 62, increased minimum benefits paid, broadened the program to include additional categories of retired persons, increased benefits to aged widows, and liberalized the retirement test.

1962   More than 160 Bills were introduced in Congress related to the aged and aging; 8 were enacted.

1964   The **Food Stamp Act** provided for improved levels of nutrition among low-income households through a cooperative federal–state program of food assistance.

1964   Formalizing a loose confederation of state administrators of aging program, the **National Association of State Units on Aging** was officially established on April 26, 1964.

1965   The **Older Americans Act** was passed and signed into law. Major provisions included establishment of the **Administration on Aging** within DHEW and grants to states for community planning, services, and training. The Act also stipulated that **State Agencies on Aging** be established to administer the program.

1965   The **Medicare** health insurance program for the elderly was legislated, financed through the Social Security system.

1965   Social Security amendments established Title XIX: "Grants to States for Medical Assistance," commonly known as **Medicaid**.

1967   Amendments to the **Older Americans Act** extended its provisions for two years and directed AoA to undertake a study of personnel needs in the aging field.

EXHIBIT 2.1   (Continued)

1967   The **Age Discrimination Act** of 1967 was passed and signed into law by President Johnson.

1967   Amendments to the Older Americans Act extended its provisions for three years and authorized the use of Title III funds to support **Area Wide Model Projects**.

1971   The Second White House Conference on Aging convened in Washington, D.C.

1972   The **Nutrition Program for the Elderly Act** was passed and signed into law by President Nixon (redesignated Title VII of the Older Americans Act, as amended in 1973).

1972   **Supplemental Security Income** is passed as a part of the Social Security Act.

1973   The **Older Americans Comprehensive Service Amendments** established **Area Agencies on Aging** under an expanded Title III. They also authorized grants for model projects, senior centers, and multidisciplinary centers of gerontology, and added a new Title IX.

1973   The **Older Americans Community Service Employment Act** authorized funding for Title VII nutrition projects and extended the Act's provisions for two years.

1973   The **Domestic Volunteer Service Act** was passed and signed into law. Major provisions included the RSVP and Foster Grandparent programs. As a result, Title VI of the Older Americans Act was later repealed.

1974   Amendments to the Older Americans Act added a **Special Transportation Program** under Title III: "Model Projects."

1974   Social Security amendments authorized TITLE XX: "Grants to States for Social Services." Among the programs which could be supported under this provision were protective services, homemaker services, adult day care service transportation services, and training: employment opportunities, information and referral, nutrition assistance, and health support.

1975   Amendments to the Older Americans Act added new language authorizing the Commissioner on Aging to make grants under Title III to American Indian tribal organizations. Priority services were mandated (transportation, home care, legal services, home renovation and repairs). Amendments also made minor changes to Title IX: "Community Service Employment for Older Americans."

1977   Amendments to the Older Americans Act authorized changes in the Title VII nutrition services program, primarily related to the availability of surplus commodities through the U.S. Department of Agriculture.

1978   The Comprehensive Older Americans Act amendments of 1978 consolidated Title Ill, V, and VII (social services, multipurpose centers, and nutrition services, respectively) into one Title III, redesignated the previous Title IX (Community Service Employment Act) as Title V, and added a new Title VI: "Grants for Indian Tribes."

1978   Amendments to the Older Americans Act extended the Act's programs for three years through September 30, 1984.

1984   The Older Americans Act amendments of 1984 clarified the roles of State and Area Agencies on Aging in coordinating community-based services and in maintaining accountability for the funding national priority services (legal access and

(Continued)

EXHIBIT 2.1   (Continued)

in-home services), provided for greater flexibility in administering programs by providing for increased transfer authority between parts B and C of Title III, and added a new Title VII: "Older Americans' Personal Health Education and Training Program" for funding grants to institutions of higher education to develop standardized programs of health education and training for older persons to be provided in multipurpose senior centers.

1987   Amendments to the Older Americans Act required coordination of in-home, access, and legal services with ongoing activities of agencies working with persons with Alzheimer's disease.

1987   In-home support services for frail elders, and disease prevention and health promotion services, were now supported under Title III.

1991   The Administration on Aging became an independent agency reporting to the DHHS.

1992   Title III C authorized school-based meals for older school volunteers and to help pay the costs of meals of older adults who volunteered in intergenerational programs.

1992   Amendments to the OAA added Part D, authorizing support for frail elders.

1992   Amendments to the Older Americans Act added Part F to Title III, entitled "Disease Prevention and Health Promotion Services."

1992   The **Office of Long-Term Care Ombudsman Programs** were established within the Administration on Aging.

1992   Title VII: the "Vulnerable Elder Rights Protection Title" was enacted, combining many of the provisions under Title III.

2000   Amendments to the Older Americans Act moved Part D: "In-Home Services," Part E: "Special Needs," and Part G: "Supportive Activities for Caretakers" to Part B: "Supportive Services"; this created Part E: "National Family Caregiver Support Program". The amendments also established a White House Conference on Aging, to be held in 2005.

2003   The **Medicare Prescription Drug, Improvement and Modernization Act** provided seniors and individuals with disabilities with a prescription drug benefit.

2006   Reauthorization of the Older Americans Act created a **National Center on Senior Benefits Outreach and Enrollment and Choices for Independence** initiative.

Source: Compiled by the authors from Ficke (1985) and OAA P.L. 89–73, as amended.

Service Retirement Act, a federal pension program, was enacted for government employees, members of Congress, and people in the uniformed and civil service. Some 15 years later, the Social Security Act (1935) was passed. Social Security—Old-Age, Survivor, and Disability Insurance (OASDI)—was created to ensure that working American families had a measure of economic security. Social Security is one of the best known legislative policies enacted for the benefit of retirees, and later for survivors, dependents, and persons with disabilities. It was the first legislation to represent a "social contract" that was "to provide protection as a matter of right for the American worker in retirement" (Ficke, 1985, p. 115). It has proved to be one of the most popular, as well as one of the most adaptable, pieces of legislation in existence.

The Social Security Act was signed into law by President Franklin D. Roosevelt on August 14, 1935. The main provision of the act was to provide a social insurance program designed to pay retired workers aged 65 or older a continuing income after retirement. The first payments began in 1937 and were made as lump sum payments averaging $58.06. Monthly payments began in January 1940. The first monthly retirement check was issued to Ida May Fuller of Ludlow, Vermont, in the amount of $22.54. Miss Fuller died in January 1975 at the age of 100. During her 35 years as a beneficiary, she received more than $20,000 in benefits (Social Security Administration, 1997). Originally, the amount received by Miss Fuller—$22.54— would be the amount she would receive for the rest of her life. Not until 1952 did Congress legislate increases in the monthly benefit. From that point, increases came only when legislated by Congress until 1972, when Congress enacted a law providing for annual cost-of-living increases, the amount to be determined by the annual increase in consumer prices.

There have been hundreds of amendments to the Social Security Act. Most have made minor adjustments to the Act; several, however, have profoundly increased the responsibility of the Act to extend benefits to previously uncovered groups (see Exhibit 2.1). One such amendment, passed by Congress in 1950, extended benefits to permanently and totally disabled workers. This was eventually broadened to cover workers under age 50 and their dependents. By 1960, some 559,000 people were receiving disability benefits, with an average benefit of $80 per month. In 2006, 6.8 million disabled workers received an average benefit of $978 per month (Social Security Administration, 2007).

Another significant amendment to the Social Security Act occurred in 1972 when, at the request of President Richard M. Nixon, the federal–state programs of Old-Age Assistance, Aid to the Blind, and Aid to the Permanently and Totally Disabled were streamlined to create the Supplemental Security Income (SSI) program. Under the SSI program, each eligible person over the age of 65 living in his or her own household and having no other income was provided, as of 2006, with an average monthly cash payment of $374 (Social Security Administration, 2007). In 2000, the Social Security Act was amended to reflect changing demographics and needs of older workers through the passage of H.R. 5, the Senior Citizens' Freedom to Work Act of 2000. Signed on April 7, 2000 by President Clinton, this law amended Social Security to eliminate the Retirement Earnings Test, which required eligible retirees to have their benefits reduced if they were also working (Social Security Administration, 2000b). Both Social Security and SSI are discussed in greater detail in Chapter 9.

Other early legislation benefiting older adults, enacted soon after the Social Security Act, included the Railroad Retirement Act of 1937 (providing pensions for railroad retirees) and the U.S. Housing Act of 1937 (enabling legislation for states to provide low-rent housing). Between 1940 and 1964, a number of other legislative and political activities occurred. In addition to the amendments added to the Social Security Act mentioned above, the Housing Act was amended and expanded, and the Food Stamp Act of 1964 was enacted.

The 1950s marked the emergence of another important influence on the evolution of aging policy—the White House Conferences on Aging. The first National Conference on Aging was held in Washington, D.C. in 1950, and the first White House Conference on Aging was held in 1961 (Ficke, 1985) and, more recently, in 2005. The conference delegates— representatives of federal, state, and local governments as well as professionals in the field of gerontology and older adults—convened to develop specific recommendations for executive or legislative action on aging policy.

The next significant date in the history of aging policy is 1965, when two major laws were enacted—Medicare and the OAA. Sixteen days after President Johnson signed the OAA, he signed Medicare, the national health insurance program for older adults, into law on July

30, 1965, through amendments to the Social Security Act. The passage of both the OAA and Medicare in the same year has marked the mid-1960s as the most politically friendly period for older Americans' programs in history. The passage of Medicare was historic not only for the health benefits that it would afford millions of older Americans but also for the sheer significance of overcoming more than 30 years of political opposition, largely from the American Medical Association, to government-funded health coverage. All along, most proponents had intended for government-funded health coverage to be universal. After years of debate, a compromise was offered that adopted an incremental approach whereby older adults would be covered first, thereby pushing universal coverage into the distant future (Rich & Baum, 1984). Today, Medicare provides partial health coverage for 42 million Americans 65 years of age and older as well as people of any age with permanent kidney failure and certain people with disabilities under the age of 65 (Centers for Medicare and Medicaid Services [CMS], n.d.). Specific benefits of Medicare are discussed in Chapter 11.

Although not the first major legislation addressing the needs of America's older adults, the OAA has become a landmark in the evolution of the nation's public policy for older adults (Bechill, 1992). Social Security represents more than 150 times the expenditures of the OAA, but the OAA is largely responsible for the development of what is frequently referred to as the "aging network." The advocacy and coordination mandates of the Act, as we will discuss later, have played a significant role in encouraging our nation's systems of human services to come together to do a better job of meeting the needs of older Americans.

In the remainder of this chapter, we discuss the history of the passage of the OAA, followed by a review of each of the Act's titles and a discussion of the impact of the OAA on the lives of older adults. We conclude by presenting some of the controversial issues surrounding the OAA.

EMERGENCE OF THE AGING NETWORK

The origin of the OAA can be traced to the 1961 White House Conference on Aging. Health care coverage was the key issue that emerged from the many state aging conferences that were held prior to the White House Conference. After the White House Conference in 1961, a special committee drafted resolutions that eventually led to the 1965 enactment of both Medicare and the OAA. The OAA was the first program to focus on community-based services for older adults and the first legislation mandated to bring together a fragmented and uncoordinated public and private service delivery system to meet the basic needs of elders at the community level (Lee, 1991). This visionary nature of the OAA sets it apart from other previous and subsequent legislative initiatives.

The passage of the OAA created a network of services that is unique to social programming. Much more than a collection of agencies, the aging network is a formidable structure, made up of a well-defined system that links the Administration on Aging (AoA), the U.S. Department of Health and Human Services (USDHHS), 10 regional AoA offices, 56 state units on aging (SUAs), 665 area agencies on aging (AAAs), Title VI grants to 243 Indian tribes, and some 29,000 providers delivering services to older Americans (see Exhibit 2.2). This network is bonded together around a central role—to support the federal government in transforming a patchwork of programs for the older population into a locally coordinated service system. Relying on partnerships among the three levels of government, education, and research institutions, and on a wide range of voluntary organizations working with older people, the aging network's emphasis on planning, coordination, and advocacy has provided an infrastructure and point of entry for other public and private initiatives that supplement OAA funding. These public–private initiatives represent an extraordinary record of achievement in making a small amount of federal money go a long way to help hundreds of thousands of older people avoid nursing home placement and remain independent in the community. Today, aging network programs are supported by an array of sources in conjunction with the AoA, including Medicaid, social service block grants, state and local governments, the private sector, and individual contributions. With this combination of resources, more than 12.4 million older adults received services or participated in programs funded under the OAA in 2004 (Administration on Aging [AoA] n.d.).

Best Practice: Linking Public and Private Partnerships

Many local area agencies on aging have worked to develop partnerships with the private sector to meet the needs of older adults in their communities. Here are a few examples.

- The Colorado Aging and Adult Services/State Unit on Aging is a part of the Governor's Older Worker Task Force, created as an interagency group of state-level government organizations providing employment services or funding to older adults. Shortly after the group was formed, members realized that they needed private sector input and created the Private Sector Advisory Council. The council provides the Colorado State Unit on Aging with knowledge, viewpoints, and information about older workers' issues. The council has developed a public education project, including a brochure about the impact of Colorado's aging workforce, a conference for employers, and an award to honor employers who do an exemplary job of hiring and retaining older employees. For more information, contact Colorado Aging and Adult Services, phone: 303–620–4147.
- The Clearfield Area Agency on Aging's "Blizzard Box Program" is a collaborative effort of the Clearfield Rotary Club and Dairy Queen Stores of Clearfield and DuBois, Pennsylvania. Volunteers deliver Blizzard Boxes—emergency food kits—along with regular home-delivered meals during the fall. The Blizzard Boxes are to be used when bad weather prevents the delivery of regular meals. The program was initially funded by the Rotary Club, but to meet increasing demand for Blizzard Boxes, local Dairy Queens donate $0.30 for every Blizzard Box sold during Labor Day. For more information, contact Clearfield County Area Agency on Aging, phone: 800–225–8571.

Source: Chicago Department on Aging (1992).

EXHIBIT 2.2 The Older Americans Act Network

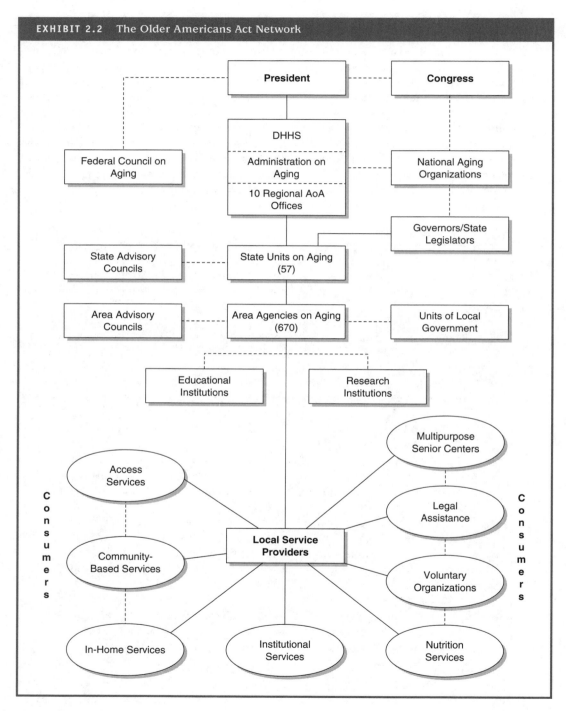

Source: Adapted from Ficke (1985).

Another notable aspect of the OAA and the network of services that has evolved from the Act is that this service network is a universal program. This universal emphasis recognizes that all older persons have needs and that programs and services should be available, as a result, to them all (Bechill, 1992). Therefore, there is no means test cutoff for programs and services funded under the Act; persons are eligible for services regardless of income or assets. Using an age-based criteria, all older persons 60 years of age or older are eligible for services. Language in the Act, however, places emphasis on helping older persons with the greatest social and economic need, particularly low-income minority persons. Amendments to the OAA in 2000 and 2006 emphasized services to older adults who are frail, in addition to low-income, rural, and racial and ethnic minority elders, including those with limited English proficiency (see Exhibits 2.1 and 2.3). In the 2006 reauthorization of the Act, Congress included language allowing programs to establish cost-sharing with participants in some circumstances (AoA, 2006a, 2006b). Cost-sharing is not permitted for information and assistance, outreach, benefits counseling or case management services, ombudsman, elder abuse prevention, legal services or other consumer protection services, congregate or home-delivered meals, or any service delivered through tribal agencies. Individuals with self-declared incomes at or below the federal poverty level would be exempt from cost-sharing. If a program is allowed to implement cost-sharing, a sliding scale based solely on income must be used; however, an older adult cannot be denied the service based on their income or failure to make a payment. The cost-share amount is based on a confidential declaration of income made by the participant. The OAA also encourages providers of services to give participants the "opportunity" to donate toward the cost of a service, but the law strictly forbids denying anyone access to a service because of an inability to donate or pay the cost-share amount. The challenges arising from the emphasis on universality, targeting, and cost-sharing in the same legislation will be discussed in more detail later in the chapter and in Chapter 20.

TITLES OF THE OLDER AMERICANS ACT

Currently, the OAA contains seven titles. *Title I* sets forth 10 broad policy objectives aimed at improving the lives of older people with regard to not only income (the principal objective of Social Security) but also physical and mental health, housing, employment, and community service. These broad objectives, listed below, continue to be the philosophical cornerstone of this Act:

1. An adequate income in retirement in accordance with the American standard of living.

2. The best possible physical and mental health that science can make available, without regard to economic status.

3. The provision and maintenance of suitable housing, independently selected, designed, and located with reference to special needs, and available at costs that older citizens can afford.

4. Full restorative services for those who require institutional care and a comprehensive array of community-based long-term care services adequate to

appropriately sustain older people in their communities and in their homes, including support to family members and other persons providing voluntary care to older individuals needing long-term care services.

5. Opportunity for employment with no discriminatory personnel practices because of age.

6. Retirement in health, honor, and dignity after years of contribution to the economy.

7. Participation in and contribution to meaningful activity within the widest range of civic, cultural, and recreational opportunities.

8. Efficient community services, including access to low-cost transportation, that provide a choice in supported living arrangements and social assistance in a coordinated manner and that are readily available when needed, with emphasis on maintenance of a continuum of care for vulnerable older individuals.

9. Immediate benefit from proven research knowledge that can sustain and improve health and happiness.

10. Freedom, independence, and the free exercise of individual initiative for older adults in planning and managing their own lives, full participation in the planning and operation of community-based services and programs provided for their benefit, and protection against abuse, neglect, and exploitation (OAA, 1965, Title I, p. 1).

These far-reaching goals are to be carried out jointly by federal, state, tribal, and local governments to achieve an adequate offering of community-based services for older adults. With a $1.3 billion budget in 2006, the programs and services funded through OAA still make the OAA one of the smallest federal programs (AoA, 2001e).

For Your Files: Policy and Planning for Disaster Preparedness

In 2005, Hurricane Katrina brought devastation to the Gulf Coast, and a disproportion number of older adults died in the storm and the chaos in the days after the storm. Although older adults aged 60 and over accounted for approximately 15% of the New Orleans population, 74% of the dead were 60 or older; nearly half were older than age 75 (The Knight Ridder News Service, cited in Glass, 2006). The emergency response that occurred afterwards often resulted in inappropriate displacements and deterioration in health and functioning (American Association of Retired Persons, 2006). Scholars have called for a re-examination of disaster preparedness policies and programs that address the unique evacuation needs of community-dwelling and institutionalized older adults, who face different risks in disasters due to physical and psychosocial limitations. The AoA responded by sending more than $1.6 million in emergency funds from its OAA FY2005 budget to aid in the reconstruction, and AoA awarded disaster assistance grants to Alabama, Mississippi, Louisiana, and Texas. The AoA entered into a Statement of

Understanding with the American National Red Cross in order to cooperate on the preparation for and response to disasters. In addition, in 2005 Association of Retired Persons (AARP) convened a diverse group of government officials at federal, state, and local levels; emergency preparedness and response experts; relief organizations; and aging and disability advocates to identify lessons learned and share promising practices in protecting older persons in disasters. The report, *We Can Do Better: Lessons Learned for Protecting Older Persons in Disasters,* can be obtained at *http://assets.aarp.org/rgcenter/il/better.pdf.* The AoA has also published a *Disaster Preparedness Manual for the Aging Network* and the *Emergency Assistance Guide 2006*, both available at www.aoa.gov/prof/disaster_assist/disaster_assist.asp.

Title II created the AoA within the Office of the Secretary of the USDHHS. AoA is headed by an Assistant Secretary on Aging appointed by the President. Through the years, there has been considerable debate about the placement of AoA within the executive branch of government. The debate has centered on whether AoA should be an independent office at the White House level, be an office of the USDHHS, or be placed under a department of the USDHHS. In 1992, President Clinton placed the AoA Assistant Secretary directly under the USDHHS Secretary—a move applauded by aging advocates because the Commissioner has the direct ear of the USDHHS Secretary and even the President when necessary.

The AoA is the federal focal point for aging issues and program planning. It has two principal roles. First, AoA is at the top of the federal–state–local hierarchy, or aging-services network, that carries out the planning, coordination, and provision of services to older adults (see Exhibit 2.2). AoA promotes training, technical assistance, and regulatory direction to help the states and local AAAs carry out their mandates. Essentially, every time the Act is reauthorized and amended, AoA must interpret Congressional intent through rule making and rule interpretation. States, local AAAs, and other interested parties may comment on the rules and frequently influence the way a particular rule is written. This is often a long and drawn-out process.

Another important role of AoA is to provide leadership on national policies affecting older adults. This is done by encouraging cooperation and coordination among the major federal agencies on federal aging policies. AoA is thus a major advocate for older adults throughout the federal government. For example, the U.S. Department of Housing and Urban Development plans and implements programs to address the housing needs of *all* low-income population groups. The Federal Transit Administration helps develop policy and funding initiatives to respond to a wide range of transit issues, including transit infrastructure. AoA is the only federal agency that has the authority to cross over agency boundaries to provide overall leadership on singularly aging issues and programs. When AoA was first established, Congress adamantly voiced its expectation that AoA have high visibility in the executive branch for developing and sponsoring a nationwide program to achieve the objectives set forth in the Act (Ficke, 1985).

The Older Americans Act amendments of 2000 required the Assistant Secretary of AoA to improve the delivery of services to rural areas by developing a "best practices" resource guide showing how rural needs can best be met and to provide training and technical assistance to help states in implementing best practices. Another significant new mandate was the requirement that AoA, in coordination with SUAs, AAAs, tribal organizations, and service providers, develop and publish before January 1, 2002, performance outcome measures for planning, managing, and evaluating activities performed under the Act. The 2000 amendments also, under Title II, established the Eldercare Locator and pension counseling as permanent programs and commissioned a White House Conference on Aging to take place before the end of 2005. One of the amendments made to the OAA in 2006 (see Exhibit 2.3) authorized the Assistant Secretary to promote an effort named "Choices for Independence," which is a $28 million demonstration project to advance consumer-directed and community-based long-term care options. This will include the creation of Aging and Disability Resources Centers in all 50 states designed to be "one-stop shops" for older adults and their families to receive information about long-term care options. Another change in the Act in 2006 was the authorization of the National Center on Senior Benefits Outreach and Enrollment program. The purpose of the program is to provide web-based support and other tools to inform older adults about the full range of federal and state benefits for which they may be eligible.

   Title III, the largest program under the Act, authorizes the development of local services to help older persons. It has been described as the heart and soul of the OAA. Title III gives authority for the development of programs to assist older persons through grants to states. States, in turn, award funds to local planning and service areas (PSAs) whose boundaries have been designated by the state. State Units on Aging (SUAs) administer the AoA grants at the state level, and the AAAs administer the AoA grants for the PSAs. An allocation formula based on the number of persons aged 60 and older residing in the state as of the most recent census determines the amount of funding each state receives. It follows, then, that Florida and California, which have large numbers of older adults 60 years of age and older, will receive larger federal allocations than states with fewer older adults, such as Colorado or Vermont. States must

---

EXHIBIT 2.3   Key Changes in the Reauthorization of the Older Americans Act, 2006

- Improve access to benefits programs for seniors with limited income through creation of a National Center on Senior Benefits Outreach and Enrollment.
- Strengthen and expand long-term care options and the availability of home and community services through the Administration on Aging's Choices for Independence initiative.
- Promote evidence-based health promotion and disease-prevention programs.
- Provide broader opportunities for seniors' civic engagement.
- Establish a program of grants and technical assistance to improve transportation for seniors.
- Establish a cabinet-level interagency coordinating committee on aging.
- Expand eligibility for the National Family Caregiver Support Program, to allow participation by a relative caregiver beginning at age 55, and to allow participation by a caregiver of any age who cares for a person with Alzheimer's disease or a related neurological disorder.
- Instruct the Assistant Secretary for Aging to designate someone to coordinate elder abuse prevention and services.
- Expand the programs on elder abuse and elder justice.
- Authorize creation of Aging and Disability Resource Centers in all 50 states.
- Target services to seniors with limited English proficiency.
- Make more explicit the inclusion of mental health as a concern and target for programming under the Act.

Source: National Council on Aging (2007, p. 1).

provide a minimum 15% match to the federal AoA grant. These matching funds vary greatly by state and help to increase the overall resources available under the OAA. SUAs keep 10% of their federal allocation for administration of the SUA. The balance is allocated to the PSAs by a more complex formula devised by the SUA using federal guidelines. The allocation formulas typically are based on census data numbers for persons aged 60 years or older, and for low-income, minority, rural, and frail individuals within this category, who reside in each PSA. AAAs must also provide local matching, which may be either cash or in-kind support, such as the value of volunteer hours or value of donated space and equipment to carry out a particular program.

The local AAA is responsible for

- developing the area plan for a comprehensive and coordinated system of services to meet the needs of older persons;
- funding service provider agencies to fill gaps in priority service areas; and
- serving as the advocate and focal point for older people within its PSA.

Throughout the country, AAAs exhibit many organizational designs and structures based on local needs and preferences. The AAA office within a PSA may be a unit of general-purpose local government, such as a county, city, or regional council of government, or a public or nonprofit private agency. In any given location, an AAA can be a part of a council of governments or regional planning commission, part of a county unit of government or city government, part of an educational institution, or a freestanding private nonprofit organization.

Under Part A of Title III, both SUAs and AAAs must develop multiyear plans describing in detail how a coordinated, comprehensive service delivery system will be provided. AAAs must also designate, where feasible, a focal point for service delivery in each community, giving strong consideration to multipurpose senior centers. The Act requires that the AAA establish a council to advise the agency on the development of multiyear plans, funding, and administration, as well as programs and services. The local councils may conduct public hearings and review and comment on all community policies, programs, and actions that affect older persons in their regions. Advisory council membership must be made up of more than 50% older persons, including older persons with greatest economic or social need, racial and ethnic minorities, and persons eligible to participate in programs assisted under the Act. Other members may represent older individuals, local elected officials, and the general public. This mandate for grassroots participation in the planning and administration of local AoA programs has given a voice to thousands of older adults on services that affect their daily lives.

Title III, Part B, of the Act is the supportive services component (see Exhibit 2.4). The mission of Part B is to develop a continuum of community-based services to assist older persons in remaining independent in the community for as long as is reasonably possible. To that end, AoA regulations state that AAAs must provide assurances that an adequate proportion of funds is allotted to service providers in their PSAs that provide

- *access services,* such as information and referral, outreach, case management, escort, and transportation;
- *in-home services,* which include chores, homemaking, personal care, home-delivered meals, and home repair and rehabilitation;

- *community services,* including senior centers, congregate meals, day care, a nursing home ombudsman program, elder abuse prevention, legal aid, employment counseling and referral, health promotion, and fitness programs; and
- *caregiver services,* such as respite, counseling, and education programs.

In most cases, AAAs do not provide these services directly. Instead, they subcontract with other organizations to deliver the services.

Title III, Part C allows for a separate federal allocation from Title III to the states and then downward to AAAs for the operation of congregate and home-delivered nutrition programs. The national nutrition program for older adults (described in more detail in Chapter 10), a result of 1972 amendments to the OAA, is a major service component under Part C. It allows AAAs to fund both congregate (group) and home-delivered meals for older adults 60 years of age and older and their spouses. The 2000 amendments gave more flexibility to transfer funds between the Supportive Services Part B budget and the Nutrition Services Part C budget. AAAs following state guidelines may now transfer up to 30% of funds between Parts B and C. This is up from the previous 20%. Also, in response to the dramatic increase in numbers of frail older adults, the OAA 2000 amendments allow AAAs following state guidelines to transfer up to 40% of funds (up from 30%) between a congregate meals budget and a home-delivered meals budget. The outline of the Title III service categories listed in Exhibit 2.4 speaks to the wide range of flexible options AAAs have locally to develop a comprehensive offering of services to meet the particular needs of their PSA.

Title III, Part D, was added to the Act in the 1992 amendments. Originally, Part D was a relatively small program that was intended to address home care needs but was never adequately funded. With the 2000 amendments, this aspect of Part D was consolidated into Part B, where home care has traditionally been an allowable service. Title III, Part D has been renamed "Disease Prevention and Health Promotion Services," which was originally Part F and was incorporated into the OAA with the 1987 amendments. First funded with the 1992 amendments to the Act, it has been minimally funded and has remained a small program. AAAs may provide disease-prevention and health promotion services and information at multipurpose senior centers, at congregate meal sites, through home-delivered meals programs, or at other appropriate sites. As with all AAA programs, disease prevention and health promotion should be targeted to the most needy. According to the Act, disease-prevention and health promotion services include

- health risk assessments;
- routine health screening;
- nutritional counseling;
- health promotion programs;
- physical fitness;
- home injury control services;
- mental health promotion;
- education concerning Medicare benefits;
- medication management screening and education;
- information on age-related diseases and chronic disabling conditions;
- gerontological counseling and counseling regarding other social services.

EXHIBIT 2.4 Community-Based Supportive Services Funded Through Area Agencies on Aging

Services to Facilitate Access

- Transportation
- Outreach
- Information and referral
- Client assessment and case management

Services Provided in the Community

- Congregate meals
- Multipurpose senior centers
- Casework, counseling, emergency services
- Legal assistance and financial counseling
- Adult day care, protective services, health screening
- Housing, residential repairs, and renovations
- Physical fitness and recreation
- Preretirement and second-career counseling
- Employment
- Crime prevention and victim assistance
- Volunteer services
- Health and nutrition education
- Transportation
- Elder abuse education and training
- Mental health education and services

Services Provided in the Home

- Home health, homemaker, home repairs
- Home-delivered meals and nutrition education
- Chore maintenance, visiting, shopping, letter writing, escort, and reader services
- Telephone reassurance
- Supportive services for families of elderly victims of Alzheimer's disease and similar disorders

Services to Residents of Care-providing Facilities

- Casework, counseling, placement, and relocation assistance
- Group services, complaint and grievance resolution
- Visiting, escort services
- Long-term care ombudsman program

Source: Ficke (1985) and the Older Americans Act of 1965, as amended.

One of the most significant developments with the 2000 amendments was the addition of a National Family Caregiver Support Program, or Title III, Part E of the OAA. This new program built upon existing services at the local level that already provided relief to families helping to care for frail loved ones. Family caregivers and relative caregivers such as grandparents of children not more than 18 years of age are now able to receive services such as information and assistance, counseling, support groups, caregiver training, respite care, and other supplemental services. Congress's addition of Family Caregiver Support as a funded service under the OAA is attributable to immense lobbying on the part of family caregivers and the aging network. An initial $125 million was allocated to this effort. The 2006 amendments allow mental health screening, outreach, and services to be funded under Title III.

In addition to service programs, AoA, under *Title IV*, awards funds to support research, demonstration, and training programs. Research projects collect information about the status and needs of various subgroups of older adults in the population that is used to plan services and opportunities that will assist them. Demonstration projects test new program initiatives that better serve older adults, especially those who are vulnerable. AoA also provides funds to educational institutions to develop curricula and training programs for professionals and paraprofessionals in the field of aging (AoA, 1995a). This title makes the OAA unique among federal programs in its ability to be a catalyst for new approaches to meeting the local needs of older persons and their families (Region VIII Office, AoA, n.d.).

As of 2006, literally hundreds of projects had been funded through Title IV. Initially, funding concentrated on the development of education and training programs to increase the number of qualified personnel in gerontology. It is difficult to believe that 30 years ago nearly all service programs faced critical shortages in trained personnel and that fewer than 10–20% of workers in the field of aging had any formal preparation for work with older people (Ficke, 1985).

For Your Files: Demonstration Projects Funded Under Title IV

The goal of the Neighborhood Elders Support Team (NEST) project is to build neighborhood capacity to identify and address the needs of frail and homebound elders through formal and informal networks of care. NEST will coordinate volunteer teams to provide in-home safety, preventive health education and screening, professional care, and social and practical support as needed to maintain independent living. Program objectives include establishing multidisciplinary case conference teams, using volunteer health and other professionals from the neighborhood, engaging student interns in care coordination and monitoring, and providing training for citywide dissemination. For more information, contact Bernal Heights Senior Services, phone: 415-206-2142; www.bhnc.org/ senior.htm.

The Legal Services of Northern California expanded its Senior Legal Hotline in Sacramento to cover the 39 northern counties in California. The expanded hotline serves low-income minority older adults and those with social and economic needs. The hotline is capable of processing more than 8,000 calls each year and relies on more than 120 private attorneys who provide pro bono or low-fee representation. For more information, contact the Legal Services of Northern California, phone: 916-551-2150; www.lsnc .info. For a complete list of all projects funded under Title IV, visit www.aoa.gov/doingbus/ comp/comp.asp.

Research and development projects were first directed to programs of practical action. For example, in 1968, 29 grants for more than $2 million were made by AoA to fund projects designed to gain new knowledge on the nutritional needs of older persons. This demonstration project laid the groundwork for the national nutrition program for older adults (mentioned earlier) funded under Title III, Part C since 1977. Between 1973 and 1977, approximately 25 new research and demonstration grants were funded to research ways to maintain vulnerable older persons (e.g., those in poorer health) in their own homes or in appropriate community settings. Later, beginning in 1984, discretionary funds under Title IV were directed to social integration of older persons, strengthening of family supports, systems improvement, outreach to minorities, and improvement of capacity through the application of knowledge (Ficke, 1985).

During those early years, multidisciplinary research centers of gerontology also benefited significantly from Title IV grants. Among the first and more prominent centers that were funded by Title IV funds were the Institute of Gerontology at the University of Michigan, Wayne State University Institute of Gerontology, the Andrus Gerontology Center at the University of Southern California, and the Center for Aging and Human Development at Duke University. These centers were specifically mandated to recruit and train personnel in the field of aging, conduct basic and applied research, provide consultation to SUAs and AAAs, serve as repositories of information on aging, and help develop training programs on aging (Ficke, 1985).

Between 1978 and 1984, AoA expanded the recipients of Title IV grants to include "special emphasis" resource centers. Six centers were funded to concentrate on the concerns of income maintenance, health, employment, housing, older women, and education and leisure. The purpose of these centers was to help AoA fulfill its role as advocate for the nation's older adults and to bridge the gap between theory and practice through education and research. The AoA continues to fund resource centers through Title IV dollars. A list of them is presented in Exhibit 2.5. Funding for support centers changes each budget year and more recently dropped from $43 million in 2005 to $24 million in 2006 (Administration on Aging, 2007). As a result of these budgetary ups and downs, many resource centers may be eliminated or their activities seriously curtailed.

During the past 15 years, Title IV funds have made numerous contributions in the areas of long-term care, home and community-based services, elder abuse, legal services hotlines, and disaster assistance. For long-term care and home and community-based services, one of the most visible examples of Title IV support is the Eldercare Locator, an effort to help local and long-distance caregivers find the information they need by calling a toll-free number (more details on the Eldercare Locator can be found in Chapter 4). Title IV was virtually the only source of funding for states that were in the initial planning stages of developing home and community-based programs for older adults needing long-term care.

Title IV demonstration projects in elder abuse prevention have brought together individuals who provide social services to the aging and to those affected by domestic violence to more effectively address domestic violence that affects older women. With Title IV assistance, statewide legal hotlines have been established in 11 states, and most recently Title IV funding has supported disaster relief programs to victims of hurricanes, earthquakes,

EXHIBIT 2.5 Resource Centers Supported by the Administration on Aging

Black Elderly Legal Assistance Support Project, National Bar Association, 1225 11th Street, N.W., Washington, DC 20001, 202-842-3900

National Legal Resource Initiative for Financially Distressed Elders, National Consumer Law Center, Inc., 11 Beacon Street, Boston, MA 02108, 617-523-8010

Legal Counsel for the Elderly, American Association of Retired Persons, 601 E Street, N.W., Washington, DC 20049, 202-434-2120

National Center on Elder Abuse, National Association of State Units on Aging, 1201 15th Street, N.W., Suite 350, Washington, DC 20005, 202-898-2586

National Center for Long Term Care, University of Minnesota School of Public Health, Institute of Health Services Research, 420 Delaware S.E., Box 197, Minneapolis, MN 55455, 612-624-5171

National Consumer Law Center, National Legal Assistance and Elder Rights, 77 Summer Street, 10th Floor, Boston, MA 02110-1006, 617-542-8010

National Legal Assistance and Elder Rights Project, AARP Foundation, Foundation Programs, 601 E Street N.W., Washington, DC 20049, 202-434-2787

National Legal Support for Elderly People with Mental Disabilities Project, Bazelon Center for Mental Health Law, 1101 15th Street, N.W., Suite 1212, Washington, DC 20005-5002, 202-467-5730

National Resource and Policy Center on Rural Long-Term Care, University of Kansas Medical Center, Center on Aging, 3901 Rainbow Boulevard, Kansas City, KS 66167-7117, 913-588-1636

National Policy & Resource Center on Housing and Long Term Care, University of Southern California, Andrus Gerontology Center, Los Angeles, CA 90089, 213-740-1364

National Long Term Care Ombudsman Resource Center, National Citizens Coalition for Nursing Home Reform, 1224 M Street, N.W., Washington, DC 20005-5183, 202-393-2018

National Minority Aging Organizations, Project Aliento, Asociacion Nacional Pro Personas Mayores, 3325 Wilshire Blvd., Suite 800, Los Angeles, CA 90010, 213-487-1922

National Resource Center on Nutrition, Physical Activity & Aging, 200 Florida International University, Miami, FL 33199, 305-348-1517

National Program on Women and Aging, Brandeis University, Heller School - Institute for Health Policy, P.O. Box 9110, Waltham, MA 02254, 617-736-3863

National Support for Legal Assistance and Elder Rights, National Senior Citizens Law Center, 11101 14th Street, N.W.—Suite 400, Washington, DC 20005, 202-289-6976

Native Elder Health Care Resource Center, University of Colorado at Denver, National Center for American & Alaskan Native Mental Health Research, 4455 East 12 Avenue, Room 308, Denver, CO 80220, 303-372-3232

Pension Rights Center, 918 16th Street, N.W., Suite 704, Washington, DC 20006, 202-296-3776

Law and Aging Project, The Center for Social Gerontology, 2307 Shelby Avenue, Ann Arbor, MI 48103-3895, 313-665-1126

University of North Dakota Resource Center on Native Americans, Office of Native American Programs, P.O. Box 7134, Grand Forks, ND 58202 701-777-4291

Source: Administration on Aging (2004a), www.aoa.dhhs.gov.

floods, and the Oklahoma City bombing. The 2000 OAA reauthorization included the following new projects: Career Preparation for the Field of Aging; Older Women's Protection From Violence Projects; Health Care Demonstration Projects for Rural Areas; and Computer Training for Older Adults. Whatever disagreement may exist about the viability of the OAA, most agree that Title IV has represented an atypical but largely successful effort by the federal government to advance knowledge on aging through applied research, training, and demonstration projects. New areas identified for funding in the 2006 OAA reauthorization include planning activities to prepare communities for population aging, including assessing the needs of the older adult population; training and technical assistance to the SUA and AAAs; development, implementation and assessment of technology-based service models; and activities that promote quality and improvement in support provided to caregivers.

Title V establishes authority for the Senior Community Service Employment Program (SCSEP) for unemployed, low-income persons 55 years of age and older. Administered initially by the Office of Economic Opportunity and later by the Department of Labor, the program was added to the OAA in 1973 but continues to be administered by the Department of Labor. During the past three decades, SCSEP has helped over half a million low-income older workers (Green Thumb, 2001). Participants work part time, typically in service areas such as education, health and hospitals, recreation and parks, and senior centers. A majority of the funds are administered through national organizations such as Experience Works (formally known as Green Thumb), the American Association of Retired Persons (AARP), the National Council on the Aging, the National Center on Black Aged, the National Council on Senior Citizens, the Asociacion Nacional Pro Personas Mayores, the National Urban League, and governors of every state. Title V projects contribute to the general welfare of communities through public service to local entities such as hospitals, senior centers, libraries, and historical sites while increasing employment opportunities for low-income older adults. Detailed information about Title V programs is provided in Chapter 8.

Title VI establishes authority for grants to Indian tribes to promote the delivery of supportive and nutrition services to American Indians and Alaska Natives that are comparable to services offered to other older persons under the Title III program. The rationale for making grants directly available to Indian tribes is to respect the needs of older Indians. Findings show that unemployment and poverty rates are much higher among Indians, housing is often substandard, and there are shortages of transportation, nursing homes, and home health care options for older Indians. Grants under Title VI to Indian tribes were first made in 1980, when AoA reported that $6 million funded 85 grants that ultimately assisted 20,000 elders. By comparison, in 2000 approximately $18.5 million funded 227 grants helping more than 134,000 elders. Although nutrition services, both congregate and home-delivered, are an important piece of these grants, other supportive services such as transportation and information and referral are funded as well (AoA, 2001a).

Title VII, on rights protection for vulnerable elders, was enacted as part of the OAA in 1992. The purpose of Title VII is to promote advocacy designed to protect the basic rights and benefits of vulnerable elders, especially those with great economic needs. According to the OAA, Title VII has a dual focus. The first is to bring together long-term ombudsman programs; programs for the prevention of abuse, neglect, and exploitation; and state elder rights and legal assistance development programs. The second is to facilitate the coordination of and linkages between the three programs in each state.

The purpose of the long-term care ombudsman program is to identify, investigate, and resolve complaints concerning the residents of nursing homes and board-and-care homes. The ombudsman program is discussed in greater detail in Chapter 19. Programs for the prevention of elder abuse, neglect, and exploitation are designed to provide public education about elder abuse and conduct outreach to help identify cases of abuse, neglect, or exploitation. These programs are also responsible for offering training and technical assistance about elder abuse to professionals working with older adults. The state elder rights and legal assistance development program requires that SUAs establish programs to provide leadership in improving the quality and quantity of legal assistance programs. Elder abuse and legal assistance programs are discussed in Chapter 13.

FUNDING FOR THE OLDER AMERICANS ACT

Exhibit 2.6 lists funding levels for selected years between 2000 and 2006 (AoA, 2001e and AoA, 2007). Small increases have been welcomed by the aging network, which sustained budget cuts in the mid-1990s.

OUTCOMES OF THE OLDER AMERICANS ACT

The OAA has been law for more than three decades. Its grand objectives, spelled out in Title I of the Act, have remained intact. The governmental structures at the federal, state, and local levels have reached mature and stable plateaus, and a wide variety of programs have been put into place nationwide. Has the OAA, then, accomplished its original goals? Little comprehensive research exists to support either a positive or a negative claim. Some say that the OAA has failed because it has not adequately served minorities. For example, a study by the U.S. Commission on Civil Rights in 1982 showed that the number of racial and ethnic minority older adults receiving services represented only a small percentage of the total number of eligible persons in six American cities. A study conducted by the Public Policy Institute of the AARP (Hasler, 1990) concluded that minority participation in AoA programs fluctuated greatly from year to year and that there was a clear problem with the reliability and validity of data being collected to report minority participation.

Another charge that has been leveled against the OAA is that those who are poor and isolated are underserved. For example, senior centers and group meals (both widely funded by local AAAs) attract primarily the healthy and active among the aged (Rich & Baum, 1984).

Other critics of the aging network hold that not enough of the federal funds intended for services to older adults ever reach them. They contend that the federal, state, and local aging network bureaucracies are self-serving and that too much of the funding is channeled into supporting these bureaucracies (Estes, 1979).

Finally, in her landmark book *The Aging Enterprise,* Estes (1979) identifies a number of shortcomings associated with the passage of the OAA. Although her comments were made more than 25 years ago, they are still being debated today. First, Estes states that the OAA

EXHIBIT 2.6 Older Americans Act Appropriations for Selected Fiscal Years 2000–2008 (dollars in thousands)

Title	Activity	FY 2000	FY 2005	FY 2006	FY 2007	President's Budget Request 2008
II	Aging Network Support Activities[1]	1,812	13,266	13,124	13,133	13,133
	Alzheimer's disease	5,968	11,786	11,660	11,668	0
III-B	Supportive Services and Centers	310,020	354,136	350,354	350,595	350,595
III	**Nutrition Services**					
	Nutrition Services Incentive Program[2]					
III-C1	Congregate Meals	374,336	387,274	385,054	385,319	383,401
III-C2	Home-Delivered Meals	146,970	182,826	181,780	181,904	180,998
III-E	National Family Caregiver Support Program		155,744	156,060	156,167	154,187
III-F	Preventive Health Services	16,120	21,616	21,385	21,400	0
IV	Research/Training/Demonstration	29,344	43,286	24,578	24,595	35,485
VI	Grants to Indian Tribes	18,457	32,702	32,353	32,375	32,375
VII	Vulnerable Older Americans	13,179	19,288	20,142	19,166	19,166
	Program Administration	16,458	18,301	17,682	17,694	18,696
	Total AOA	932,664	1,240,225	1,361,916	1,334,829	1,335,146

Source: Administration on Aging (2001c, 2007).

Notes:

1. Aging Network Support Activities, or Title II, currently consists of the Eldercare Locator and Pension Counseling. These programs, previously funded under Title IV, were moved to Title II and made permanent in the 2000 reauthorization of the Older Americans Act.

2. The funds for the Nutrition Services Incentive Programs were previously housed in the United States Department of Agriculture (USDA) and transferred to the OAA budget in 2001

does nothing to alleviate the economic and social conditions that determine the quality of life of older Americans. Indeed, securing a "brown bag" of groceries for older adults who have limited food does nothing to help them escape the poverty that causes daily worry about obtaining food. Moreover, the social structures that have led some older adults into marginal economic status, such as providing mechanisms for ensuring adequate retirement income for lifelong homemakers, are not addressed. Estes contends that existing social policy for aged persons simply preserves the existing social class distinctions. Second, Estes argues that the insistence on age-segregated programs creates tension between social groups and makes older adults targets of blame for the country's economic hardships. The rise in groups such as Americans for Generational Equity and the current discussion about rising health care costs associated with Medicare seem to offer support for this concern. Finally, Estes notes that funding the OAA reassures the public that aged persons are adequately being cared for while nothing is being done to change the functioning of social class. She recommends that structural changes be made in income, retirement, and employment policies that accentuate class differences; that universalist policies be adopted which, among other things, would facilitate intergenerational bonding; and that universal health care be enacted.

Those who support the OAA point to hundreds of thousands of older adults who receive services through OAA programs. These services are important for maintaining current levels of wellbeing as well as for assisting those who have low levels of functioning. Thus the programs and services supported by the OAA help elders with better levels of wellbeing maintain their physical and social vitality as well as assist those at risk of physical decline and social isolation. Services available under the OAA help people such as the Wrights, described at the beginning of the chapter; to whom would they turn if the aging network ceased to exist? Moreover, locally based AAAs must be responsive to the needs of the people they are directed to serve. For example, as the population has aged and there are increasing numbers of frail elders, local AAA funding has shifted to concentrate more on programs that help meet the needs of these individuals. One example of a program that has improved the lives of frail elders is the nutrition program. A study of the national nutrition program for older adults conducted in 1994 showed that the nutritional wellbeing of participants has measurably improved (Ponza, Ohls, & Millen, 1996). Others point to the success of many AAAs in leveraging other resources, both public and private, to support needed services.

Should the success of the OAA be measured against the degree to which it accomplishes its goals stated in Title I? Such lofty aspirations are laudable, but they are impossible to reach given the Act's limited resources. We will revisit the OAA in Chapter 20 and consider the future of the Act. In the next chapter, we examine some of the factors associated with service use by older adults and some theoretical models that can be used to explain why some older adults choose not to seek services.

3

Patterns of Service Use and Theories of Help-Seeking Behavior

Katherine Hahn is an 80-year-old retired physician who lives alone with her two dogs in a condominium in Phoenix. She never married, and her only living relative is her brother, who lives in Germany. Recently, she has not been well, and dirty laundry, trash, and old newspapers have begun to accumulate in the entryway into her apartment, where there is a terrible stench. She has become increasingly frail and unable to descend her stairway safely to get outside. As a result, she is unable to take her dogs outside, so the dogs wear diapers. The neighbors are starting to complain to the building's management. She refuses all attempts to help her.

Most older adults enjoy good health, are active well into later life, and are content with retirement; the role changes that accompany later life, however, have the potential to be quite disruptive unless adequate support is available. For example, widowhood is often associated with a decrease in income, a loss of emotional support, and a decline in physical health that can complicate simple daily tasks such as shopping and preparing meals. Most communities offer a number of community and social support services to help older adults cope with their changing social, personal, and financial circumstances.

Community and support services can improve the wellbeing of recipients, but how many older adults use the services available to them? A review of the literature about the use of community service programs reveals a common theme: only a small percentage of older adults report using services (Krout, 1983b; Mitchell, 1995; Spense, 1992; Starret, Wright, Mindle, & Van Tran, 1989). Consider Katherine Hahn's situation. She could use the assistance of a home health aide or homemaker. Certainly, she could use a volunteer to walk her dogs. But she refuses any assistance. How can we explain this paradox? Moreover, many older adults in our communities need assistance. But on whom do they rely most often to meet those needs? In this chapter, we present information about the social care older adults receive from informal and formal networks, and look at how the informal and formal networks interact to assist older adults. Next, we examine possible reasons why older adults might not be inclined to use community services and present some social psychological theories that help explain help-seeking behavior. We end this chapter with a discussion about how social theory can be used to help understand patterns of service use among older adults.

SOCIAL CARE FOR OLDER ADULTS

When we encounter a problem, need help getting something done, or just need someone to talk to, what do we do? Most of us probably first seek help or advice from someone we know in our *informal network*—a friend or family member—rather than from a resource in the *formal network*. Older adults also show a preference for turning to the people with whom they are familiar and who are involved in their daily lives. Researchers have discovered that older adults turn to their informal network of family and friends for help before they turn to the formal network (Cantor, 1983, 1991; Horowitz, 1985; Litwak, 1985; Suitor & Pillemer, 1990). When seeking help from members of the informal network, older adults exhibit a hierarchical preference for assistance from spouses and children first, and then friends and neighbors (Cantor, 1979; Horowitz, 1985; Palley & Oktay, 1983). The care given by persons in the informal network is generally long term, is motivated by a desire to reciprocate for past assistance, is offered free of charge, and generally requires a low level of knowledge or training (Doty, 1986; Travis, 1995). Spouses, children, siblings, and other family members provide older adults with personal care, emotional support, and social support services such as meal preparation, transportation, and mediation with bureaucracies (Brody, 1981; Matthews & Rosner, 1988; Sangl, 1985; Shanas, 1979; Stone, Cafferata, & Sangl, 1987). A voluminous amount of research exists documenting that family caregivers of older adults assume this significant role at great expense to their financial, psychological, and physical wellbeing (e.g., Biegel, Sales, & Schultz, 1991; Montgomery & Kamo, 1989; Scharlach & Boyd, 1989; Strawbridge & Wallhagen, 1991). Siblings, as well as friends, also provide support to one another in later life, but their help is more likely to comprise emotional support and companionship rather than assistance with the tasks of daily living (Bedford, 1989; Jones & Vaughan, 1990; Wellman & Wortley, 1989).

In contrast to the informal network, the *formal network* consists of agencies that operate within a bureaucratic structure, generally have no prior emotional relationship with their clients, and provide care for a limited or specified amount of time (Lipman & Longino, 1982; Litwak & Misseri, 1989). The community resources that we discuss later in this book represent the formal network that exists to enhance the well-being of older adults. As Travis (1995) points out, the formal network also consists of agencies that are nonservice in nature and includes religious, ethnic, and social groups. When families become caregivers to frail older adults, they in essence become gatekeepers to the use of formal services. There has been considerable interest regarding when and how the informal network interacts with the formal network.

INFORMAL AND FORMAL INTERACTION

Although families offer a tremendous amount of care to older family members, there are occasions when older adults and their families turn to the formal network for assistance.

Because the informal network plays such an important role in delivering and securing assistance for older adults, researchers have been interested in creating conceptual approaches to aid in understanding the interaction between the informal and formal network.

Litwak (1985) proposed the *dual specialization model,* suggesting that informal and formal networks carry out responsibilities that are best suited to each. For example, the informal network can respond to unscheduled or unplanned needs, and the formal network can offer scheduled, structured care provided by trained professionals. Being available to assist a frail older adult with frequent trips to the bathroom in the middle of the night is best provided by a caregiving spouse or child; checking on vital signs once a day is a task better suited to a trained individual in the formal network. According to Litwak's model, both the informal and formal networks work best when they perform the tasks to which they are most suited.

The *supplemental model* (Stoller, 1989; Stoller & Pugliesi, 1988) acknowledges that the informal network is the primary source of social care but that formal services are used to supplement assistance provided by the informal network when its resources are not able to meet the caregiving needs. The informal network relies on formal services to augment, rather than replace, its caregiving activities.

To date, the research on the interplay between the formal and informal networks has been sparse. Clearly, more longitudinal research is needed to determine the patterns of formal network use during the course of the caregiving career. The conceptual models discussed here can alert the practitioner to be cognizant of the different ways in which the informal network reaches out to the formal network and to realize that the formal network frequently assists both the older adults and their informal network. We turn next to a review of the factors associated with service use.

Service Use by Older Adults

Researchers have identified a number of factors related to service use, but studies often report conflicting results regarding which factors predict service use. These differences are in part due to the use of dissimilar independent variables when predicting service use and the different community resources studied. Despite these methodological limitations, we can make some generalizations about the variables associated with service use. Characteristics such as age, transportation, gender, marital status, living arrangement, geographical location, race and ethnicity, health status, and awareness of services have all been found to be associated with the use of community services. Specifically, as age increases, so does service use (Chappell & Blandford, 1987; Krout, 1985b; McCaslin, 1989; Webber, Fox, & Burnette, 1994). Older women are more likely to use services than are older men (Coulton & Frost, 1982; McCaslin, 1989). Those with access to transportation are more likely to use services (Krout, 1983b; McCaslin, 1989; Mitchell, 1995). Older adults living in rural communities are less likely to use community resources than are their urban counterparts (Krout, 1983b; Spense, 1992). Older adults who are married are less likely to use services than are older adults who live alone (Krout, 1983b; Spense, 1992). Whites are significantly more likely to use community services than are their non-White counterparts (Carlton-LaNey, 1991; Fellin & Powell, 1988; Guttman, 1980; Spense, 1992), and those whose health needs are greater are more likely to use services (Calsyn & Winter, 2001; Coulton & Frost,

1982; Strain & Blandford, 2002). Finally, not surprisingly, higher levels of awareness are linked to greater service use (Burnette, 1999; Strain & Blandford, 2002).

Currently, much of the research investigating service use by older adults has focused on the relationship between demographic and social characteristics and service use. More research is needed to indicate the reasons *why* older adults do or do not use community services.

Psychosocial Barriers to Service Use

Studies of help-seeking behavior have identified several social-psychological barriers that might explain why older people do not use programs that could help them. Some years ago, Lipman and Sterne (1962) suggested that older adults are reluctant to use services because they wish to maintain an image of self-reliance and competency. A person's image of self-reliance may be compromised when he or she experiences a decline in physical health and is unable to continue some activities. When the perception of self-reliance and competency is compromised, asking for formal assistance only verifies this personal shortcoming. Moen (1978) found that respondents in her study were reluctant to admit needs and did not want to use services that they associated with "welfare" programs. Furthermore, American culture puts a high value on independence and self-reliance and, as a result, people feel uncomfortable when they "impose" on others for assistance. In addition, older adults from different cultural backgrounds and experiences may have varying views of the appropriateness of seeking assistance from formal service providers.

Along with the cultural norms and values people hold about self-reliance, their self-perceptions and social comparisons with others can influence the act of seeking assistance. For example, many older adults do not see themselves as old. At age 93, the grandfather of one of the authors stated that he did not want to go to the senior center to socialize with those "old" people. Perhaps, like many other older adults, his view of himself did not fit his image of who uses services or attends programs designed for older adults. Similarly, Powers and Bultena (1974) suggest that older respondents in their study might have been reluctant to use services because they perceived that programs were meant for older adults who were worse off than themselves.

Another barrier to seeking help is the desire to avoid embarrassment (Shapiro, 1983). The act of asking someone for assistance implies having problems that one cannot resolve on one's own. For the current cohort of older adults, who survived such hardships as the Depression, this admission might be difficult. Moreover, when recipients seek formal services, they are forced to make their personal problems public (Williamson, 1974).

These psychosocial variables (i.e., independence, self-reliance, and embarrassment), although illuminating, are somewhat limited because they do not explore the help-seeking context in greater detail. Below we discuss theoretical models that can help explain service use among older adults.

PSYCHOSOCIAL THEORIES OF SERVICE USE

Within the fields of gerontology, sociology, and psychology, several theories or models can be used to help explain who is likely to use services and why some older adults might not be willing to seek assistance. Although researchers have not specifically applied some of these models and theories to older adult populations, they offer a way to think about the factors that might be associated with service use. These theories are psychosocial in that they draw on social as well as psychological dimensions.

Continuity Theory

Continuity theory (Atchley, 1971, 1989, 1997) is a theory of adult development based on the premise that, as adults develop, they become invested in mental pictures that organize their ideas about themselves and their external environment. Moreover, these ideas are actively constructed as people age. As adults reach middle age, they have a good idea of their strengths and weaknesses and use these ideas to make choices that take advantage of their strengths. Thus Atchley (1997) states that, when making choices in life,

> people will be attracted to past views of self . . . the coping strategies that have been successful, ways of thinking that have been effective, people that have been supportive and helpful, and environments that have met the need for security and predictability. (1997, p. 272)

Application of continuity theory to help-seeking behaviors suggests that the coping strategies used by older adults throughout their lives are likely to predict the circumstances under which they will seek or accept help. Remember the story of Katherine at the beginning of the chapter? She refused all attempts to help improve her health and living arrangements. No doubt, spending her life as a doctor—especially at a time when there were few women physicians—fashioned her self-perception and ways of contending with difficulties. She was probably an independent, self-sufficient woman and found that she could successfully cope with most of life's challenges by herself. On the basis of this assumption about her past ways of handling difficult situations, the application of continuity theory to her situation evokes no surprise at her reluctance to accept assistance. Longitudinal research on help-seeking behavior and the use of formal services employing the continuity theory would help to better clarify how past views of self and coping strategies developed throughout the life course can influence help-seeking behavior in later life.

Social Behavior Model

Anderson and Newman (1973) developed the social behavior model in an attempt to explain why individuals use health services. More recently, researchers have relied heavily on this model for guidance when investigating the use of social services. The model (shown in Exhibit 3.1) suggests that using services is a function of older adults' predisposition to use the service, enabling factors that either facilitate or impede use of a service, and the need for the service (Anderson, 1995; Anderson & Newman, 1973).

According to the social behavior model, certain individuals are more inclined than others to use services because of personal characteristics that are present before the need for a service arises. These predisposing characteristics include the demographic factors of age and gender. They also include social structure characteristics of marital status, education, occupation, ethnicity, and social networks that are thought to determine the status of a person in the community, his or her ability to cope with the problem at hand, and the resources available to deal with the problem. General beliefs or attitudes about support services might also predict service use.

Even those who are predisposed to using services will not do so unless they can access those services. Enabling characteristics that facilitate the use of services include personal and family characteristics of income level, insurance coverage, access to transportation, and awareness of service. At the community level, enabling characteristics include the availability of the service and the distance to the service. Finally, service need can be either an individual's subjective assessment of need or an evaluated need provided by a professional. Researchers have found that predicting service use cannot be influenced by need alone unless the person is predisposed to use the service and then has the necessary enabling resources.

Let us illustrate how we can use this model to predict whether an older adult will attend a congregate meal site. Walter is 78 years old and has lived alone since his spouse of 45 years died two years ago. His monthly income is $850 a month, and he lives in a small one-bedroom apartment. Although he is in good health and able to drive, he does not go out much and easily becomes despondent when thinking of his spouse. Walter has found that he is uncomfortable with shopping and cooking because his wife was responsible for most of those duties. As a result, he often skips breakfast and lunch. After learning about his plight, a friend tells him about the congregate meal program offered three times per week at the senior center and invites Walter to go with him. Walter steadfastly refuses and states, "I do not need to eat like I used to, and I am getting along just fine." How can we explain Walter's reluctance to attend the congregate meal program? At first glance, he has many characteristics presented in the social behavior model that should be related to attending the program. He has the resources that would enable him to pay the suggested donation for the meal, he has transportation to the site, and he is aware of the service. Walter does not, however, perceive that he has an unmet nutritional need. In his mind, he can do without going to the congregate meal program, and he does not see how he could benefit from attending. Unless there is a change in Walter's perceived need for the program, he probably will not attend.

The social behavior model has had varying success in predicting actual community service use. Researchers using this model have found that the predisposing characteristics of being older, female, unmarried, and more highly educated, and the enabling characteristic of income, are associated with increased likelihood of service use (Krout, 1983b; Peterson, 1989). But these characteristics do not explain use as well as awareness and need. Although awareness of services is strongly related to service use, it is often not sufficient to predict use. Researchers have reported that even when respondents were aware of community programs, their use of programs continued to be low (Krout, 1984; Mitchell, 1995; Powers & Bultena, 1974). Overall, perceived need is most often the best predictor of service use. Researchers using the social behavior model should also investigate the role cultural barriers play in facilitating or inhibiting service use. In this next section, we describe some theories designed to predict help-seeking behavior developed primarily from the field of psychology.

EXHIBIT 3.1   Social Behavior Model

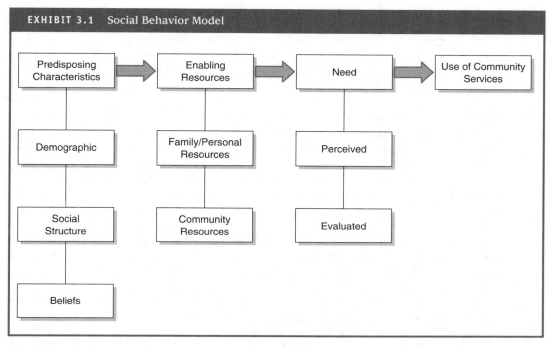

Source: Adapted from R. Anderson (1995, pp. 1–10). Copyright American Sociological Association. Used with permission.

THE PSYCHOLOGY OF HELP-SEEKING BEHAVIOR

People probably can remember a time when they were sick enough to see a doctor but did not do so until a friend or family member cajoled them into going. Or perhaps they can recall a time when they drove around hopelessly lost but refused to stop and ask for directions. Why do individuals refuse to ask for help when clearly they would be better off if they did? According to the psychology of help-seeking behavior, seeking assistance is more complicated than might be expected.

Decisions about whether to seek help involve weighing the psychological costs of asking for assistance against the benefits that might occur. In contrast to the social behavioral model, the help-seeking theories we discuss here take into account the psychological processes of a person who is considering seeking assistance. In this next section, we present a summary of the reactance theory, the attribution theory, the equity theory, and the threat-to-self-esteem model. We base this summary on the work of Fisher, Nadler, and Whitcher-Alagna (1983), who provide an in-depth review of how each of these theories can be used to predict help-seeking behavior.

Reactance Theory

The reactance theory (Brehm, 1966) suggests that people value certain states such as freedom of choice and autonomy. When these states are threatened, a negative psychological state (reactance) occurs, and people respond in ways that attempt to restore the valued states. The degree of reactance experienced by an individual depends on how important the freedom is to the individual, the number of freedoms lost or threatened, and the strength of the threat (Brehm, 1966; Brehm & Brehm, 1981). Thus, when recipients perceive that the aid or assistance will threaten their freedom or autonomy, they are likely to react negatively (Fisher et al., 1983). Some researchers have shown that reactance can occur even if there is no direct personal threat to freedom. For example, Fisher et al. suggest that individuals may refuse aid if they think there are "strings attached" that could compromise freedom. Furthermore, as recipients seek to reestablish their freedom or autonomy, they may also form a negative impression of the person who is trying to provide the assistance (Gergen, Morse, & Kristeller, 1973).

How can we use reactance theory to explain why an older adult might choose not to seek assistance? Consider the case of Lydia, an 82-year-old widow living alone in a mobile home that she and her husband bought some years ago. Her monthly income consists of a Social Security check of $225 that she receives as a surviving spouse. An outreach worker informs Lydia that she is probably eligible for SSI, which would provide her with additional income as well as Medicaid coverage for her health care needs. She refuses, and states that she does not want to give any information about her personal affairs to a government worker. She fears that once she gives them any personal information and begins to receive SSI, the government could invade other aspects of her personal life or restrict what she does with her money. According to the reactance theory, even though a direct threat to Lydia's autonomy does not exist, she does not want to go through a process that she perceives will indirectly cause harm to her autonomy. As a result, she chooses not to accept any financial assistance.

Attribution Theory

Think about the last time someone helped you out of a difficult situation. Do you recall asking yourself why that person decided to help you? When contemplating whether to ask for help, did you wonder why you needed help with that problem? Attribution theory states that individuals formulate attributions to understand, predict, and control their environment and help explain why certain events occur (Kelley, 1967). Individuals assign attributions to both internal (self) and external (environment) factors to help them understand the occurrence of events or behaviors.

Let us examine the first question: why did that person help you? If you have been on the receiving end of some assistance recently, you might have pondered for a moment *why* the person helping you chose to do so. What was the person's real motivation for helping you fix your flat tire or assisting you to solve a computer problem? How we formulate an answer to this question plays an important role in whether we will allow someone to help us.

According to the attribution theory, a recipient of assistance will want to know what motivated the helper's behavior (Fisher et al., 1983). In deciding what the helper's motive is, the recipient can attribute the helping person's behavior to three possible motives. Fisher et al. suggested that the recipient might think that the person providing the assistance (a) acted from genuine concern; (b) acted for ulterior motives; or (c) performed the action because his or her role demanded it. These possible inferences readily apply to seeking assistance from helpers in the older person's formal network. If the older adult believes that the person providing assistance does so because that person's role requires it or that the helper acts from genuine concern, chances are that the older adult will be less hesitant about seeking assistance from a formal source.

Another application of the attribution theory is its use in answering another important question linked to seeking help when people need it—why do we need help? Remember, the basic premise of the attribution theory is that individuals scan their environment to explain some of their behaviors or actions. According to the theory, if individuals cannot explain their behaviors by external (environmental) factors, then they will look inward for internal factors (personal disposition). In the process of trying to determine why they need help, they will look for three types of information: the *distinctiveness* of the behavior (does the behavior always occur?), *consensus* (are others responding similarly?), and *consistency* (how often the behavior occurs).

The recipient assesses each of these dimensions in any help-seeking situation. An internal or external attribution depends on the combination of different levels of distinctiveness, consensus, and consistency (Fiske & Taylor, 1991). For example, if you decide that you *always* have trouble with computers (low distinctiveness), that you have had difficulty using computers ever since you first started working on them (high consistency), and that other people do not seem to have the same trouble you do with computers (low consensus), then you are likely to attribute your computer trouble to an internal attribute (you cannot learn new things). In contrast, if you have experienced difficulty with only one particular computer in the computer lab (high distinctiveness), you infrequently have trouble using computers (low consistency), and you notice others in the computer lab having the same difficulty (high consensus), then you will probably attribute your troubles to an external factor (the computer is a lemon).

This reasoning process is an important determinant in the decision to seek assistance. For example, if recipients feel that they need assistance because of a personal inadequacy (internal attribution), then their self-perception will be low and help seeking may not occur (Fisher et al., 1983). On the other hand, if individuals perceive that many people need help for a similar condition (high consensus), they will make an external attribution and will be more likely to accept assistance (Gerber, 1969; Tessler & Schwartz, 1972).

How can the attribution theory be used to understand why a caregiver might not use the services of an adult day program? Consider the situation of Jacque, an adult daughter. Her mother, Olivia, is 82 and has lived alone since her spouse died 11 years ago. In the past six months, Jacque has seen her mother's physical condition steadily worsen—she is becoming more forgetful, and her unsteady gait causes her to fall frequently. Jacque has helped with shopping, meals, and other errands along with working and caring for her own two children. Her work and family obligations make it impossible to constantly supervise her mother during the day, and she is becoming increasingly worried about Olivia's wellbeing. A friend tells Jacque about the local adult day program and suggests she take Olivia. What are the chances that Jacque will use the services of the adult day program?

If we apply the attribution theory to this situation, we can expect that when Jacque is deciding whether to take her mother to the program, she will think about why she would need to use the services of an adult day program. She may come to the conclusion that taking her mother to the program demonstrates that she does not have the personal fortitude to take care of her (an internal attribution). She may, on the other hand, attribute the need for assistance to her mother's condition (external attribution). If her reasoning follows this latter line of thinking, she will probably be more likely to use the adult day program. If she formulates an internal attribution, she will be less inclined to use the service.

Equity Theory

Social exchange theories suggest that individuals interact with one another through the exchange of valued objects or sentiments. Several similar versions of exchange theories exist, including Walster, Berscheid, and Walster's (1973) equity theory. This theory is based on the premise that individuals strive to maintain equity within their relationships (Adams, 1965). Individuals who feel they are getting more than they should and who feel indebted to others react negatively to these situations in which equity is compromised (Rook, 1987). When inequities occur, individuals experience a certain degree of distress and attempt to rectify the imbalance either by altering the tangible elements of the interaction process or by psychologically reformulating the interaction context. Furthermore, equity theory states that the greater the degree of inequity, the greater the degree of stress experienced because of the inequity (Hatfield & Sprecher, 1983). In a help-seeking situation, recipients will feel inequality when they have a higher ratio of outcomes to inputs (Walster et al., 1973).

A number of researchers reported that individuals on the receiving end of assistance who were unable to reciprocate were less likely to seek or ask for assistance (DePaulo, 1978; Greenberg & Shapiro, 1971; Manton, 1987). When researchers introduced reciprocity into an inequitable situation, recipients reported feeling better about the assistance they were receiving (Wilke & Lazette, 1970). In situations in which introducing reciprocity is not possible, changing a recipient's perception of the helping context can be just as useful in restoring a sense of equity (Greenberg & Westcott, 1983; Roberto & Scott, 1986). If we apply this idea to receiving assistance from the formal network, older adults may avoid feeling indebted by differentiating between programs in which they are entitled (i.e., Social Security) and those that are needs-based (i.e., food stamps; Lipman & Sterne, 1962). There is a sense of equity in programs such as Social Security because older adults have *paid* into the program—and they perceive that they are receiving financial benefits to which they are entitled. In contrast, the number of older adults who participate in programs in which recipients are always on the receiving end and provide nothing in return for those benefits may be low.

Equity theory also can be used to explain help-seeking behavior. Consider the situation of Hanna, 72, who suffers from rheumatoid arthritis that severely limits her ability to attend activities outside her home. Before her arthritis limited her activities, she worked part time and was a volunteer at the local hospital. Although she enjoyed working, she always remarked on how much satisfaction she experienced when helping patients. She describes herself as an independent person, having always provided for her own needs. Because her arthritis keeps her from volunteering and getting out as much as she would like, she finds herself becoming more and more isolated. She reads in the newspaper about a friendly visiting program, a service in which a volunteer provides social companionship and assistance with errands. She wonders how she could ever compensate someone for coming and spending time with her—she feels that she has nothing to give the volunteer in return. If Hanna feels she will be unable to reciprocate the help she receives, it may be difficult for her to accept the assistance of the volunteer.

Threats-to-Self-Esteem Model

The threats-to-self-esteem model (Fisher et al., 1983) is based on the assumption that most help-seeking situations contain a mixture of both positive and negative elements (see Exhibit 3.2). Whether the helping situation is perceived as positive or negative depends on the characteristics of the (a) aid, (b) helper, (c) recipient, and (d) context. If recipients perceive the aid as highlighting their inferiority or dependency, they will view the aid as *self-threatening*. In contrast, if they see the aid as positive, they will perceive the assistance as *self-supportive*. If the helper is similar in age or status to the recipient, or has a higher status than that of the recipient, the recipient is likely to see the aid as highlighting their inferiority, and the helping situation becomes self-threatening (Fisher & Nadler, 1976; Nadler, Fisher, & Streufest, 1976). Recipient characteristics also can influence how the help-seeking episode can influence the perception of the help-seeking behavior. Researchers have found that recipients who were ego-involved in the task and who valued autonomy were more threatened by receiving the assistance (DePaulo & Fisher, 1980; Nadler, Sheinberg, & Jaffe, 1981). Evidence suggests that those with high self-esteem are more reluctant to receive help than those with low self-esteem (Nadler & Mayseless, 1983).

Best Practice: Equity Theory in Action

Partners in Care is a service credit exchange program in Severna Park, Maryland, designed to create community by linking frail elderly and disabled adults with neighbors who volunteer their time to help with occasional tasks and errands. Participants may provide services, receive services, or both. For each hour of service donated by volunteers, an hour of service credit is earned. That credit may be used at a later time or donated back to the program for frail elderly who cannot volunteer themselves.

Volunteer services are matched to individual needs and may include providing grocery shopping, transportation, handyman help, yard work, or friendly visits. Volunteers are encouraged to utilize their individual talents, interests, and creativity as Partners in Care. The goal of these services is to help seniors and adults remain in their own homes. Each hour of volunteer work earns an hour of credit for the volunteer. Groups of volunteers are encouraged to collaborate efforts for larger projects.

For more information about Partners in Care Partnerships and/or services, call 410–544–4800, or toll free 1–800–227–5500, www.partnersincare.org.

Source: Fisher et al. (1983). Used with permission.

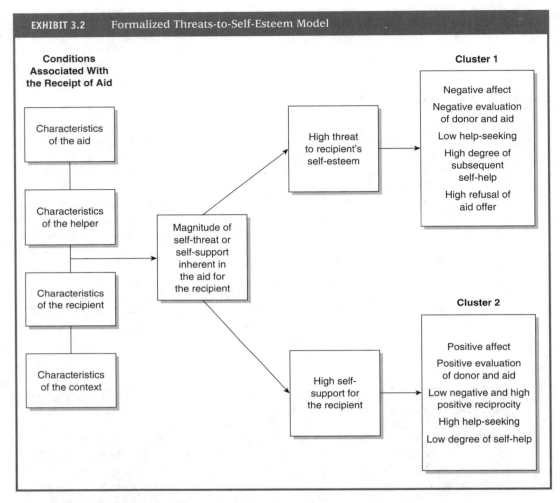

EXHIBIT 3.2   Formalized Threats-to-Self-Esteem Model

Source: Adapted from Fisher et al. (1983).

Accordingly, the recipient will perceive the characteristics associated with the receipt of aid as either self-threatening or self-supporting. This, in turn, will influence the recipient's decision to seek assistance. If the recipient perceives the help as predominantly self-threatening, the recipient's reaction will be negative (Cluster 1 in the model shown in Exhibit 3.2). On the other hand, if the recipient views the assistance as primarily self-supportive, the recipient's reaction will be positive (Cluster 2 in the model).

Let us look at how the threats-to-self-esteem model can help predict help-seeking behavior. Consider Mabel and John, who have lived in a small rural community for

25 years. Mabel is 75 and still works at the local school district as a secretary. She is quite proud of the many years she has worked and is well known in the community. John, 84, retired 15 years ago and has remained healthy until recently. John has begun to experience back problems, high blood pressure, and arthritis that limit his mobility. He has successfully recovered from angioplasty for clogged arteries in his heart and neck. Because of John's health problems, Mabel thinks it is time to look into additional insurance that will supplement their Medicare coverage. Mabel has collected information from various insurance companies but is having trouble determining which policy is best. The local area agency on aging has trained a number of older adults who live in the community to be insurance counselors and assist other older adults in comparing Medigap policies. Mabel refuses to use the service because she does not want to "look stupid" in front of the people she knows. In this situation, Mabel perceives that both the situation and the characteristics of the donor are self-threatening and most likely will not seek the assistance of an insurance counselor.

APPLICATION OF THEORY IN PRACTICE

Theories can be powerful tools in understanding and predicting the patterns and behaviors of others. The theories and models described in this chapter, summarized in Exhibit 3.3, can give practitioners and students a better understanding of why older adults may or may not use the services and programs that would enhance their wellbeing. If service providers are aware of the different models and theories of help-seeking behavior, they can work to deliver their services in a way that addresses issues of equity or self-esteem. Using attribution theory, adult day program directors can convey a message to overworked caregivers that can help them reformulate the attributions they construct about using the services of an adult day program. Changing caregivers' internal attribution that using adult day care services is an indication that they are personal failures to an external attribution will increase the likelihood of program use. Simply informing older adults of the services that exist in communities will not guarantee that they will use the services. Understanding and acknowledging the psychosocial and cultural barriers to accepting help will increase the use of community-based services by older adults in times of need.

SUGGESTIONS FOR FURTHER READING

In this chapter we have provided only a brief overview of different psychosocial theories that can help in understanding service use among older adults. Some suggested readings about each of the theories are listed below if you would like to learn more about each of these theories.

EXHIBIT 3.3   Summary Table of Psychosocial Theories

Theory	Author(s)	Summary
Continuity Theory	Atchley	Continuity theory holds that, in making adaptive choices, middle-aged and older adults attempt to preserve and maintain existing internal and external structures; and they prefer to accomplish this objective by using strategies tied to their past experiences of themselves and their social world. Change is linked to the person's perceived past, producing continuity in inner psychological characteristics as well as in social behavior and in social circumstances. Continuity is thus a grand adaptive strategy that is promoted by both individual preference and social approval Atchley (1989, p. 183).
Social Behavioral Model	Anderson and Newman	Using services is a function of predisposing (e.g., age, race/ethnicity, marital status, and gender), enabling (e.g., income, access to transportation, awareness of services), and need (e.g., subjective assessment or professional evaluation) variables.
Reactance Theory	Brehm	Individuals value states such as freedom and autonomy and when these valued states are threatened, a negative state occurs (reactance).
Attribution Theory	Kelley	In order to understand, predict, and control one's environment, individuals assign attributions to themselves and the external environment.
Equity Theory	Walster, Berscheid, & Walster	Individuals strive to maintain equity within their relationships, and when perceived inequities occur, individuals react negatively and attempt to rectify the imbalance.
Threats to Self-Esteem	Fischer et al.	Help-seeking situations are a combination of positive and negative perceived characteristics of the type of aid being provided, the person helping, the recipient, and the context.

Continuity Theory

Atchley, R. C. (1989). A continuity theory of normal aging. *The Gerontologist, 29*(2), 183–190.
Atchley, R. C. (1999). *Continuity and adaptation in aging: Creating positive experiences*. Baltimore, MD: Johns Hopkins University Press.

Social Behavioral Model

Phillips, K. A., Morrison, K. R., Andersen, R., & Aday, L. A. (1998). Understanding the context of health-care utilization: Assessing environmental and provider-related variables in the behavioral model of utilization. *Health Services Research, 33*(3), 571–596.
Wolinsky, F. D., Coe, R. M., Miller, D. K., Prendergast, J. M., Creel, M. J., & Chavez, M. N. (1983). Health services utilization among the noninstitutionalized elderly. *Journal of Health and Social Behavior, 24*, 325–337.

Reactance Theory

Brehm, S. S., & Brehm, J. W. (1981). *Psychological reactance: A theory of freedom and control*. New York: Academic Press.
Dillard, J. P., & Shen, L. (2005). On the nature of reactance and its role in persuasive health. *Communication Monographs, 72*(2),144–168.
Woller, K., Buboltz, M. P., Walter, C., & Loveland, J. M. (2007). Psychological reactance: Examination across age, ethnicity, and gender. *American Journal of Psychology, 120*(1), 15–24.

Attribution Theory

Martinko, M. J., & Thomson, N. F. (1998). A synthesis and extension of the Weiner and Kelley attribution models. *Basic & Applied Social Psychology, 20*(4), 271–284.
Stajkovic, A. D., & Sommer, S. M. (2000). Self-efficacy and causal attributions: Direct and reciprocal links. *Journal of Applied Social Psychology, 30*(4), 707–737.
Weiner, B. (2000). Intrapersonal and interpersonal theories of motivation from an attributional perspective. *Educational Psychology Review, 12*(1), 1–14.

Equity Theory

Argyle, M. (1992). Receiving and giving support: Effects on relationships and well-being. *Counselling Psychology Quarterly, 5*(2), 123–133.
Lu, L. (1997). Social support, reciprocity, and well-being. *Journal of Social Psychology, 137*(5), 618–628.
Messick, D. M., & Cook, K. S (eds.) (1983). *Equity theory: Psychological and sociological perspectives*. New York: Praeger.
Jung, J. (1990). The role of reciprocity in social support. *Basic & Applied Social Psychology, 11*(3), 243–253.

Threats to Self-Esteem

Nadler, A. (1987). Determinants of help-seeking behaviour: The effects of helpers' similarity, task centrality and recipient's self esteem. *European Journal of Social Psychology, 17*(1), 57–67.

Goodwin, R., Costa, P., & Adonu, J. (2004). Social support and its consequences: 'Positive' and 'deficiency' values and their implications for support and self-esteem. *British Journal of Social Psychology, 4*(3), 465–474.

Schütz, A. (1998). Coping with threats to self-esteem: The differing patterns of subjects with high versus low trait self-esteem in first-person accounts. *European Journal of Personality, 12*(3), 169–186.

PART II

The Continuum of Services

4

Information and Assistance

Gary was panicked. His mother, Ruth, was coming home from the hospital in two days. Ruth, 81, had suffered her third stroke. She was confused and weakened on her right side but not paralyzed. Gary knew that his mother could not return to her apartment at this time, but he could not imagine Ruth living with him. With his bachelor's lifestyle and two jobs, he simply could not provide the care and attention she needed. His girlfriend suggested that he look in the community services section of the phone book for help. There he found Carelink listed under senior services. He didn't know what to expect, but he knew he had to start somewhere. Pete, the Carelink information and referral specialist, spent 20 minutes suggesting several options for Gary. When Gary talked with his girlfriend that evening, he told her that he still felt overwhelmed but that he had had no idea there were so many services for seniors with problems such as his mother's.

It is easy to see why Gary was overwhelmed with the idea of caring for his mother. Who would supervise her during the day? Who would cook her meals and administer her medications when he was at work? What about rehabilitation therapy? Although people such as Gary know that there must be services and programs in their community that can help, they often do not know where to begin to look. Not knowing who to call for assistance can result in leaving a personal or familial crisis unresolved; finding help, however, can be extremely difficult. As Levinson (1988) points out, the volume of services is so great that the result is a complex and fragmented network that makes finding information problematic for the average person. Information and referral/assistance (I&R/A) services are designed to help older adults and their families to access the services they need. Chelimsky (1991) defines I&R/A as "the active process of linking someone who has a need or problem with an agency that provides services meeting that need or solving that problem" (1991, p. 2). In this chapter, we review the policies that helped create I&R/A services, describe the different types of programs and the people they serve, and look at the challenges that lie ahead for I&R/A services.

POLICY BACKGROUND

Information and referral services trace their origins to a social support agency created in the 1870s called the Social Service Exchange. Social Service Exchanges were created to prevent duplication of relief giving and increase the efficiency of screening "worthy" from "unworthy" applicants (McCaslin, 1981). By 1946, there were 320 exchanges, but the number had dropped to 97 by 1963 (Long, Anderson, Burd, Mathis, & Todd, 1971).

During this period, the Social Service Exchanges were being replaced by different I&R/A systems. In the 1940s, Britain and the United States set up information centers to assist World War II veterans in finding appropriate resources. By 1949, however, the majority of these centers had shut down as well (Long et al., 1971). Also during this time, the United Community Funds and Councils of America, the predecessor to the United Way, began to provide information about social welfare resources and, with the creation of the Public Health Service, began to expand I&R/A efforts into health and aging resources (Levinson, 1988; Long et al., 1971).

A boost to the concept of I&R/A services came in the 1960s with the increase in public and private sector programs, which included legislation promoting the creation of I&R/A services to persons who were chronically ill, mentally ill, and aged (Levinson, 1988). In addition, the Older Americans Act (OAA) of 1965 instructed the Administration on Aging (AoA) to create a network of I&R/A services. Amendments to the OAA in 1978 provided that the AoA would act as a clearinghouse for all information related to the needs and interests of older persons and would provide access to services that included transportation, outreach, and I&R/A (Lowy, 1980). I&R/A services are currently funded along with other programs under Title III-B (Support Services and Senior Centers) of the OAA. Because I&R/A services are funded in this manner, the total amount of Title III dollars spent in delivering I&R/A services to older adults is unknown.

The OAA defines I&R/A as a service for older adults that (a) provides individuals with current information on opportunities and services available to the individuals within their communities, including information relating to assistive technology; (b) assesses the problems and capacities of the individuals; (c) links the individuals to the opportunities and services that are available; (d) to the maximum extent practicable, ensures that the individuals receive the services they need and that they are aware of the opportunities available through the establishment of adequate follow-up procedures; and (e) serves the entire community of older individuals, particularly older individuals with the greatest social and economic need and those at risk for institutional placement.

In part because the OAA requires the AoA to establish I&R/A as a priority service, the AoA has actively been involved in promoting and enhancing I&R/A services. For example, the National Association of State Units on Aging received a grant from the AoA in 1990 to establish the National Information and Referral Support Center (NIRSC) to strengthen the capacity of I&R/A activities under the OAA. The support center has served as the focal point for education and training of I&R/A providers across the country. During the first three years of the project, the support center developed a series of guides designed to promote consistency and improve the quality of I&R/A services. More recently, the NIRSC offers technical assistance documents that educate I&R/A specialists in areas of diversity, Medicare, communication skills, best practices for I&R/A, and information technology support. In addition, the support center is encouraging the exchange of information about I&R/A services through an online "Strategy Exchange," the compilation of existing I&R/A materials, and the publication of the *eBulletin,* which is a monthly newsletter that features public policy updates, resources, tools, strategies, and emerging trends to promote aging I&R/A professionalism. In collaboration with the National Alliance of Information and Referral Systems (AIRS), NIRSC has developed a certification for I&R/A Specialists in Aging. The certification is a documentation of one's ability in the field of I&R/A, reflecting specific competencies and related performance criteria which describe the knowledge, skills, attitudes, and work-related behaviors needed by practitioners to successfully execute their duties.

Another national initiative to enhance I&R/A services is the AoA's creation of the National Eldercare Locator. This nationwide I&R/A service, created in 1991, is administered by the National Association of Area Agencies on Aging and the National Association of State Units on Aging. The service links callers or online users with I&R/A networks of state and local organizations that assist older adults and their families. These policy initiatives have been instrumental in providing technical support to I&R/A services. Under the 2006 amendments to the OAA, the AoA is also charged with building awareness of programs that provide benefits to older adults and to work with states and local area agencies on aging to carry out outreach and benefit enrollment assistance. The AoA will be establishing a National Center on Senior Benefits Outreach and Enrollment that, among other activities, is to maintain web decision-support and enrollment tools, develop and maintain a clearinghouse on best practices in enrolling older adults with the greatest economic need, and collaborate with federal partners administering federal programs to provide training on the effective outreach strategies.

Another I&R/A initiative, called the National 211 Initiative, has been underway since 1997. It was developed by a national partnership between AIRS and United Way and is modeled after the 911 phone number for emergencies. The 211 number is a way for individuals and families to search for health and human services information and referral services in their communities. In 1997, the I&R/A United Way of Metropolitan Atlanta created the nation's first 211 initiative that provides a free 24-hour telephone information and referral service, using a database of over 2,000 agencies to match callers to social services, and volunteer and donation opportunities (United Way of Connecticut, 2001). In 2000, the Federal Communications Commission authorized the 211 number to be used across the country for information and referral for human service information and referral. As of July 2006, 211 serves over 172 million Americans—over 57% of the entire population—through 192 active 211 systems covering all or part of 39 states (including 16 states with 100% coverage) plus Washington DC and Puerto Rico. In Canada, 211 currently covers over 20% of the population (Alliance of Information and Referral Systems, 2007). In this next section, we examine the I&R/A program structure and services and provide a profile of users of I&R/A services.

USERS AND PROGRAMS

Although I&R/A services play an important role in linking older adults with needed services, few scholarly evaluations of I&R/A services have been conducted during the past 25 years. Moreover, local studies that have evaluated I&R/A services are unpublished and not readily accessible (McCaslin, 1981). As a result, who uses I&R/A services and the outcomes of such use remain unclear. The few studies that have been conducted on I&R/A programs are reported below.

In 1975, the AoA embarked on a six-year research and demonstration project to develop a more useful and comprehensive system of I&R/A centers (Long, 1975). An evaluation of services provided by a demonstration project—the Wisconsin Information Service (WIS)—was conducted. Thirteen I&R/A sites were created and evaluated throughout Wisconsin from 1972 to 1974. Researchers found that 90% of inquiries were made by telephone and that slightly less than half (40%) of the respondents said that they had found out about the service through word of mouth. More than 75% of respondents who were informed about WIS through outreach efforts followed through with a contact to a recommended agency. A similar percentage of callers followed through with a call to a recommended agency; when referral appointments were made, however, 82% followed through with the recommended contact. All the WIS centers in the study served a high proportion of older adults. In addition, a higher percentage of older adults (55.6%) than younger adults (18.8%) received escort and/or transportation services.

For Your Files: Eldercare Locator

The Eldercare Locator is sponsored by the Administration on Aging, the National Association of Area Agencies on Aging, and the National Association of State Units on Aging. Fully operational since November 1992, the Eldercare Locator is a nationwide directory assistance service designed to help older persons and caregivers locate local support resources for aging Americans. This service links callers with the I&R/A networks of state and local area agencies on aging. The Locator receives 130,000 calls annually and the website receives, on average, 15,000 visits monthly and can handle 150 different languages.

When contacting the Eldercare Locator, callers speak to a friendly, trained professional who has access to an extensive list of I&R/A services. The Eldercare Locator will provide the names and phone numbers of organizations within a desired location, anywhere in the country. Anyone may call the toll-free number, 800–677–1116, Monday through Friday, 9:00 a.m. to 8:00 p.m. Eastern Time. Callers should have the following information ready: (a) county and city name or zip code and (b) a brief description of the problem.

Source: National Association of Area Agencies on Aging (n.d.).

Two years later, Mark Battle Associates (1977) provided additional information about I&R/A services for the AoA by conducting a national study of 62 I&R/A programs across the country. The researchers collected data from I&R/A directors and staff, state units on aging (SUAs) or area agencies on aging (AAAs), and users about the organizational structure, type of services offered, and client satisfaction. They reported that I&R/A services that were age segregated were more likely to provide a more comprehensive array of services than I&R/A services that were age integrated. The average number of calls about or from older adults was 179 per month, and the range of callers was from 2 to 11,000. Of the users, 75% indicated that the I&R/A staff had fully or partially resolved their problems, and almost all users (97%) indicated that they were pleased with the way in which their interviews were conducted. A similar percentage (92%) indicated that the I&R/A service did a good job in assisting them. The most common problems of older callers were related to financial matters and Social Security, transportation, health problems and care, and home health care. Housing maintenance and repair, food and nutrition, and homemaker services were also frequently mentioned.

The different nuances of I&R/A programs with regard to data collection make it difficult to identify consistencies across programs. In addition, simply collecting the data can be problematic. For example, to protect the caller's identity, some I&R/A agencies do not collect information about the caller's race, income, or other demographic information (U.S. General Accounting Office [USGAO], 1991b). This makes it hard to generalize about the type of older adults who use I&R/A systems and the problems for which they are seeking assistance. The studies that have been conducted, however, can inform us about the types of older adults seeking services and can serve as a starting point for more rigorous empirical investigations.

Coyne (1991) examined the demographic characteristics and use patterns of 257 callers to a statewide I&R/A service specializing in Alzheimer's disease and related dementia. Results indicated that the average age of respondents was 50 years and that the majority were women (78%). In addition, the majority were married and working full time (71% and 58%, respectively). Slightly fewer than half the callers were direct caregivers (44%), and 31% were family members of caregivers. The majority of callers also indicated that they were pleased with the services they received. For example, 96% reported that they had received the information they requested and thought the information was helpful. Of callers who received referrals to specific community agencies, 65% reported that they had contacted or used the referral.

Researchers have also investigated the effectiveness of various outreach efforts by I&R/As, such as direct mailings of resource directories and door-to-door canvassing in targeted neighborhoods. For example, Cherry, Prebis, and Pick (1995) examined the effects of a mass-mailed *Senior Access Directory* to 35,000 older adults over the age of 60 living in northwest Indiana. To evaluate the effectiveness of the mailing in increasing service awareness and use, staff asked all callers 9 days before the mailing and 10 days after the mailing how they had found out about the agency and whether they had used the directory. More than 80% of the respondents indicated that the directory had increased awareness of services. Moreover, 44% reported that receiving the directory had prompted some action, such as talking to family members or calling an agency listed in the directory. Finally, calls to United Way more than doubled, increasing from 52 before to 122 after the distribution.

Best Practice Information and Referral/Assistance Services—Medicare Information Outreach

The National Association of Area Agencies on Aging (N4A) received a $1.9 million grant for fiscal year 2001 to fund the Medicare Empowerment and Collaboration Initiative in collaboration with the National Association of State Units on Aging

(NASUA). The overall goal of the Initiative was to enhance the capacity of Information & Referral/Assistance (I&R/A) programs and other aging network programs to provide information about Medicare options to beneficiaries and their caregivers. Twenty-six projects representing 24 states and the District of Columbia were funded through the Initiative. Here are two examples of outreach activities funded by these grant dollars:

Inter Tribal Council of Arizona, Inc., Phoenix, Arizona

The Inter Tribal Council of Arizona, Inc. (ITCA) developed the Medicare Education and Training (MET) project to provide education, information and referral, and outreach services to existing and potential Medicare beneficiaries, their caregivers and persons with disabilities living on six tribal reservations in remote areas of Arizona. Two project goals were achieved by ITCA. It successfully developed several strategies for increasing accessibility to entitlement programs for American Indian elders and individuals with disabilities. With the help of 33 new volunteers from 10 different tribes, eight Medicare workshops held in Phoenix and at each participating tribe, and six outreach visits, 228 clients were given information about Medicare, and door-to-door outreach was conducted at the Hopi Tribe.

For more information, contact Inter Tribal Council of Arizona, Inc., 2214 North Central Ave. Suite 100, Phoenix, AZ 85004, Contact Person: Lee Begay, 602-258–4822, lee.begay@itcaonline.com (Source: National Association of State Units on Aging, 2006, p. 3).

Boulder County Aging Services Division, Boulder, Colorado

Boulder County Aging Services Division (BCASD) empowered Spanish-speaking elders, low-income elders, homebound elders, and elders living in sparsely populated areas of Boulder County to maximize their health care choices by targeting Medicare education, counseling, and ombudsman services to these groups. A new person hired through this grant successfully conducted outreach to the Hispanic community throughout Boulder County, provided counseling and ombudsman services, made educational presentations in both English and Spanish, trained providers to make referrals, and distributed Spanish-language resources to health and human services organizations, senior center staff, and church leaders. Additionally, BCASD enhanced the technological abilities of project staff by providing laptop computers for PowerPoint presentations and on site access to internet resources. Project staff made over 150 outreach efforts over the course of the year and conducted 41 educational presentations reaching 1,186 people. Partnerships were established with community groups, various communities of faith, veterans' organizations, and civic community groups, affording the project greater visibility and credibility than had resulted from previous outreach efforts.

For more information contact the Boulder County Aging Services Division, Boulder, Colorado, PO Box 471, Boulder, CO, 80306. Contact (303) 441–1170, flag@co.boulder .co.us (Source: National Association of State Units on Aging, 2006, p. 4).

CHARACTERISTICS OF PROGRAMS

Where and how do older adults and their families access I&R/A services? The location of the agency responsible for providing I&R/A services, the target population served, and the scope of information and services provided all vary by community. For example, I&R/A programs can be located in government offices, public or private agencies, voluntary associations, public libraries, or community centers (McCaslin, 1981). Local AAAs may directly deliver I&R/A services or may contract with other agencies to deliver I&R/A services to older adults. Moreover, I&R/As may target services to the general population or to a specific population, such as older adults, families with children, or persons with disabilities or chronic conditions. They may provide information about all types of community resources and services or may specialize in one information area, such as services for persons with Alzheimer's disease. I&R/A services may have information about national, state, or local services (Levinson, 1988). Despite these myriad differences, all I&R/A programs have the same goal: to link individuals to appropriate services. A well-designed I&R/A will provide the following elements:

- *Information Provision.* Information is given to an older person, caregiver or another provider in response to an expressed need concerning opportunities and services available to them.
- *Referral Provision.* Referral is made when the individual's needs are determined through an assessment and the person is directed to a particular resource or choice of resources.
- *Advocacy/Intervention.* Advocacy can involve helping an individual explain his or her situation in the "agency's language" in an effort to obtain a needed service. Or advocacy can involve articulating the needs of a specific group of older persons to community policy makers, planners, and service providers in order to develop new services, expand existing services, modify service delivery, or secure financial resources.
- *Follow-Up.* Follow-up is conducted with an older person, his/her caregiver, and/or the service provider or agency to which the individual was referred, to determine whether the inquirer has received the appropriate service(s), and whether the service(s) provided were useful in meeting the individual's assessed need (National Aging I&R/A Support Center, 2001, pp. 2–3).

DEVELOPING AND MAINTAINING A RESOURCE FILE

The foundation of a good I&R/A service is its resource database. It must be accurate and up-to-date and must include detailed information about community agencies. According to the guidelines established by the National Information and Referral Support Center, the database should include the following information about community agencies:

- unique record identification number;
- code to identify the organization responsible for maintaining the record (to facilitate combination, in a single database, of records maintained by different organizations);

- organization name (legal name), and AKAs including former name(s), popular names and popular acronyms;
- program name, if applicable;
- street and mailing addresses (main location and branches);
- telephone number(s) including TDD/TTY, fax, website address and electronic mail addresses for the agency, its sites and specific services, if applicable;
- hours and days of operation;
- services provided and target populations served;
- eligibility requirements and exclusions (e.g., age, gender);
- documents which may be required by the organization for application (such as birth certificates);
- geographic area served;
- application process;
- languages other than English in which the service is offered (bilingual staff or interpreter services);
- legal status (e.g., nonprofit, government, for-profit, unincorporated group);
- fee structure for service, if any (the phrase "sliding scale" may be sufficient; use "none" or the equivalent when applicable);
- method of payment accepted (e.g., Medicaid, Medicare, private insurance);
- name and title of the organization's administrator/director; and
- date the information was last verified (Alliance of Information and Referral Systems, 2005, p. 16).

The Alliance of Information and Referral Systems (AIRS) (2005) recommends that I&R/A services also collect information about the characteristics of the inquirer. Collecting information about the inquirer's socioeconomic status and demographic characteristics, including language requirements, the nature and extent of the problem, and the level of assistance needed can assist in problem-solving activities as well as provide valuable information about gaps in community resources.

PROMOTION OF INFORMATION AND REFERRAL SERVICES

The functions of an I&R/A program are useless unless older adults and their families know how to access I&R/A services. Unfortunately, studies of awareness of community resources consistently identify I&R/A services as the least known by older adults (Krout, 1983b). Clearly, if I&R/A programs want to empower persons who are "information poor," older adults and their families must be made aware of I&R/A services and benefits (Levinson, 1988). The *National Standards* document (Whaley & Hutchinson, 1993a) recommends that I&R/A services promote their agencies through personal contact, public service announcements, news stories, printed materials, telephone directories, and displays. In addition, I&R/A systems should network with other community agencies to encourage interagency linkages and target subpopulations of older adults such as foreign-language groups, low-income persons, minorities, persons who are socially isolated, and persons with hearing or vision impairments. Canvassing targeted neighborhoods is another strategy often used to inform older adults about I&R/A services. When canvassing neighborhoods, outreach workers can make contact with older adults who may be unaware of the help that community services can provide (Cushing & Long, 1974).

FUNCTIONS OF INFORMATION AND REFERRALS

As shown in Exhibit 4.1, I&R/A programs can provide a range of services within each I&R/A function. The functions of an I&R/A include basic I&R/A activities, support services that facilitate use of needed services, and advocacy (Levinson, 1988; Whaley & Hutchinson, 1993b). Within each function, a range of services is provided to older adults. Ideally, all I&R/As should offer services along the I&R/A continuum to inquirers, and the I&R/A specialists should conduct interviews to determine the extent of I&R/A assistance that inquirers need.

EXHIBIT 4.1 Extent of Provider Intervention in Information and Referral/Assistance Services		
	Extent of I&R Intervention	
I&R Function	*Less Intervention*	*More Intervention*
Basic I&R components	Information giving → Referral giving →	Follow-up
Support services	Translation services → Transportation →	Escort services
Advocacy	Individual advocacy → Family advocacy →	Group advocacy

Source: Adapted from Levinson (1988, p. 44). Used by permission.

INFORMATION AND REFERRAL PROCESS

Exhibit 4.2 illustrates the I&R/A process. When inquirers contact the I&R/A service, an I&R/A specialist determines the needs of the caller, the appropriate resources needed to address the identified needs, and whether referral giving or simply information giving is necessary. The specialist also provides follow-up and assesses the need for advocacy. Each of these steps is discussed below.

Information Giving

At the least, an I&R/A service responds to the request of an inquirer about a particular agency or service by providing basic information about the appropriate agency. The I&R/A staff member gives the inquirer the agency's name, address, and phone number or an explanation of the agency's application process (Whaley & Hutchinson, 1993b). For example, if a caregiver calls and requests information about local adult day programs, the I&R/A service will give the caller the name, address, and phone number of all local adult day programs. Other information that could be helpful to the caller, such as hours of operation or type of service provided, will also be given.

EXHIBIT 4.2 Delivery Process of Information and Referral/Assistance Services

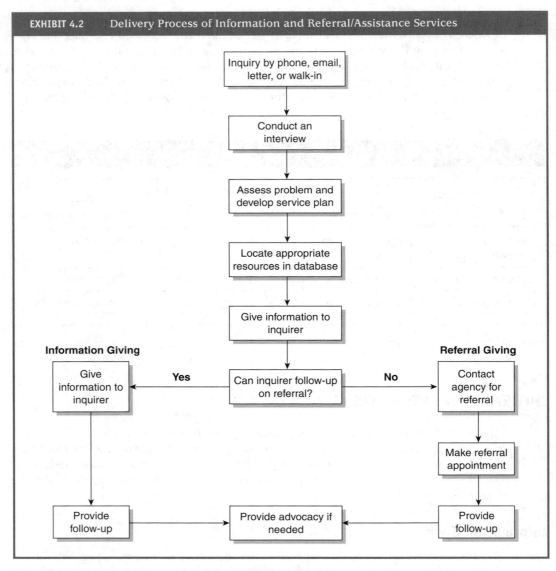

Source: Adapted from Levinson (1988, pp. 147–149). Used by permission.

Referral Giving

Referral giving is a more involved process than information giving. In referral giving, the I&R/A staff are actively involved in assessing the needs of the caller, matching those needs with the appropriate agency, and linking the caller to the appropriate agency either by providing the caller with agency information or by calling the agency and arranging for services (Whaley & Hutchinson, 1993b).

Let's use Gary and his mother as an example of how referral giving works. When Gary calls the I&R/A service, he explains that his mother, who has suffered a series of strokes, will be coming to live with him. Because Gary has no idea what services could help him, the I&R/A specialist must assess the needs of Gary and his mother. After assessing the nature and extent of their problem, the I&R/A specialist can give Gary options for keeping his mother at home. He may be able to care for his mother with help from in-home health services, Meals on Wheels, and the use of an adult day program. The I&R/A specialist may also determine whether Gary's mother qualifies for help in paying for community-based long-term care services. Finally, the I&R/A specialist determines whether it would be appropriate to contact these agencies directly to notify them of Gary's forthcoming contact or to make an appointment on his behalf.

Contacting the agency on behalf of the caller is especially critical in situations in which the caller does not speak English, is hesitant or uncertain about dealing with bureaucracies, or does not have the personal resources needed to negotiate through the process. The complexity of the problems that the inquirer has might require that the I&R/A specialist make multiple referrals, repeated contacts with the inquirer, and numerous contacts with appropriate agencies (Levinson, 1988). I&R/A programs that help inquirers access the services they recommend are commonly referred to as *information and assistance (I&A)* or *enhanced I&R/A* programs, rather than I&R/A programs.

Follow-Up

All I&R/A programs should follow-up on referral cases, including those who received only information, to determine whether inquirers contacted the recommended community service and, if not, why they did not; what assistance was given; and any additional needs that may have arisen (Whaley & Hutchinson, 1993b). Follow-up allows the I&R/A specialist an opportunity to provide additional assistance securing other services if needed. Moreover, follow-up can provide the I&R/A with valuable information about waiting lists or other problems (e.g., eligibility requirements) that inquirers encountered in trying to access recommended services (Huttman, 1985).

Advocacy and Intervention

In some instances, the I&R/A specialist will need to act as an advocate on behalf of an individual or groups of clients. The I&R/A specialist may need to act as an advocate when clients have difficulty receiving services for which they are eligible, when they have been mistreated, or when they are unable to effectively represent themselves (Whaley & Hutchinson, 1993b). The I&R/A specialist also can act as an advocate on behalf of a group of older adults by articulating service gaps and needed policy changes to community and government leaders.

Best Practice: Information and Referral/Assistance Services

The National Information and Referral Support Center identified a number of state and local agencies on aging that used unique strategies to promote the use of I&R/A services. Here are three examples of best practice in I&R/A activities.

White River Area Agency on Aging, Batesville, Rural Arkansas

The White River Area Agency in Aging promoted the concept of "one-stop shopping" to older persons and their caregivers in a 10-county rural area by developing a colorful, attention-getting flyer mailed to each of 69,900 households in the service area. The flyer explained services available; directed persons to call the I&R/A for service information; featured a peel-off label containing the agency's name and toll-free telephone number; and contained information to target low-income and minority group older persons on benefits such as SSI, food stamps, qualified Medicare beneficiaries, and person care services. The objectives of this project were to improve access to information and to increase visibility and use of the I&R/A service. For more information, contact White River Area Agency on Aging, phone: 870–612–3000, www.wraaa.com.

Oklahoma Aging Services Division, Oklahoma City, Oklahoma

Working with national, state, and local agencies, the state of Oklahoma developed a training manual featuring techniques for conducting outreach to Black older adults. Increasing outreach efforts and service use among Blacks was the primary goal of the proposal. Demographic data and proceedings from the 7th Annual State of Oklahoma Minority Outreach and I&R/A Conference were digested and compiled into a comprehensive outreach manual. The benefits of the project are the collaboration with other groups, meeting an I&R/A systems improvement plan objective, and creating an outreach manual that can be replicated. For more information, contact the Aging Services Division at 405–521–2281.

Bucks County Area Agency on Aging, Pennsylvania

The Bucks County Area Agency on Aging conducted a cable television project to offer an alternative way for TV viewers to think about when to call the I&R/A. The project was an effort to improve existing I&R/A services by using new strategies for outreach and building a new relationship with cable TV in Bucks County. Volunteers produced three 30-second informational videos for cable TV and a how-to manual for replication. Benefits of the project include the enhancement of current I&R/A capabilities, increased visibility of the I&R/A, and opportunities for older volunteers to develop new skills that are on the cutting edge of the communications industry. For more information, call Bucks County Area Agency on Aging, 215–348–0510.

Source: Quirk, Whaley, and Hutchinson (1994).

INFORMATION AND REFERRAL SERVICES WITH A NATIONAL SCOPE

As previously mentioned, the Eldercare Locator is an I&R/A service funded by the AoA and sponsored by the National Association of State Units on Aging and the National Association of Area Agencies on Aging. It is a nationwide directory service designed to help older persons and caregivers locate services. Inquirers can call a toll-free number to receive assistance. Callers are asked to provide the information specialist with the county and city name or zip code and the type of problem or service desired. The Eldercare Locator also can be obtained from the National Aging Information Center's Web site, www.aoa.gov/naic. Publications such as the *Resource Directory for Older People* (National Institute on Aging and AoA, 1996) are available from the National Aging Information Center.

CHALLENGES FOR INFORMATION AND REFERRAL SERVICES

As the number of private and public programs and services for older adults continues to grow, it will become more and more difficult to locate the appropriate service in a time of need. I&R/A services will need to respond to a variety of challenges.

For Your Files: **The Alliance of Information and Referral Systems**

The Alliance of Information and Referral Systems (AIRS) is an agency which was formed in 1973 to improve the access to services through the use of I&R/A systems. It currently has a professional membership association of over 1,000 organizations, supporting over 30 state and regional affiliates. AIRS provides training and support of I&R/A activities and offers a certification process for I&R/A practitioners. AIRS also provides publications about I&R/A, conducts national training conferences, and acts as a clearinghouse for I&R/A. AIRS publications include a newsletter, the *Journal of the Alliance of Information and Referral Systems*, and the *National Directory of I&R/A Services in the United States and Canada*. Inquirers can reach AIRS by calling 703-218-AIRS (2477) (or e-mail info@airs.org). The AIRS website is a great place to start when you are looking for more information about I&R/A: see www.airs.org.

Enhancing Information and Referral Services

At the request of the Special Committee on Aging, the USGAO (1991b) examined 12 I&R/A programs that experts believed were illustrative of the promising ways in which I&R/A systems served older adults. The USGAO's research revealed effective methods of delivering I&R/A services used by the programs. On the basis of these findings, the USGAO made four recommendations for I&R/A programming. The first was locating I&R/A services where older populations live or frequently visit, such as grocery stores, drugstores, and shopping centers. For example, the Waxter Center for Senior Citizens in Baltimore, Maryland, has located 14 I&R/A offices in neighborhood senior centers; of those, 6 are located in minority neighborhoods. The second recommendation was to hire professional staff, including minorities, to serve diverse cultural populations. The AAA in Billings, Montana, uses Native American I&R/A workers to make home visits to isolated older adults at six Indian reservations. The effectiveness of using minority I&R/A staff to work with racial and ethnic communities was documented by the Office of Senior Information, Referral, and Health Promotion in San Francisco. They found that in the year after hiring a Black outreach worker, the program served 405 more Black clients. Employing a Chinese American outreach worker also increased the number of Chinese clients served by the program.

The third recommendation was the use of automated information resources and telephone technology to effectively provide information. Strategies included the use of automated information booths at sites throughout the community, multilingual telephone message lines, and computer bulletin boards. Indeed, I&R/A services have begun to appear on the internet. For example, Exhibit 4.3 shows the I&R/A home page of the Minnesota Board on Aging, www.minnesotahelp.info/en/mn/cgi-bin/location.asp. Posting information on the internet provides an additional avenue for older adults and their caregivers to access information. Inquirers can access information anytime and anywhere they have access to the necessary computer technology. As internet access becomes the norm for most households, the number of older adults and their families who are accessing information via the internet is increasing.

Publicizing I&R/A services to older adults and their caregivers through active outreach methods was the fourth recommendation. Suggestions for active outreach included publicizing services in locations such as convenience and video rental stores. Many programs distribute printed materials publicizing I&R/A services throughout their communities. Examples of such efforts include monthly agency newsletters mailed to 19,000 older adults in Manhattan, Kansas, and the distribution of a senior magazine called *Lifetimes* to doctors' offices, nutrition sites, and service providers in Indianapolis and to seniors in an eight-county area.

Future efforts of increasing access to information must include locating I&R/A services in nontraditional places and providing options for multiple entry points to information. Nontraditional places include the workplace, restaurants, and schools. Multiple entry points would assist clients because service providers not associated with I&R/A programs are often the first point of contact for older adults. Hence, staff must be familiar with I&R/A programs as well as services available in communities. It should not matter where older adults start their inquiry for assistance; persons working with older adults must know where to send their clients for further assistance.

Enhancing Information and Referral Databases

Additional empirical evaluations are needed to provide a profile of I&R/A programs and services as well as the effectiveness of I&R/A and outreach services. I&R/A studies could examine the problems that inquirers have, the short- and long-term outcomes of I&R/A intervention, and training needs of staff. In addition, if most people receive information outside a formal I&R/A service, such pathways to service access need to be identified.

EXHIBIT 4.3   Home Page of the Minnesota Board on Aging

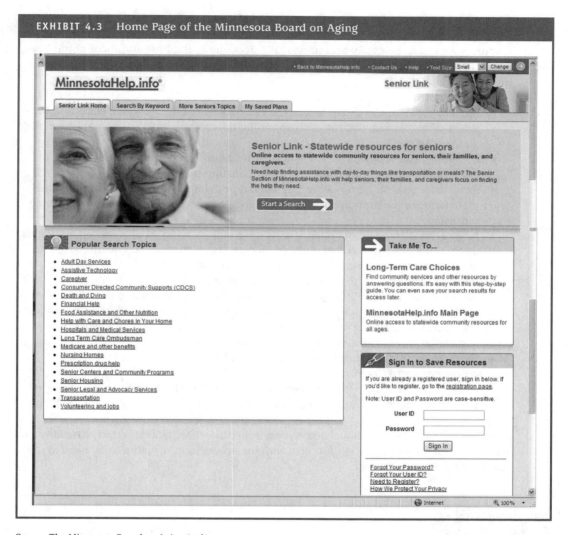

Source: The Minnesota Board on Aging (n.d.).

Supporting the Future of Information and Referral

Although none of the 45 resolutions put forth by the delegates of the 2005 White House Conference on Aging specifically identified I&R/A, I&R/A was included as a means of achieving proposed actions. For example, the delegates proposed to support working caregivers by encouraging and offering incentives for employers to provide information and referral services and to educate Employee Assistance Programs about Eldercare Locator and other information resources. The National Association of State Units on Aging (NASUA) (2000) published a position paper about Information and Referral entitled

Vision 2010: Toward a Comprehensive Aging Information Resource System for the 21st Century. NASUA believes that, in order for the Older Americans Act information and resource system to be easily and universally accessible, the best and most comprehensive source of information for older Americans, their families, and the public, the following are needed:

- *Leadership*. With the Older Americans Act network at the national, state, and local levels taking a proactive role in responding to increases in demand for information and related services.
- *Comprehensiveness*. So that the aging information resource system becomes, in essence, a one-stop shopping source for consumers.
- *Responsiveness*. To better serve the diverse population of older consumers and their families by attending to the wide range of special needs and interests they represent.
- *Integration*. Establishing linkages with programs in aging, health and educational institutions, state and community service agencies, the federal government, and business to promote seamless information delivery.
- *Adequate Funding*. With increases commensurate to increasing needs and demands for services by a growing number of older persons and their families.
- *Skilled Personnel*. Sufficient in number to meet the anticipated number of requests for information and to provide counseling, decision-support, and advocacy assistance appropriate for empowering consumers.
- *Technology*. To maximize communication and reach greater numbers of user audiences cost-effectively.
- *Marketing*. To ensure that older persons and their families across America have an understanding of and access to the information resource system (NASUA, 2000, p. 7).

Indeed, the challenge remains how to best utilize the information highway to inform and empower older adults and their families with the access to information they need to make choices and solve problems.

CASE STUDY

Finding and Asking for Help

Frank is an 83-year-old Hispanic man who has had several small strokes during the past three years. The strokes have weakened him, and on occasions he is mildly confused. He and his wife, Maria, have been married for 35 years. Maria is Frank's second wife and is 26 years younger than Frank.

When Frank retired, they moved to a large urban community in which both have relatives. Although Frank and Maria do not have children, Frank has three daughters from his first marriage, who he rarely sees. Maria attends her neighborhood church regularly and does some volunteer work for the parish. Otherwise, they lead a quiet life.

Since Frank's retirement, Maria has worked at a nursing home as a laundry assistant. Eventually, the many years of hard field work and an injury from lifting laundry culminated in a serious lower back condition. She had two back surgeries; neither surgery was successful. The arrangements for the second surgery were bungled because the surgery was not approved by her health maintenance organization (HMO). The HMO refused to pay for the surgery, and Frank and Maria are now responsible for a $20,000 medical bill that they are unable to pay.

Maria is no longer able to work. She would like to take over the payments of the HMO insurance that the nursing home gave her as a benefit. These payments are $326 per month. The local hospital charity fund has made the payments for a couple of months but cannot continue the assistance much longer. Fortunately, Frank is covered by Medicaid. A detailed examination of their financial condition shows that they are barely able to make ends meet. They have expenses of $625 per month and income of $623 per month, derived from the $494 per month Social Security received by Frank and $129 per month received by Maria. Now that Frank is no longer able to drive, transportation is a serious problem for the couple. At Frank's insistence, Maria never learned to drive. With her own health in jeopardy, no health insurance coverage, and little income of her own, Maria worries constantly about how she will take care of Frank and what she will do if something happens to him. Maria's good friend from church decides to take matters into her own hands and call a senior I&R/A number that she heard about on the radio.

Case Study Questions

1. Would you agree that Maria's friend is calling an appropriate resource with regard to Frank and Maria's situation? Why or why not?

2. List and describe each factor that has a role in justifying Maria's concern about Frank's future and her own.

3. If you were the I&R/A specialist assigned to this case, what additional information about Frank and Maria's situation would you want to know?

4. What do you think is Maria's greatest concern? What do you believe is her greatest problem? If not the same, which problem should be addressed first? Defend your answer.

5. What community resources would you recommend for Frank and Maria? List at least five.

6. How comfortable would you be as an I&R/A specialist that Maria and her friend could follow through on their own with the information that you have provided them? If concerned, what might you do to ensure that some of the suggested resource agencies were contacted?

Learning Activities

1. Watch your daily local newspaper for a week. How many aging network agencies advertise their programs or services during that time? What are the pros and cons of using newspapers as a source of information about aging services and programs? Call the newspaper to determine how much it would cost programs to advertise.

2. Using the case study in this chapter about Frank and Maria, identify the resources you think they need. Go to the library and select two phone books—one of an urban city and one of a rural community in your state. If possible, select unfamiliar cities, and try to identify the community resources you would call that could assist them. What problems did you encounter in locating those services in the phone book? Were there noticeable differences between the rural and urban locations?

3. See if you can locate a senior resource book in your community. How many calls did you have to make before you located a copy? Examine the resource book closely. How is it organized? How much detailed information does the resource book provide about each service or program? What changes would you recommend?

4. Log on to the internet. What type of community resources does your community have online? (If your community does not have any information online, select a city in your state.) How easy or hard was it to find information and services for older adults? Do you think the internet will become a viable resource for older adults and their families to find out about services and programs?

For More Information

National Resources

1. Aging Network Services, 4400 East-West Highway, Suite 907, Bethesda, MD 20814; phone: 301-657-4329; www.agingnets.com.
   The network provides comprehensive assessment of older adults in their own settings with recommendations for appropriate services.

2. B'nai B'rith, 1640 Rhode Island Avenue N.W., Washington, DC 20036; phone: 202-857-1099; www.bnaibrith.org.
   B'nai B'rith is the world's oldest and largest Jewish service organization. The Caring Network is a fee-for-service program that offers information, referrals, and advice to older persons and their families throughout the United States.

3. National Asian Pacific Center on Aging, Melbourne Tower, 1511 3rd Avenue, Suite 914, Seattle, WA 98101; phone: 206-624-1221; www.napca.org.
   This private organization works to improve the delivery of health and social services to Asian Pacific older adults and maintains a national network of service agencies.

4. National Information and Referral Support Center, 1225 I Street N.W., Suite 725, Washington, DC 20005-3914; phone: 202-898-2578; www.nasua.org/informationandreferral/index-ir.cfm.
   The support center provides technical assistance to those who deliver I&R/A and I&A under the OAA. It publishes the *Information and Referral Reporter* quarterly.

Web Resources

1. Boulder County: Human Services Center, Boulder, Colorado: http://bcn.boulder.co.us/human-social/center.html.

    This site has extensive information about and links to local, state, federal, and international human service agencies.

2. USA.gov is the official information and services from the U.S. government. The Senior Citizens' Resources page has a number of different links for more information on education, housing, consumer protection, health, taxes and travel: www.usa.gov/Topics/Seniors.shtml.

3. Community Information and Referral, Phoenix, Arizona: www.cir.org.

    Visitors can search this community I&R/A home page by selecting either an alphabetical listing of community service agencies or a listing of community service categories.

4. Administration on Aging, Washington, DC: www.aoa.dhhs.gov.

    The AoA's home page has an extensive number of links to other national organizations and programs of interest to older adults and their families.

5. Senior Link Online: www.seniorlink.com.

    Senior Link is an elder care resource website that offers referral and consultation for older adults, their families, and providers. Visitors can access elder care professionals, programs, providers, facilities, and agencies that are involved in caring for older adults.

6. Alliance of Information and Referral Systems (AIRS): www.airs.org.

    AIRS functions as a clearinghouse for issues related to managing and using I&R/A services. Its website provides visitors with access to information about professional development opportunities, an information resources library, and a calendar of events.

7. National Aging Information Center: www.aoa.gov/naic.

    The Eldercare Locator can be obtained from this website. The information center also has publications available such as the Resource Directory for Older People.

5

Volunteer and Intergenerational Programs

Twice a week, 88-year-old Hazel volunteers at a local adult day care center. She helps with the hands-on care of participants. Her volunteer duties include helping people to eat, walking with them to the bathroom, and just sitting and talking with them. She also does what the director calls "tender loving pushing." Hazel enjoys volunteer work. When interviewed by a local newspaper, Hazel said, "I hope if something happens to me, there will always be someone to care."

With the growth of the older population and the decline in resources, community agencies often seek assistance from seniors in delivering their programs and services. In many communities, senior volunteerism has developed into a highly organized and often large-scale activity. It is not uncommon to find older volunteers, such as Hazel, working within their local churches, civic or religious groups, hospitals, nursing homes, schools, and human service agencies. According to a national survey, approximately 50% of persons aged 55 to 64, 47% of adults aged 65 to 74, and 43% of persons aged 75 and older volunteer (Saxon-Harrold & Weitzman, 2000). In addition, volunteer rates for older adults have increased over time. In 2004, over 23% of older adults volunteered compared with about 14% in 1974 and 17% in 1989 (Corporation for National and Community Service, 2006).

However, participation in formal volunteer opportunities represents only part of the picture. Older adults also volunteer informally, without support or direction from formal organizations (Corporation for National and Community Service, 2006; Kutner & Love, 2003; Zedlewski & Schaner, 2006). Informal volunteering includes self-initiated activities such as providing transportation, helping around the house, and providing companionship to individuals outside of the household (Zedlewski & Schaner, 2006). Findings from the 2002 National Health and Retirement Study indicate that 60% of all adults aged 55 and older engage in some form of volunteer activity (Johnson & Schaner, 2005). Approximately 10% engage in formal volunteer activities only, 23% are involved in both formal and informal activities, and slightly more than 38% engage in informal volunteer activities only. Estimates of the dollar value of volunteerism suggest that in 2002, $44.3 billion was donated through formal volunteer activities and another $17.8 billion by volunteering time through informal channels (Johnson & Schaner, 2005).

Despite the need for volunteers and the willingness of many seniors to volunteer, many are never asked; thus, older adults are often an untapped resource for volunteer positions. Just 17% of adults aged 55 and older volunteer on their own; among those who were asked to volunteer, 83%—or four times as many—volunteered (Civic Ventures, 2006).

Most individuals give multiple reasons when asked why they volunteer. A 2003 AARP survey of community service and charitable giving practices of 2,069 persons aged 45 and older found that 40% or more of volunteers were motivated to do so because (a) they believed it was a personal responsibility to help others; (b) it made life more satisfying; (c) the organization had an established track record; (d) it helped their own community and made a difference on issues; (e) it helped keep them active; (f) someone they knew was affected by the issue; (g) it was an expression of their religious beliefs; (h) it provided an opportunity to use their skills; and (i) it was something family and friends can do together. Differences in motivations do not appear significant across racial and ethnic groups. Blacks, Hispanics, Asian-Americans, and non-Hispanic Whites identified the main motivation behind volunteering as a personal responsibility to help others.

The manner in which people volunteer, however, does appear to vary across racial and ethnic groups. According to the findings of the AARP (2003) study, Black elders volunteered an average of 17 hours per month and were more likely to engage in informal volunteering than other groups. They tended to volunteer through religious organizations focusing on meeting the needs of the homeless, problems in their neighborhood, advancing the rights of minorities, and tutoring or mentoring others. Eighty-five percent of Asian-American adults volunteered an average of 15 hours a month with a primary focus on advancing minority rights and supporting the arts. Hispanics reported giving the most time of all minority groups: 22 hours a month. Helping other Hispanics—considered very important in their culture—was the focus of their volunteer activities. Non-Hispanic Whites, the largest group, were more likely to engage in volunteer activities to help animals, protect the environment, assist public servants, and support the arts.

Other study variables that distinguished among older adults' motives for volunteering were gender and age (AARP, 2003). Women identified a greater number of motivations as being very important to them than did men. Volunteers aged 70 and older were much more likely than volunteers aged 45 to 69 to view keeping active as a very important motivation for volunteering.

Organizations need to consider a variety of factors when recruiting older volunteers, including the individuals' experience, their perceptions of need, and personal interests (Fischer & Schaffer, 1993). Older adults who have volunteered before are easier to recruit than inexperienced volunteers. Thus it is important for organizations to recruit baby boomers as volunteers prior to their retirement. The good news is that boomers are willing to participate in volunteer activities as long as they can balance their work, leisure, community responsibilities, and other pursuits (Corporation for National and Community Service, 2006).

In this chapter, we begin by examining federal support for volunteer programs. Next, we profile senior volunteers and describe the various volunteer programs designed specifically for older adults, including those with an intergenerational focus. We conclude with a discussion of the current and future issues facing senior volunteer programs.

POLICY BACKGROUND

The idea of structured programs to promote senior volunteerism first emerged in 1963 when President Kennedy pushed for the establishment of a National Service Corps.[1] This organization was to "provide opportunities for service for those aged persons who can assume active roles in community volunteer efforts" (Special Committee on Aging, 1963, p. 14). Although Congress defeated the proposal for the Corps, there was strong pressure from the Senate to include senior participation in programs (e.g., VISTA) sponsored by the newly created Office of Economic Opportunity.

President Johnson supported his predecessor's idea of using the experiences and talents of older adults within their local community but with a new focus on engaging poor people in service endeavors. His vision was to create new roles and functions for older people while providing them with income support via employment and providing services to local communities. In 1965, the first service program targeting low-income seniors, the Foster Grandparent Program emerged. Seniors who enroll in this program provide one-on-one assistance to children with special and exceptional needs (ACTION, 1992). Initially, the Office of Economic Opportunity administered the program. In 1968, the Foster Grandparent Program moved to the Department of Health, Education, and Welfare, where it stayed for three years until it was incorporated into the then newly created agency ACTION (the federal domestic volunteer agency).

In 1971, ACTION became the new administrative home of the Foster Grandparent Program and several other service-oriented programs, including the largest and most versatile program for older adults, the Retired and Senior Volunteer Program (RSVP). This program differs from the Foster Grandparent Program in that older adults have the opportunity to volunteer in a variety of community projects. They are not limited in their participation by income guidelines, they do not receive a stipend, and participation does not require a minimum time commitment. A third senior-specific service program, the Senior Companion Program, began in 1974. Modeled structurally on the Foster Grandparent Program, this program recruits low-income seniors to serve frail and homebound elders. We will discuss each of these programs in greater detail later in the chapter.

Through the early 1990s, ACTION funded, monitored, and supported local public and private nonprofit organizations that sponsored these service projects. In 1993, President Clinton worked with Congress to pass the National and Community Service Trust Act. This Act created the AmeriCorps initiative and established its administrative entity, the Corporation for National and Community Service (CNCS). ACTION programs became part of this umbrella organization.

Although the federal government provides primary funding sources for these larger-scale senior volunteer programs, foundations, the private sector, and private donations also offer financial support for program development. They also support volunteer programs specifically designed to meet the needs of local communities (Wilson & Simson, 1993). For example, funds from the Elvirita Lewis Foundation created the first intergenerational child care center and other intergenerational programs (Struntz & Reville, 1985). Funds from a foundation in South Carolina supported a statewide public and private partnership to develop and evaluate seven rural intergenerational programs that focus on the needs of at-risk children and youth

(Newman, Ward, Smith, Wilson, & McCrea, 1997). The National Institute of Senior Centers also offers funding to projects that make a substantive contribution to knowledge and understanding of senior programs and stimulate questions for further research in the field. For more information see http://aging.wisc.edu/funding/funding.php.

USERS AND PROGRAMS

Characteristics of Older Volunteers

Several background characteristics distinguish among older volunteers. For example, the likelihood of volunteering declines with advancing old age and increasing health concerns (Zedlewski & Schaner, 2006). Approximately 20.0% of persons aged 70 to 74 years, compared with 17.3% of persons aged 75 to 79, 12.7% of persons aged 80 to 84, and 7.2% of persons over age 85, participate in volunteer activities (Federal Interagency Forum on Aging-Related Statistics, 2000). On average, older persons under the age of 75 volunteer 3.6 hours per week, whereas individuals 75 years of age and older average 3.1 volunteer hours per week (Saxton-Harrold & Weitzman, 2000).

Although it is commonly believed that women are more likely to volunteer than men, the existing research does not substantiate this perception (Independent Sector, 2001; Zedlewski & Schaner, 2006). We do know, however, that gender plays an important role in understanding the experiences of volunteers in later life. Older men have been found to volunteer informally more often than women once differences in work status, education, and health between the sexes are taken into account (Zedlewski & Schaner, 2006). An investigation of volunteerism among 1,113 middle-aged and older women living in Washington found that the majority of women (73%) volunteered for a group or organization at some time in their lives; 39% were currently volunteering at the time of the survey (Bowen, Andersen, & Urban, 2000). Current volunteers were more likely to be White, married, better educated, and in better health than non-volunteers or past volunteers. Four motivations—values, social expectations, increased knowledge, and enhanced esteem—were endorsed more highly by current volunteers than by past volunteers.

Race and ethnicity affects the likelihood of volunteering. Both White and Black older adults volunteer formally and informally more often than Hispanic elders (Zedlewski & Schaner, 2006). Although the helping tradition is strong in Hispanic and other minority communities, volunteers often provide help informally rather than as members of formal volunteer programs (AARP, 2003). Individuals also are inclined to volunteer for groups that bring people of their own race and ethnic background together and provide service to individuals who are similar to themselves. For example, Black adults aged 45 and older focus the majority of community service efforts on advancing the rights of minorities and those in their neighborhood. Hispanic adults, many of whom are immigrants themselves, are most likely to be providing volunteer help to other immigrants (AARP, 2003).

Social class is strongly associated with volunteerism in later life. Individuals with higher incomes and more education are more likely to have been connected to volunteer activities through employment and are more likely to volunteer in their retirement years than those with less education and lower incomes (Harvard School of Public Health, 2004; Kutner

& Love, 2003; Zedlewski & Schaner, 2006). These individuals are also more likely to stay with their volunteer assignments and to report more satisfaction with the volunteer experience than individuals who have less volunteer experience (AARP, 2003).

Other personal characteristics associated with volunteerism in later life include health, marital status, and employment status. Older individuals who perceive themselves to be in good health are more likely to volunteer than those in poorer health and married older people are more likely to volunteer than elders who are not married. Nearly 72 % of adults between the ages of 65 and 74 who continue to work for pay volunteer compared to 60 % of individuals not working. Of the adults 75 years and older who continue to work for pay, more than 66 % volunteer compared with approximately 45 % of their non-working peers. This supports the adage, "If you want to get something done, ask someone who is busy" (Corporation for National and Community Service, 2006).

The most common organizations for which older volunteers work are religious organizations, social and community services, and health-related organizations (U.S. Department of Labor, 2007; see Exhibit 5.1). While most older adults (67.5 %) volunteer for one organization, 20.5 % volunteer for two organizations, and 11.8 % volunteer for three or more organizations. The most common types of responsibilities they assume within these organizations include collecting, preparing, distributing, or serving food; providing professional or management assistance; providing general office services; and raising funds.

Federal Senior and Volunteer Programs

As previously discussed, several volunteer programs receiving federal support can be found throughout cities and towns nationwide. In this section, we describe the activities of four well-known programs: the Retired and Senior Volunteer Program (RSVP), Senior Companions, the Foster Grandparent Program, and Counselors to America's Small Business (SCORE).

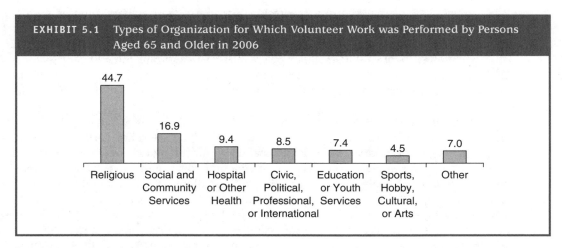

EXHIBIT 5.1   Types of Organization for Which Volunteer Work was Performed by Persons Aged 65 and Older in 2006

Source: U.S. Department of Labor (2007).

Retired and Senior Volunteer Program (RSVP)

The RSVP offers men and women aged 55 and older the opportunity to put their talents and experience to work in community-defined, community-supported projects. Although RSVP is one of the largest federally funded volunteer organizations in the country (Senior Corps—RSVP, 2005), the program represents a true partnership between federal, state, and local government and the private sector in each community. In 2004, RSVP received $55.9 million in federal funds and $48.4 million in nonfederal funds in support of its programs (Senior Corps—RSVP, 2005). The federal government awards grants to community sponsors of RSVP for program operation. This support may amount up to 70% of a program's total budget. Individual RSVP project sponsors are public agencies, private nonprofit organizations, and institutions that promote vital local interests and offer financial support to the project. The sponsor has full responsibility for the development and management of the project.

RSVP projects respond to community needs by matching the interests and abilities of seniors with rewarding part-time opportunities. The volunteers choose their assignments from a broad list of possibilities provided by the local RSVP office. They serve without compensation, but may receive transportation or reimbursement for program-related out-of-pocket expenses. RSVP provides all volunteers with appropriate accident and liability insurance when on assignment at their host stations. Examples of organizations that serve as host agencies for the volunteers include health centers, hospitals, schools, libraries, crisis centers, correctional facilities, senior centers, nursing homes, government agencies, universities, and community service programs. Among the many services provided by RSVP volunteers are tax aid, Medicare counseling services, home renovation, telephone reassurance, shopping assistance, mentoring and tutoring programs, home visitation, disaster relief, and respite care (Senior Corps—RSVP, 2005).

In 2004, there were 755 RSVP grantees across the nation (Senior Corps—RSVP, 2005). They managed 467,000 volunteers who contributed 78 million hours of service. Approximately 58% of the volunteers were women. The majority of RSVP workers were White (83%), 8% of the volunteers were Black, and 4% were Asian. Volunteers help people through 65,000 individual organizations of which nonprofit organizations comprise 20%, followed by social service agencies (18%), and senior centers (15%). Approximately 20% of volunteer stations were in rural areas. Using Independent Sector's (2001) valuation of volunteer labor at $15.39 per hour, the estimated value of services provided in 2000 was approximately $1.2 billion, representing a 35-fold return on the federal dollar.

Findings from the 2004 Senior Corps Accomplishments Survey reveal that RSVP volunteers help their volunteer stations to meet a wide variety of needs and serve millions of people across nine primary service areas: health and nutrition (49% of volunteer hours; 32.2 million people served); community and economic development (15% of volunteer hours; 24.6 million people served); education (6% of volunteer hours; 17 million people served); housing (1% of volunteer hours; 4.4 million people served); the environment (1% of volunteer hours; 4.1 million people served); public safety (3% of volunteer hours; 3.8 people million served); disaster preparedness/relief (1% of volunteer hours; nearly 900,000 people served); homeland security (< 1% of volunteer hours; 500,000 people served); and other human needs services (24% of volunteer hours; 14.4 million people served) (Senior Corps—RSVP, 2005).

According to a majority of volunteer station supervisors, RSVP volunteers help the volunteer stations better serve the community "to a great extent" by improving the quality of services and helping free up paid staff time (Senior Corps—RSVP, 2005). In addition, a majority of station supervisors credited the RSVP volunteers with helping to expand the types of services available to clients, increasing the number of clients served, increasing public support for the program, recruiting non-RSVP volunteers, and reducing the time and effort needed to recruit volunteers.

In 1984, RSVP went international (RSVPI), receiving sponsorship from organizations such as Rotary and the Red Cross (Garson, 1994). In 2000, the University of Maryland's Center on Aging assumed administration of the RSVPI program (RSVPI, 2001). Since its inception, RSVPI has carried out projects in 30 countries, including Australia, Colombia, Ireland, Italy, Japan, and West Africa. Objectives of RSVPI include increasing the number of volunteers age 50 and older, creating sustainability in volunteer current forces, and developing networks of collaborative partnerships to improve community awareness and establish mechanisms for problem-solving. RSVPI volunteers serve as mentors in schools, provide support to hospitals, businesses, and government agencies, act as translators, and help older adults to remain living in their homes.

Best Practice: The Nevada Rural Counties Retired and Senior Volunteer Program

In Nevada, the Nevada Rural Counties Retired and Senior Volunteer Program serves 15 of the state's 17 counties. In 2006, over 1,500 RSVP volunteers in rural Nevada provided more than 260,000 hours of volunteer service to over 250 public and nonprofit community agencies and individual older adults. RSVP plays a vital social services leadership role for the communities it serves and continues to expand its role of assisting not only the low-income and homebound seniors in the service areas, but serving all persons in need and enhancing the quality of life of all citizens.

One of the volunteer opportunities in which older adults are engaged is the Senior Farmer's Market Nutrition Program. The goal of the Farmer's Market program is to increase the consumption, production, and distribution of locally grown fruits, vegetables, and fresh unprocessed herbs, while supplementing nutritional needs for seniors. Free coupons for fresh fruit and vegetables are provided to older adults living in six counties who have individual incomes of less than $14,700 per year and $19,800 for a couple. The program is a cooperative effort by the United States Department of Agriculture, RSVP, the Nevada Department of Administration—Commodity Food Distribution Program, the Nevada Department of Agriculture, the Nevada Certified Farmers' Market Association, and the Nevada Division for Aging Services.

For more information, contact Nevada RSVP, P.O. Box 1708, Carson City, NV 89702. Phone: 775-687-4680, http://nevadaruralrsvp.org.

Senior Companion Program

The guiding premise of the Senior Companion Program is that the best way to help people is to help them help each other (ACTION, 1990b). Senior companions provide emotional support and assistance to primarily older adults who are frail, homebound, and living alone. They usually serve two to four clients on a weekly basis. They serve 15 to 40 hours a week, often as members of a comprehensive care team, helping homebound older adults live independently. For example, senior companions may provide physical and emotional assistance to individuals with physical disabilities or cognitive limitations, those recovering from substance abuse problems or major medical interventions, and older adults who are frail. Senior companions are a "safety net" for their clients, providing an extra set of eyes and ears and being ever alert to their changing needs (Senior Corps—Senior Companion, 2005).

Senior companions are low-income individuals, 60 years of age and older. They receive a stipend of $2.65 an hour, accident and liability insurance and meals while on duty, reimbursement for transportation, and monthly training (Senior Corps—Senior Companion, 2005). Senior companions receive 40 hours of preservice training. Volunteer stations provide four hours of in-service training monthly for the senior companions. Senior companions are recognized for their work at award luncheons and other special recognition events.

In 2004, Senior Companion programs received $45.2 million in federal funds and $24.7 million in nonfederal funds (Senior Corps—Senior Companion, 2005). Local communities sponsor the Senior Companion Programs; project directors must raise at least 12% of their project funds from nonfederal sources. Most of the nonfederal funding comes from state and local governments, private social service agencies, United Way, private businesses, and fundraising campaigns. Each project has an advisory council whose members act as liaisons between projects and their communities.

In 2004, there were 224 senior companion projects across the nation (Senior Corps—Senior Companion, 2005). The projects employed 15,037 volunteers; 85% of the volunteers were female. Approximately 40% of the volunteers were from minority groups, with Black elders constituting the largest percentage (33%). The volunteers contributed 14 million hours of service, helping more than 56,000 frail older adults live independently through 5,000 public, nonprofit, and faith-based community volunteer stations. Social service organizations and human needs agencies comprise 25% of all volunteer stations, followed by multipurpose centers (23%), and community development nonprofit organizations (21%). About 14% of volunteer stations were in rural areas. The National Senior Service Corps (1997b) estimated the value of Senior Companions' service at about $150 million, representing a fivefold return on federal dollars invested in the program.

Senior Companion activities impact the lives of older adults across multiple venues. These include health and nutrition (37% of volunteer hours; 275,000 people served), community and economic development (4% of volunteer hours; 77,000 people served), education (1% of volunteer hours; 22,000 people served), housing (<1% of volunteer hours; 5,400 people served), public safety (<1% of volunteer hours; 1,100 people served), disaster preparedness/relief (<1% of volunteer hours; 1,800 people served), and other human needs services (58% of volunteer hours; 111,000 people served) (Senior Corps—Senior Companion, 2005).

According to the majority of volunteer station supervisors, Senior Companions help the volunteer stations better serve the community "to a great extent" by expanding the types of services available to clients and improving the quality of services (Senior Corps—Senior Companion, 2005). Senior Companions improve the quality of their clients' lives by providing social and emotional support to their clients. In addition, they serve as additional pairs of "eyes and ears" to watch over clients. As noted by one station supervisor, Senior Companions serve as "a safety net through their observational and reporting skills to catch residents early in a decline so treatment intervention comes prior to a significant decline" (2005, p. 6). In addition, a majority of station supervisors credited the Senior Companions with helping to increase the number of clients served, helping free up the time of paid staff, increasing public support for the program, recruiting non-Senior Companion Program volunteers, and reducing the time and effort needed to recruit volunteers.

Foster Grandparent Program

The Foster Grandparent Program initiated its first 21 demonstration projects in 1965 (ACTION, 1990a). The first Foster Grandparent Program served very young children in institutions such as pediatric hospital wards and public homes for children with mental retardation, orphans, and other children without families. Today, foster grandparents help a broader array of children who experience academic or personal problems. Depending on the needs of the community and the skills and interests of the foster grandparents, these volunteers may be found in a variety of settings, including reading and literacy programs, teen pregnancy and parenting programs, juvenile correctional centers, homeless shelters, and drug treatment centers. In 2004, there were 337 projects established throughout the United States, which served 1 million children and youth. Of the 31,000 volunteers, 90% were female; 56% were White elders and 38% were Black elders. The volunteers contributed 28 million hours and carried out the program at 10,000 volunteer stations. Public and private primary schools comprised 45% of all volunteer stations followed by Head Start centers (19%) and non–Head Start educational preschools (16%). About 16% of volunteer stations were in rural areas and 10% were associated with faith-based organizations. The National Senior Service Corps (1997a) estimated the value of this service at $286 million, representing more than a fourfold return on federal dollars invested in the program.

As with the Senior Companion Program, sponsors of Foster Grandparent Programs must provide at least 12% of the project's funding themselves or through other nonfederal sources. In 2004, Foster Grandparent Programs received $109.3 million in federal funds and $36.5 million in nonfederal funds (Senior Corps—Foster Grandparents, 2005). An independent advisory council, consisting of professional and lay members of the immediate community, assists each project. Project directors assign volunteers to a volunteer station. Each volunteer station formally agrees to supervise and assist the foster grandparents serving under its direction.

To be eligible for the Foster Grandparent Program, volunteers must be at least 60 years old, low income (eligibility guidelines vary from state to state), no longer in the regular workforce, and capable of serving children with exceptional or special needs without detriment to themselves or the children served. Individuals must commit to serving the program 15 to 40 hours per week. In return for their service, Foster Grandparents receive a stipend of $2.65 an hour, accident and liability insurance and meals while on duty, reimbursement for transportation, and training (Senior Corps—Foster Grandparents, 2005). Before beginning their volunteer work, all foster grandparents receive a minimum of 40 hours of training. They also receive four hours of in-service training per month that builds on and enhances their skills and knowledge relative to their volunteer assignments. In addition, each foster grandparent annually receives recognition of his or her services to the community at a formal public recognition event—acknowledgment perhaps as important as the monetary rewards.

The 2004 Senior Corps Accomplishments Survey documented the service activities of the Foster Grandparent Program (Senior Corps—Foster Grandparent, 2005). Foster grandparent activities focus primarily on four areas: education (80% of volunteer hours; 935,000 children and youth served), health and nutrition (12% of volunteer hours; 234,000 children and youth served), human needs services (6% of volunteer hours; 214,000 children and youth served), and public safety (2% of volunteer hours; 95,000 children and youth served). According to volunteer station supervisors, Foster Grandparents help the agencies better serve the community "to a great extent" by improving the quality of services, helping expand the types of services to the children and youth, and increasing support for the organization and/or improving community relations.

Senior Corps of Retired Executives

SCORE, "Counselors to America's Small Business," is a nonprofit association dedicated to entrepreneur education and formation of small businesses. Formed in 1964, SCORE is funded through a $5 million grant from Congress that is administered by its resource partner, the Small Business Administration (SCORE, 2006a). SCORE volunteers, who include retired CEOs of large corporations, former small business owners, computer consultants, doctors, lawyers, government officials, and university professors, provide real-world knowledge to entrepreneurs through counseling, educational training workshops and seminars, and online assistance. In 2005, some 10,500 counselors volunteered 1.07 million hours, providing face-to-face counseling at 389 chapter offices and more than 800 branch locations across the nation, 93,691 online sessions, and 6,746 workshops and seminars (SCORE, 2006b). In addition, entrepreneurs can find dozens of online guides, in both English and Spanish, and templates for business plans, loan requests, and more. In 2005, SCORE's website received more than 59 million hits and 6.3 million page views from 1.3 million unique visitors (SCORE, 2006a).

Public and Private Volunteer Programs

In addition to volunteer programs funded by the federal government, many public and privately sponsored programs involve older adults in service to their communities. Although less is written about the participants and outcomes of these programs, they provide seniors with the opportunity to give back to their professions and communities. For example, the American Bar Association developed the Second Season of Service Network, which links lawyers transitioning from full-time practice with organizations that can use their volunteer services (see www.abanet.org/dch/committee.cfm?com = BG110800). In Idaho, at the Kootenai Medical Center, retired nurses volunteer in the general medical unit where they discuss diagnoses with patients, listen to their worries, help them prepare questions for their doctors, and smooth their departures from the hospital (Taggart, 2005). The Volunteer Patrol, a law enforcement program in Oceanside, California, where volunteers perform patrol duties (Corder, 1991; www.oceansidepolice.com/Senior_volunteer.asp), is yet another example of programs that rely on the assistance of senior volunteers in meeting the needs of their communities.

Intergenerational Programs

Many senior volunteer programs are intergenerational.[2] These programs bring together two or more independent agencies or organizations that serve different client populations. Persons served by intergenerational programs come from diverse economic, ethnic, and cultural backgrounds. The children represent mainstream, special needs, or at-risk individuals from infancy through college age. The older adults are well or frail; they may be living independently or in a supportive environment such as a retirement community or a long-term care facility (Goyer, 1998–99; Hirshorn & Piering, 1998–99; Kaplan, 1997; Middlecamp & Gross, 2002). Most intergenerational programs focus on bringing the generations together to promote the development of relationships and to provide support and services. Although intergenerational programs are structured so that all age groups benefit from the interactions, in the vast majority of programs one age group is the provider of services or support and another age group is the recipient of services (AARP, 1994).

The establishment of the Foster Grandparent Program formally introduced intergenerational programming to the American public. Since its origination, the number of intergenerational programs has continued to grow exponentially throughout the United States. In this section, we will highlight intergenerational programs and opportunities in the areas of education, recreational activities, and support programs.

Best Practice: Aetna Life and Casualty Senior Volunteer Program

In the past 10 years, the business sector has emerged as a valuable source of volunteers. Through public–private partnerships, alliances have been created between business and the aging network to solve problems jointly in more efficient and effective ways. Aetna Life and Casualty, based in Hartford, Connecticut, is an excellent example of how a large corporation can connect with a community to serve the needs of older adults. Beginning in 1980, Aetna started using corporate attorneys, paralegals, and support staff to assist older adults in a wide range of cases. The program was initiated in response to publicity about the legal needs of older adults regarding public benefits, wills, probate, age discrimination, landlord–tenant rights, consumer credit, divorce, and victim assistance.

Aetna is recognized as one of the first to use corporate lawyers to provide pro bono services to individuals. This program serves a definite need for clients who do not meet the guidelines of other legal programs funded through federal and state governments. Aetna reports that lawyers who donate time for this program experience a high level of satisfaction because they are greatly appreciated by their clients.

For more information, contact Connecticut Lawyers Legal Aid to the Elderly, phone: 860-273-8164 or visit their website at www.ctelderlaw.org/legal-asst.asp.

Educational Programs

From preschool through college, students and older adults are working together to enhance their learning opportunities. In Chicago, for example, seniors work in preschool programs, helping young children prepare for reading (Lowenthal & Egan, 1991), whereas elementary students in Ohio provide one-on-one computer instruction to older adults (Drenning & Getz, 1992). Through the University of Pittsburgh intergenerational studies program, Generations Together, older low-income adults and African American college students who are the first generation of their families to attend college participate as co-learners in a one-credit seminar that examines community services and housing options for older adults (Manheimer, Snodgrass, & Moskow-McKenzie, 1995). Southern Illinois University (SIU) at Carbondale sponsors a mentoring program that pairs retired faculty members with first-term students who do not meet the criteria of high school rank and admission test scores but have instead been admitted to the university on the basis of their academic potential (Bedient, Snyder, & Simon, 1992). The mentors help the students identify their academic deficiencies and guide them through appropriate exercises to enhance their skills (for more information, visit www.siu.edu/offices/iii). The situation is reversed in Philadelphia, where Project SHINE (Students Helping in the Naturalization of Elders, www.projectshine.org) and Project LEIF (Learning English through Intergenerational Friendship) mobilize college students to address the language, naturalization, and everyday needs of elderly refugees and immigrants (Skilton-Sylvester & Garcia, 1998–99; http://phillyshine.org).

With funding from the Corporation for National Service, Generations Together and the Association for Gerontology in Higher Education established a partnership to promote and support the development of intergenerational service learning models at colleges and universities throughout the United States. This innovative method of teaching and learning integrates community service activities into academic curricula; intergenerational service learning focuses specifically on the issues affecting the community's older adults. As a result of this project, a variety of intergenerational courses and service projects are being implemented nationwide (McCrea, Nichols, & Newman, 1998, 1999, 2000).

Recreational Activities

Parks and recreation centers, senior centers, and fitness clubs are but a few organizations offering joint recreational activities and programs for younger and older adults. For example, as a result of society's focus on exercise, intergenerational fitness programs link youth and college students with older adults (Colston, Harper, & Mitchener-Colston, 1995; Duquin, McCrea, Fetterman, & Nash, 2004). These programs allow older adults to participate in leisure and fitness programs while providing the opportunity for students to learn about the aging process. Gardening is another recreational activity easily shared between older adults of all functional levels (e.g., nursing home residents, homebound elders with physical disabilities, and healthy elders) and children or young individuals (Gigliotti, Jarrott, & Yorgason, 2004; McKee, 1995) Roots&Branches Intergenerational Theater grew out of New York's Jewish Association for Services for the Aged Theater Ensemble (Roots&Branches Theatre, 2001; http://muse.jhu.edu/journals/theatre_topics/v014/14.2vorenberg.html). While training young actors to work with older adults, it builds understanding and respect between generations by challenging stereotypes about age and aging through original theater, workshops, and other projects. The work of Roots&Branches springs from interactions that transcend age, culture, religion, and class.

Support Programs

Probably the most popular model of intergenerational support programs is having older adults providing formal care for young children (Newman & Riess, 1992; Smith & Newman, 1992, 1993). The Whitney Young Child Development Center in San Francisco operates three full-time child-care sites to meet the needs of the working poor in an industrial area of the city. Older volunteers serve more than 400 children from infants to sixth grade, providing a broad spectrum of multicultural and developmentally appropriate activities (Larkin, 1998–99; www.whitneyyoungcdc.org/home.htm). The Friendly Listener Intergenerational Program (FLIP) pairs third, fourth, and fifth graders with older active and homebound volunteers who call children who are home alone after school at preappointed times to check in and to talk (National Eldercare Institute on Health Promotion, 1995). Seniors, however, are not the only ones providing care and support. Teens and college students across the United States who participate in the Adopt an Elder Program (Waggoner, 1996) serve as junior interns in facilities that serve older adults (e.g., senior independent living, adult day services, skilled nursing homes, and Alzheimer's centers). Participants provide companionship and some minimal physical support to their assigned elder. Information about many of the local programs is available through the Internet. A unique program in Honolulu trains volunteers to provide spiritual, emotional, and physical support to older adults who are frail and homebound (Takamura, 1991). Project Dana (which means "selfless giving" in the Buddhist belief system) volunteers are of all ages and are drawn primarily from within the Buddhist community and from the Moiliili Hongwanji Mission (visit the mission's website at www.moiliilihongwanji.org/Project_Dana_.htm).

For Your Files: The Illinois Intergenerational Initiative

The Illinois Intergenerational Initiative is a coalition of individuals and organizations committed to enhancing education through intergenerational efforts, involving young and old in solving public problems and promoting vital communities through service and learning. The initiative is a Higher Education Cooperation Act partnership composed of statewide education and aging organizations such as the AARP, the Illinois Retired Teachers Association, the University of Illinois and Southern Illinois University systems, and the Illinois Association of School Boards. Accessing the initiative's website allows individuals to download publications on starting intergenerational programs, aging across the curriculum, and ideas for intergenerational projects. Individuals can also access the quarterly intergenerational newsletter, *Continuance,* online. For more information, visit the organization's website at www.siu.edu/offices/iii.

CHALLENGES FOR VOLUNTEER AND INTERGENERATIONAL PROGRAMS

Many successful volunteer programs provide thousands of hours of volunteer services; without these volunteers, many nonprofit community organizations would not be able to maintain their current level of services. Because senior volunteers are critical to the delivery of services, programs need effective strategies to recruit and retain volunteers. Volunteer coordinators face many challenges as they attempt to staff and carry out their programs, including finding volunteers to work during the day, coordinating volunteer efforts efficiently, and identifying new sources for recruiting volunteers (Substance Abuse and Mental Health Services Administration [SAMHSA], 2005; Urban Institute, 2004).

Tapping Untapped Potential

Many older people currently do not participate in any formal volunteer program. Barriers to volunteering include employment and family obligations, health, lack of knowledge of volunteer programs, perceived lack of skills, lack of transportation, and a belief that programs should pay people for their work. Agencies must implement aggressive and systematic recruitment efforts to recruit older individuals (Caro & Bass, 1995). Programs must also make a greater effort to recruit older adults from diverse ethnic and cultural backgrounds. Initiatives targeting nonreligious adults, Hispanics, and the more disadvantaged (those with low education levels and low incomes) might yield big payoffs because these individuals report the lowest levels of volunteer activity (Zedlewski & Schaner, 2006).

In addition, the current corps of senior volunteers is aging. Greater efforts need to focus on the recruitment of young-old individuals to supplement, and at some point replace, older volunteers. Programs must develop new positions and opportunities for those elders who may be growing older but who still wish to give their time to support community programs and initiatives.

Training Volunteers

Training volunteers to complete their assignments efficiently and effectively remains a challenge for charities and nonprofit organizations. Recognition of this important dimension to retaining volunteers is a capacity-building option not yet embraced by most organizational cultures. Only three of out five charities and one out of three congregations report employing a staff person to coordinate services and train volunteers. In that group, only 66% report possessing the skills they feel they need to train and manage their volunteer corps. Yet, most would agree that making an ongoing investment in maintaining volunteers benefits program recipients, which in turn justifies greater volunteer investment (Urban Institute, 2004).

Retaining Volunteers

The first three to six months are crucial in the life cycle of a volunteer. During this time, agencies are most likely to lose senior volunteers. To enhance retention of volunteers, agencies must be selective in their recruitment efforts. Once volunteers are recruited, retention is higher when programs match their interests and skills with appropriate assignments. Volunteer positions should offer intrinsic rewards, and the volunteers should perceive their experiences as successful.

Long-term volunteers who experience feelings of burnout also may leave their volunteer positions. These feelings result from grief (especially for individuals working with persons who are seriously ill or who are dying), frustration, intrusion on their private lives, and the time demands of their assignments. Volunteer leaders need to protect their volunteers by setting limits on both the type and amount of service asked of them.

Funding Volunteer Programs

Some federally sponsored programs have experienced cutbacks in funding in the past several years. Volunteers are not free. They require investments in training and supervision. Thus, the effective use of volunteers is a necessity for operating a cost-effective volunteer program (SAMHSA, 2005). A lack of adequate resources also limits the scope and effectiveness of many volunteer programs for older adults. Financial and technical support that enhances the recruitment and retention of volunteers would greatly expand the scope of services offered by many programs.

Evaluating Volunteer Programs

Most volunteer and intergenerational programs put only minimal effort into evaluating their programs (Fischer & Schaffer, 1993; Jarrott, 2005). Regular system-wide evaluations are necessary to identify both the strengths and weaknesses of existing programs and the effectiveness of the services that the volunteers provide. Often, when evaluations are conducted, they are published as final reports submitted to the administration of the national program or to the individual projects. Evaluation information needs to be made more available and accessible to increase public knowledge about volunteer and intergenerational programs, garner community support for intergenerational programs, and secure funding for expansion and/or maintenance of these programs (Jarrott, 2005; Ward, 1997).

Supporting the Future of Senior Volunteer Programs

Among the top 50 resolutions put forth by delegates of the 2005 White House Conference on Aging, two gave specific attention to volunteer programs. Specifically, delegates called for

- the development of a national strategy for promoting new and meaningful volunteer activities and civic engagement for current and future seniors; and
- reauthorization of the National and Community Service Act to expand opportunities for volunteer and civic engagement activities.

The numerous strategies outlined for implementing these resolutions included the following:

- Establish a broadly representative National Commission to develop a blueprint for capturing baby boomers in significant sustained volunteer service to their communities.
- Establish a fund for innovation to foster the growth of promising practices and program models that foster volunteering by older adults to address critical human and community needs.
- Authorize and fund the AmeriCorps Program to establish the Silver Scholarship initiatives for older adults and establish incentives for organizations to engage greater numbers of older adult volunteers.
- Include civic engagement in the Older Americans Act (OAA) through senior centers and aging network initiatives.
- Support the expansion to 1 million volunteers in Senior Service Corps and support this program being a part of Corps for National and Community Service with increased funding to support the Foster Grandparent Program, RSVP, and Senior Companion Program.

Clearly, when policies support the use of older volunteers, everyone benefits.

CASE STUDY

Reconnecting With the Community

Maggie is a 79-year-old woman whose husband, Warren, died of cancer three years ago. Maggie and Warren were a close couple. They had many interests in common and were known in their neighborhood for their activities with the local Audubon chapter. A county wetland area was preserved largely because of their efforts. Warren was the advocate, and Maggie quietly helped with the organizing and details. This was the way they approached everything in which they were involved. When Warren died, Maggie was completely devastated. It was as if she had lost her right arm. Warren had been the outgoing person in their relationship, and she felt lost.

Maggie is a bright woman and would have gone to college if finances had permitted. Her daughters, Kathy and Michelle, did further their education and currently teach in nearby communities. For the past year, the daughters have watched their mother become ever more detached and isolated from the community. She stopped attending the Audubon chapter meetings, which she had always enjoyed. She dropped out of her bridge club, and even stopped going to church. Maggie was literally pining away. Nothing seemed to get through to Maggie, no matter how many conversations her daughters had with her about the importance of getting on with her life. It seemed that the normal grieving process had continued for too long and was having a dramatic impact on their mother. Kathy and Michelle regarded their mother as a healthy, vital woman whose quality of life was deteriorating needlessly.

Case Study Questions

1. Maggie's daughters are urging her "to get on with her life." On the basis of your reading of the chapter, what benefit would volunteering bring to Maggie's situation?

2. What personal characteristics of Maggie's would be important for someone to consider when proposing volunteer opportunities to her? Why?

3. Think about the volunteer programs discussed in this chapter and any others of which you are aware. What volunteer situations might appeal most to Maggie?

4. Ultimately, it will be Maggie's decision whether she will become reinvolved in her community as a volunteer. What role could her daughters play in helping to direct their mother toward an interest in a volunteer program or activity?

5. Drawing on your own personal experiences and observations, discuss with the class examples of older adults as volunteers who impressed you. Why?

6. The chapter pointed out that recruiting and retaining older volunteers is a great challenge. What suggestions do you have that could increase recruitment and retention of older volunteers?

Learning Activities

1. Interview the director of a senior volunteer program. Find out who volunteers, in what type of programs, and in what type of activities.

2. Meet with one or a group of older adult volunteers. Find out what they do, why they do it, and how volunteering has affected their lives. What are the benefits of volunteering? What did you learn about their programs, experiences, and the impact of senior volunteers? After this experience, do you see yourself volunteering when you are older? What types of volunteer activities interest you?

3. Interview staff members at a program that has older adult volunteers. What type of benefits do they see in having the volunteers? What types of activities or duties are assigned to volunteers? What would be the effect on their program if they did not have the volunteers?

4. Attend an inservice training that is designed for older volunteers and/or those working with them. What was the emphasis of the training?

5. Observe or volunteer for an intergenerational program. Was one age group the focus of service more than the other? What types of activities or services were there? Did the participants seem to enjoy themselves? Were there problems or issues that arose? What was your overall impression?

For More Information

National Resources

1. Corporation for National and Community Service, 1201 New York Avenue N.W., Washington, DC 20525; phone: 202-606-5000; www.nationalservice.org.

    The corporation oversees AmeriCorps, the National Senior Service Corps, the Foster Grandparent Program, the Retired Senior and Volunteer Program, and the Senior Companion Program. Information about each of the programs is available on request.

2. National Caucus and Center on Black Aged, 1220 L Street N.W., Suite 800, Washington, DC 20005; phone: 202-637-8400; www.ncba_aged.org.

    The National Caucus and Center on Black Aged is a nonprofit organization that works to improve the quality of life for older black Americans. One of its programs includes the Living Legacy Program, which promotes intergenerational dialogue between older and younger blacks.

3. Volunteers of America, 1660 Duke Street, Alexandria, VA 23314; phone: 800-899-0084; www.voa.org.

    Volunteers of America is a national nonprofit organization that offers programs and services to meet the needs of local communities. The organization offers services that assist the young and old, persons with disabilities, and persons with alcoholism. It sponsors foster grandparent and senior volunteer programs and publishes a quarterly newsletter, *Volunteers Gazette*.

4. *Journal of Intergenerational Relationships: Programs, Policy, and Research*, The Haworth Press Inc. 10 Alice St. Binghamton, NY 13904; phone: 800-429-6784; www.haworthpress.com/store/product .asp?sku=J194.

    This is the only international journal focusing exclusively on the intergenerational field from a practical, theoretical, and social policy perspective. It provides readers with information about the latest intergenerational research and program development.

Web Resources

1. Illinois Intergenerational Initiative: www.siu.edu/offices/iii.

    The home page of the Illinois Intergenerational Initiative offers information on how to begin intergenerational programs or service learning experiences, intergenerational conferences and workshops, intergenerational ideas and resources (that can be downloaded), and fundraising strategies for intergenerational programming. Visitors can also access its newsletter, *Continuance*.

2. Generations Together: An Intergenerational Studies Program: www.gt.pitt.edu.

    Generations Together: An Intergenerational Studies Program is an intergenerational program in the University of Pittsburgh's Center for Social and Urban Research. The home page offers information about the development and evaluation of intergenerational programs, as well as information about the development of intergenerational studies as an academic discipline.

3. Center for Intergenerational Learning: www.templecil.org/index.htm.

    The home page of Temple University's Center for Intergenerational Learning offers information about cross-age programs, training and technical assistance, and other resources for intergenerational programming. The site also has links to other resources for intergenerational programmers.

4. Retirement and Intergenerational Studies Laboratory's Intergenerational Entrepreneurship Demonstration Project: www.strom.clemson.edu/teams/risl/howe-to.html.

    This home page explains the Intergenerational Entrepreneurship Demonstration Project, a pilot program that uses new retirees as volunteer mentors to at-risk youth. The retirees help the young people operate their own country market in a renovated dairy barn. Website visitors can access the newsletter and barn catalog online.

5. The Virtual Volunteering Project: www.serviceleader.org/new/index.php.

   This website offers information to agencies that wish to expand their volunteer efforts to the internet and provides resources to volunteers who wish to volunteer online. Examples of helpful information provided by this website include how to involve volunteers through the internet, how to set up a virtual volunteering program, and how to include people with disabilities in online volunteering.

6. AARP's Volunteer Website: www.aarp.org/about_aarp/community_service.

   AARP's volunteer website provides information about volunteer activities and programs in AARP chapters throughout the country and provides resources for those interested in volunteering nationally or locally.

7. Corporation for National Service: Senior Corps: www.seniorcorps.gov.

   This site is the home page for the Senior Corps organization, which provides information about the Foster Grandparent Program, the Retired and Senior Volunteer Program (RSVP), and the Senior Companion Program. It also gives information for other organizations that want to become partners with Senior Corps.

NOTES

1. Unless otherwise noted, the information in this section comes from a discussion of the origins of senior service by Freedman (1994).
2. For more in-depth information about the history, development, and outcomes of intergenerational programs, see Brabazon and Disch (1997), Kuehne (2000), and Newman et al. (1997).

6

Education Programs

Jim and Donna Wagner retired to a small rural community of 3,000. They chose the community for its geographical location, climate, and proximity to relatives. Although they enjoy small-town living, they miss the many educational and cultural opportunities that larger communities offer. Six months after they settled into their new home, Donna decided to visit the tiny Senior Center on Main Street. After lunch, she remained with a group of seniors for a class on famous women of the World War II era. The other seniors told Donna that the local community college had brought many classes to their center through the years. They liked that the classes were noncredit and affordable. They also mentioned that the county extension agent frequently came to town and offered classes on health, self-care, and financial management for retirees.

Educators recognize now, more than ever before, that learning does not stop when adults enter the later stages of life. Although the process of learning changes during the life course (e.g., older adults take longer to assimilate information and are less likely to use memory schemas), study after study confirms that humans maintain the capacity for learning throughout their lives (Schaie, 1994). Like Donna and her new friends at the Senior Center, many seniors find participating in educational programs to be an enriching experience. Most older adults, however, prefer attending classes outside traditional academia. They want the opportunity to actively participate in classes that are of interest to them and relevant to their lives now and in the future.

The idea of lifelong education first appeared in the research literature in the 1930s. By definition, lifelong education implies a cradle-to-grave approach to learning and recognizes that people can be learners at 18 or 80 (Manheimer et al., 1995). It differs from the traditional lockstep model of education that assumes one's life path extends in a straight line. A lifelong education model provides a more fluid perspective that considers individuals as learners and, often simultaneously, as teachers who have a broad range of needs throughout their life course (Feldman, 1991).

EDUCATIONAL LEVEL OF OLDER ADULTS

Contributing to the lifelong learning phenomenon is the current education level of older adults and the future increase in the overall level of formal education achieved by

Americans. Exhibit 6.1 shows the educational attainment of men and women aged 65 years and older in 2006. Overall, 71% of older adults had completed high school; about 21% of older men and 11% of older women reported having a bachelor's degree or higher (U.S. Bureau of the Census, 2006a). Education levels among older adults, however, vary considerably by race and ethnicity. Approximately 80% of non-Hispanic White elders, compared with 70% of Asian elders, 55% of Black elders and Native Hawaiians/Pacific Islanders, 52% of American Indians/Alaska Natives, and 39% of Hispanic elders had completed high school (U.S. Bureau of the Census, 2006a).

Older non-Hispanic Whites are more likely to be high school graduates than are Blacks, Asians, Hispanics, Native Hawaiians/Pacific Islanders, or Native Americans/Alaska Natives (U.S. Bureau of the Census, 2006a) (see Exhibit 6.2). In 2006, approximately 30% of Asian elders and 20% of non-Hispanic White elders, compared with 11% of Black elders and 9% of Hispanic elders, had completed a bachelor's degree or higher (U.S. Bureau of the Census, 2006a).

The educational status of future cohorts of older adults will be dramatically different. It is anticipated that there will be more older adults with college degrees than older adults with less than a high school education. By the year 2030, more than 85% of older

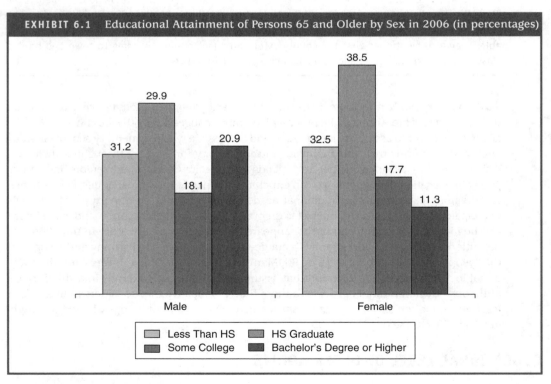

EXHIBIT 6.1   Educational Attainment of Persons 65 and Older by Sex in 2006 (in percentages)

Legend:
- Less Than HS
- HS Graduate
- Some College
- Bachelor's Degree or Higher

Male: Less Than HS 31.2, HS Graduate 29.9, Some College 18.1, Bachelor's Degree or Higher 20.9

Female: Less Than HS 32.5, HS Graduate 38.5, Some College 17.7, Bachelor's Degree or Higher 11.3

Source: U.S. Bureau of the Census (2006a).

adults will have at least a high school education. As shown in Exhibit 6.3, approximately 87% of older men and 88% of older women will have completed high school and approximately 31% of older men and 28% of older women will have attained a bachelor's degree (He, Sengupta, Velkoff, & DeBarros, 2005). In addition, the difference between the percentages of Asian, non-Hispanic White, Native Hawaiian/Pacific Islanders, and Black older adults with a high school education will grow smaller. Approximately 94% of Asians, 93% of non-Hispanic Whites, 93% of Native Hawaiian/Pacific Islanders, and 87% of Blacks aged 25 to 29 have graduated from high school; however, only 69% of American Indians/Alaska Natives and 63% of Hispanics aged 25 to 29 have graduated from high school (U.S. Bureau of the Census, 2006a). Of persons aged 25 to 29, 61% of Asians, 34% of non-Hispanic Whites, 21% Native Hawaiian/Pacific Islanders, 14% of Blacks, 10% of American Indian/Alaska Natives, and 9% of Hispanics have a bachelor's degree (U.S. Bureau of the Census, 2006a). These differences in educational levels will no doubt influence the types of educational programs offered to older adults. In addition to basic education programs, there will be a renewed interest in the concept of lifelong education.

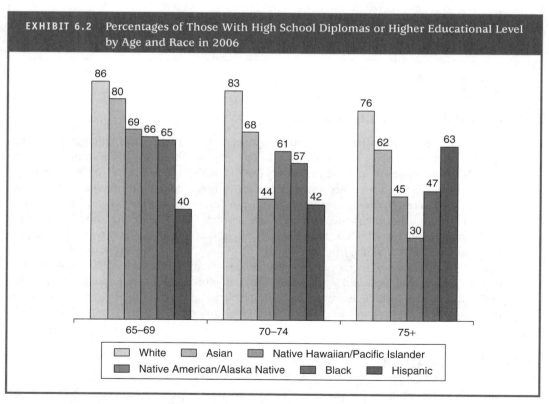

EXHIBIT 6.2 Percentages of Those With High School Diplomas or Higher Educational Level by Age and Race in 2006

Source: U.S. Bureau of the Census (2006a).

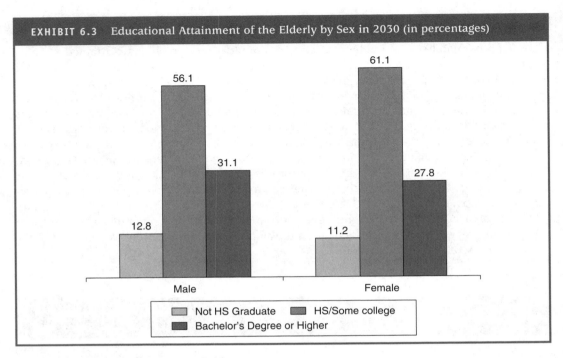

EXHIBIT 6.3 Educational Attainment of the Elderly by Sex in 2030 (in percentages)

Male: Not HS Graduate 12.8, HS/Some college 56.1, Bachelor's Degree or Higher 31.1
Female: Not HS Graduate 11.2, HS/Some college 61.1, Bachelor's Degree or Higher 27.8

Legend: Not HS Graduate ▪ HS/Some college ▪ Bachelor's Degree or Higher

Source: He, Sengupta, Velkoff, & DeBarros (2005).

Literacy in the Older Adult Population

Although literacy proficiencies tend to increase as level of education increases, a significant percentage of older adults continue to have limited literacy skills. Findings from the 2003 National Assessment of Adult Literacy (NAAL), which measures the English literacy of America's adults aged 16 years and older living in households and prisons, suggest that, although the average literacy of adults aged 65 and older increased between 1992 and 2003, adults in this age group had the lowest average literacy of any age group and accounted for the largest percentage of adults with below basic prose (i.e., no more than the most simple and concrete literacy skills) (Kutner, Greenberg, & Baer, 2005). Among adults aged 65 and older, 23% had levels of literacy below basic prose literacy, 27% had levels below basic document literacy, and 34% had levels below basic quantitative literacy. Older adults' literacy skills and abilities influence every aspect of their lives and are of major concern to government agencies, health care entities, and social institutions.

LIFELONG EDUCATION

Moody (1976, 1988) contends that society's focus on lifelong education has emerged through five chronological stages indicative of changes in attitudes toward later life. In the late nineteenth and early twentieth centuries, education for older adults was in the *rejection stage,* with the prevailing belief being that older adults neither needed nor deserved more learning opportunities. Society viewed education as the preparation of children and youth for the future, an investment not justifiable for older adults. From the late 1950s through the mid-1970s, beliefs about education moved through the *social services stage.* During this time, society viewed education for older adults as worthwhile if it had a special thera-peutic value. Education programs focused primarily on the problem areas of growing older and the responsibility of social institutions to meet elders' needs through service programs (Peterson, 1985). By the mid-1970s, a shift began from the segregationist "social problem" per-spective to an assumption that older adults should remain active and involved in their com-munities and in society. In this *normalization stage,* educators and practitioners minimized the differences between older and younger adults. Older adults seeking educational opportuni-ties were placed in existing educational pathways. A decade later, the *self-actualization stage* emerged, in which learning in later life held special transformative possibilities for personal growth. Practitioners emphasized psychological and spiritual concerns as part of the edu-cational milieu for older adults. Most recent is the *emancipation stage,* in which personal growth is intertwined with current community events. The focus is on the empowerment of older adults to actively participate in all realms of life.

In this chapter, we explore the opportunities for lifelong learning for individuals living throughout the United States. We begin by examining the federal government's support for education programs for older adults. Next, we present a description of the types of educa-tional programs available for seniors and a profile of older adults who attend these pro-grams. In the final section of this chapter, we discuss the challenges facing education programs currently and in the future.

For Your Files: Seniors and Literacy

The Centre for Literacy of Quebec is home to one of Canada's largest and most comprehen-sive special collections on literacy and related topics. In 2004, staff developed the *Seniors and Literacy* annotated bibliography, which provides references and annotations of research arti-cles, project reports, resource guides, and other documents that address the issue of seniors' literacy levels and practices. It includes websites from a range of governmental and nonprofit agencies in Canada and around the world. The annotations are descriptive and do not analyze or evaluate. To download a copy, go to the Centre's website: www.centreforliteracy .qc.ca/Publications/lacmf/v0117n02/32–33.htm.

POLICY BACKGROUND

Historically, support specifically for the education of older adults represents only a small fraction of the total federal expenditures for education. Provisions made under Title I of the Higher Education Act of 1965 provided colleges and universities the opportunity to direct some of their resources and staff to program development for older people. Most of the sup-port for educational programs for older adults during the late 1960s through the mid-1970s, however, came from demonstration projects funded by federal agencies such as the National Endowment for the Arts and the National Endowment for the Humanities (Manheimer, 1992). Despite enthusiastic claims of success, these projects usually terminated at the end of their grants. Without outside money, most institutions closed older adult education programs because attending to the education needs of older adults was not high on the priority lists of traditional colleges and universities.

Following the gradual recovery from the post–Vietnam War recession, an increasing number of non-traditional-aged adults began to go back to school. Continuing education and lifelong learning became popular concepts. In 1976, Congress passed the Lifelong Learning Act. Hailed as "a landmark of social legislation" (Weinstock, 1978), it had the goal of providing lifelong learning opportunities for all citizens "without regard to restrictions of previous education or training, sex, age, handicapping condition, social or ethnic background, or economic circumstances" (1978, p. 16). The Act was the first legislation to specially mention older adults and retired persons as potential recipients of educational resources. Unfortunately, Congress did not provide funding for the Act.

Although state and local governments have the responsibility for developing public and continuing education, the federal government, through the office of Vocational and Adult Education, has been instrumental in setting national priorities for education opportunities for persons of all ages. For example, under the Adult Education and Family Literacy Act, Title II of the Workforce Investment Act of 1998, federally funded, state-administered adult education programs address the needs of older adults by emphasizing functional competency and grade-level progression from the lowest literacy level, with provision of English literacy instruction, through attainment of the General Education Development (GED) Certificate. States operate special projects for older persons through individual instruction, use of print and educational technology, home-based instruction, and curricula focused on coping with daily situations. In 1998, a total of 246,067 adults 60 years of age or older were served in the adult education programs (U.S. Department of Education, 1998). In addition to adult literacy programs, a variety of federal programs have supported informal educational activities of interest to older adults, including consumer education, older reader services, community schools, continuing education, and health education.

The Administration on Aging (AoA), under the provisions of the Older Americans Act (OAA), also plays an important role in encouraging older adults to seek educational opportunities and in developing educational programs for older adults. The 1987 amendments to the OAA instructed local Area Agencies on Aging (AAAs) to identify the postsecondary schools in their area that offered tuition-free education to older adults and to distribute the findings to senior centers and other locations (U.S. Senate Special Committee on Aging, 1991b). State and local AAAs also are involved in a number of grassroots education programs aimed at providing older adults with the knowledge they need to enable them to lead more productive lives by broadening their occupational, cultural, and social awareness. For example, AAAs sponsors educational programs in health and nutrition, injury prevention, preretirement and legal concerns, employment, and consumer education.

USERS AND PROGRAMS

There is great diversity among learners within the older adult population. Like any age group, older adults are heterogeneous and multidimensional in learning needs and abilities. They come from all educational levels and have interests in a variety of subjects from the liberal arts to programs more focused on issues of aging (e.g., health care and finances). Variation also exists in the educational programs designed to meet the needs of the aging population. In this section, we examine three primary settings for formal education programs for older adults: (a) institutions of higher education, (b) community-based organizations, and (c) at-home programs. For each setting, we describe the types of programs available and the older adults who participate in them.

Institutions of Higher Education

In 2005, 14,000 Americans 65 years of age and older were enrolled in undergraduate credit programs at four-year institutions of higher education throughout the United States (U.S. Bureau of the Census, 2005). Women constituted 64% of the "older" undergraduate population. The institutions classified all of the older students as part-time students. In addition, 29,000 older adults were enrolled in graduate programs. Men made up 76% of this population of graduate students. Of older students, 69% were pursuing their graduate degrees on a part-time basis (U.S. Bureau of the Census, 2005).

For Your Files: Leadership Training for Older Persons

Leadership Training for Older Persons is a program for underserved adults aged 50 years and older from low-income or minority communities. The program is designed to enable participants to gain the skills, knowledge, and confidence necessary to become effective leaders and to advocate for their peers in the community. Through classroom sessions and time spent on community projects, participants learn practical skills such as how to organize and lead meetings, public speaking, utilizing community resources, teamwork, and advocacy strategies. Since its inception, over 50 new community leaders have "graduated" from the program. For more information, contact North Carolina Center for Creative Retirement, Reuter Center, CPO # 5000, The University of North Carolina at Asheville, One University Heights, Asheville NC 28804-8516; phone: 828-251-6140; www.unca.edu/ncccr/index.htm.

Most states have established guidelines within their statutes for tuition waiver programs for older adults. State requirements vary with respect to minimum age, number of credits for which a person may enroll, the type of course (i.e., credit or noncredit), and the availability of space. In some states, policies for tuition waiver programs also vary by institution. Few older adults, however, take advantage of the tuition waiver policy. Many older adults are unaware of it, and others find the campus environment intimidating and are not really interested in the type of learning offered by conventional higher education departments (Moody, 1988). Finally, some colleges encourage older adults to return to school by offering credit for life or work experience. For example, the Assessment of Prior Experiential Learning program at American University in Washington, D.C., allows older students to translate their work or life experience into as many as 30 credit hours toward a bachelor's degree.

Community Colleges

Community colleges are major providers of educational programs for older adults. In 1970, community colleges became the focus of the expanding instructional network on aging. The AoA awarded a grant to the American Association of Community and Junior Colleges to encourage the organization "to develop an awareness of the needs of older Americans and to explore ways in which these community-oriented institutions might contribute to an improvement in the quality of life in the nation's elderly population" (Korim, 1974, p. 5). Because of this project, community colleges developed many new programs for older people in the mid-1970s. In 2005, 18,000 older adults enrolled in courses or programs taught through community colleges (U.S. Bureau of the Census, 2005). Virtually all of the older adults were part-time students.

At several community colleges around the country, Next-Chapter or life-options programming is being developed to respond to the educational and social needs of aging baby boomers (Goggin & Ronan, 2004). Such programs are designed to help adults approaching the traditional age of retirement make a successful transition to the next phase of their lives. A theme common to these programs is that they are not modeled on traditional seniors programs; their focus is derived from market research and opinion surveys that clearly indicate baby boomers are not attracted to the retirement options that traditionally have been available for aging adults. To adapt to and capitalize on the changing demographics and emerging social trends, Goggin and Ronan (2004) propose a number of things that community colleges need to do to address the educational needs of the aging boomers:

- Develop a clear understanding that this new student cohort has explicit desires and expectations.
- Prepare new programs and services based on the expressed desires of adults at this life stage.
- Adapt existing service learning, leadership training, and workforce development models to the needs and interests of post-midlife adults.
- Create a simple and specific access point for existing and new programs that will appropriately serve this group.
- Partner with other community organizations such as libraries, community centers, other community-based organizations, and government agencies to build a collaborative network for life planning, meaningful engagement, continued learning, and community connections.
- Educate the workplace and the nonprofit sector about the ways they will need to change in order to take best advantage of the contributions these experienced adults can make.

Lifelong Learning Institutes

Lifelong Learning Institutes (LLIs), formerly known as Learning in Retirement (LIR) programs, are community-based organizations of retirement age people dedicated to meeting the educational interests of its members. The first LLI was established in 1962 at the New School in New York City. Throughout the 1960s and 1970s, other colleges and universities replicated or adapted the educational model. During the 1980s, several national conferences introduced the concept to a wider audience and spurred the development of many more groups. In 1988, 24 LLIs collaborated with Elderhostel, Inc. to form the Elderhostel Institute Network, with a mission to strengthen and support the effectiveness of their programs and spread the LLI concept to new communities. Today, the Network links independent programs at more than 400 institutions of higher learning across North America (Lifelong Learning Institute [LLI], 2006a, 2006b, 2006c). Although every LLI is unique and independent, most LLIs are sponsored by a college or university and have an open membership for all retirement-age learners regardless of previous education (LLI Overview, 2006). Located at institutions large and small, private and public, and in communities both urban and rural, LLIs provide unique, noncredit academic programs developed and attended by the members themselves. A typical LLI has 200–300 members, offers 10–20 courses per term, and has two or three terms each year. Most members take two or three courses per term (LLI Factsheet, 2006a). The members are local people who commute to the program, and who participate regularly year after year. An LLI program is structured like a typical college program, with regular semesters and often homework. In addition, many LLIs provide volunteer services to their sponsoring institutions or to the community at large.

Some LLIs are institution-driven programs with a paid college staff coordinator who manages the program and college faculty members who teach the courses (Young, 1992). However, most LLIs are member-driven programs, governed by their own members, with members leading the courses in lieu of professional faculty. Regardless of type, the most successful LLI programs share several characteristics. These programs are designed to serve the learning needs and interests of the local older adults involved in the program; offer a broad-ranging educational program; are nonprofit, charging a modest tuition or membership fee; often have a need-based scholarship program; publicly commit themselves to affirmative action goals; use volunteer teachers or course leaders who are members of LIR; offer social, cultural, and physical experiences that complement the curriculum and are appropriate for the program participants; and provide for participant involvement in planning, evaluating, teaching, and, where appropriate, administering the program (Young, 1992).

Elderhostel

Conceived as a means of getting older adults directly involved with stimulating activities and with each other, Elderhostel combines the excitement and challenge of travel with the enrichment of academic courses on substantive subjects.[1] The founders offered the first program during the summer of 1975. Throughout that summer, 220 older individuals came to one of five New Hampshire colleges to participate. By 1980, all 50 states and several Canadian provinces offered Elderhostel programs. In 1981, Elderhostel offered its first international programs in Great Britain and Scandinavia. Today, Elderhostel offers nearly 8,000 programs in every American state, Canada, and 90 other countries, with nearly 160,000 participants per year (Elderhostel, 2006a).

Elderhostel is a nonprofit educational organization; its national office is in Boston. There are five U.S. area offices, a U.K. office, and headquarters program staff that support and guide travel organizations and program coordinators in developing and maintaining individual Elderhostel programs. The travel organizations and program coordinators who are, to hostelers, the most visible part of the Elderhostel organization, develop and host the individual Elderhostel programs under the guidelines of the administrative offices. They are responsible for all aspects of running a program, from lodging and meals to courses and instructors.

Elderhostel is a network of educational and cultural sites, including colleges and universities, state and national parks, museums, and environmental/outdoor educational centers. Coordinators at each site design and operate individual Elderhostel programs. They must decide what courses to offer, select the instructors, develop the weekly schedule, and determine where to house and serve meals to the hostelers. Most institutes of higher education offer their programs during the off-season and vacations, thereby taking advantage of the low-cost room and board, and the availability of classrooms.

The standard Elderhostel program brings together a group of 15 to 45 persons over the age of 55 to a college campus, conference center, or retreat. During their five- or six-night stay, they take noncredit courses accompanied by field trips and extracurricular events. The courses do not carry college credit, and there are no tests. The intent is that students delve into the subject matter for the sheer joy of learning. The cost of a five-night program in the continental United States in 2006 starts at around $600 per person; programs in Hawaii and Alaska are slightly more expensive (Elderhostel, 2006a).

Although most program sites offer varied programs from year to year, they typically include at least one course about the cultural or historical significance of their geographic location. In recent years, "full immersion" programs have developed in which students spend their whole time studying one topic. For example, Elderhostelers enrolled at Yavapai College in Prescott, Arizona, spend a week living on the Hopi reservation where the instructors are all Hopi (Pierce, 1993; see www.elderhostel.org/Programs/programdetail.asp?RowId = 1%2B2SH%2B454).

For individuals wishing to expand their educational horizons, Elderhostel offers international programs in more than 90 countries. Course-related field trips and excursions providing a variety of opportunities for learning about and experiencing the culture and traditions of the country and its people complement the classroom studies. International programs usually are two or three weeks long, with hostelers spending time at several different study sites. Depending on the location, the all-inclusive cost of a two-week program is as low as $3,000 (plus travel expenses to the U.S. city from which the trip departs). In 2005, some 2,000 international programs enrolled more than 22,000 hostelers (Elderhosel, 2006b).

Older adults attend Elderhostel because they want to expand their knowledge. They are a self-selecting group of highly motivated individuals. Most hostelers are single women. In general, they are a privileged group. Primarily White Americans and Canadians, almost two-thirds of the participants report an annual income of $30,000 or more and substantial prior education. More than 80% of hostelers have attended college.

Many Elderhostel participants wish to spend time with their grandchildren and share the wonders and experiences Elderhostel programs provide. In response, intergenerational programs have been developed. In 2007, over 125 programs were offered across the United States. Trip options included visiting national parks, camping, participating in outdoor activities, and expanding cultural experiences. To facilitate the intergenerational experience, programs are designed for one adult to be paired with one child in attendance. Check it out at www.elderhostel.org/programs/intergenerational_default.asp.

Elderhostel recently created a new kind of learning-travel adventure to serve the burgeoning new generation of independent, active, culturally inquisitive travelers—Road Scholar. Road Scholar is an exciting travel-study opportunity structured to meet the interests and capabilities of participants in their 40s, 50s, and 60s (Roadscholar, 2006). While Road Scholar programs share the Elderhostel focus on learning, as well as inclusive packages of educational lectures, field trips, transportation, meals, and accommodations, Road Scholar takes participants off the beaten path to hidden or little-known places such as private vineyards, rural villages, ancient monasteries, and wilderness research stations located in the United States and abroad. Groups are small, limited in size to 23 participants. Programs run from five nights to two weeks, with a price range of about $700 to $4,000.

Community-Based Organizations

Many community-based agencies and organizations also provide educational programs for older adults. Several favorable characteristics account for the popularity of community-based education programs with older students, including their location, the schedule of program offerings, and the format of the offerings (Courtenay, 1990). Because the primary mission of the sponsoring organization is to be responsive to all the residents, these educational programs generally are dispersed throughout the community. Senior centers, hospitals, community centers, churches, and libraries often provide educational programs and/or the physical space for such programs. Almost without exception, older adults prefer educational programs offered from late morning to mid-afternoon during the week. The availability of alternative scheduling makes community-based organizations especially accommodating to the needs of the older learner. They also have an advantage over colleges and universities in that they are not under educational accreditation/standards requirements, do not need extensive registration procedures, and have nearby parking or free transportation. Although they typically do not have the resources to offer every type of educational experience, community-based organizations do have the flexibility to provide a wide range of subject matter.

Libraries have established a variety of onsite education programs specifically for older adults (Manheimer et al., 1995). Participants take part in learning activities such as mini-courses, book and film discussions, forums on consumer and health issues, and life enrichment programs. For example, the Queens Borough Public Library in Queens, New York (www.queenslibrary.org) offers programs on topics related to disabilities and aging, including information about community resources for older adults and health and wellness programs.

The Older Adult Service and Information System (OASIS, 2006) is a public–private partnership offering programs through a national network of community-based sites. The OASIS Institute is the headquarters, overseeing educational, cultural, health, and volunteer outreach programs at OASIS sites for adults aged 55 and older. Sponsored by the Federated Department Stores and multiple corporate and nonprofit agencies, OASIS centers provide participants an opportunity to remain independent and active in community affairs. The program, administered nationally from St. Louis, has centers operating in 26 cities with more than 350,000 members. Membership is free, and older adults from all socioeconomic, cultural, and educational backgrounds participate in the programs. Courses in areas such as visual arts, music, drama, creative writing, contemporary issues, history, science, exercise, and health occur usually once a week for 1 to 12 weeks.

The Shepherd's Center is a nationwide nonprofit interfaith community organization providing services and programs to more than 175,000 older adults in 25 states (Shepherd's Centers of America, 2006). One program, Adventures in Learning, provides college-type classes in an environment in which older adults share their knowledge, talents, skills, and interests with peers. They are the teachers, students, planners, and participants in the program. Other educational programs include computer classes, defensive driving classes, and intergenerational programs. The centers charge a nominal fee for participation. Classes are held through affiliate locations nationwide and cover a wide range of topics, including workplace etiquette, leadership, business practices, personal wellbeing, health, and travel.

For Your Files: Women Work!

Women Work! educates displaced homemakers—women who have lost their principal means of self-support through events such as widowhood or divorce—to assist them in achieving economic self-sufficiency. Local programs based in community organizations (e.g., community colleges and employment centers) offer vocational testing, employment training, tuition assistance, and job referral services. The program also produces *Network News*, a quarterly newsletter for displaced homemaker advocates; *Women Work!* a biannual newsletter for displaced homemakers; and *Women Work! Program Directory*, a listing of job training and education programs nationwide. For more information, contact WomenWork! at the National Network for Women's Employment, 1625 K Street, Suite 300, Washington, DC 20006, 202-467-6346; www.womenwork.org.

The Cooperative Extension System also provides community-based education programs for older adults focusing on family, health, aging, and caregiving issues as well as leisure and home-based activities. This nationwide educational network established through legislation is a partnership of the U.S. Department of Agriculture, and over 100 state land grant universities and colleges (U.S. Department of Agriculture, 2006a). For a listing of aging programs and resources offered through Cooperative Extension in each state, see www.csrees.usda.gov/nea/family/pdfs/aging_resources.pdf.

Best Practice: The Close Up Foundation

The Close Up Foundation, in cooperation with AARP and other corporate and civic organizations, is a nonprofit, nonpartisan civic education organization dedicated to helping citizens of all ages better understand the important role they play in U.S. democracy. While most of Close Up's programs focus on educating and inspiring middle and high school students to participate in the democratic process, the foundation offers a Lifelong Learning Series Program for Older Americans over 50. For example, a program offered in cooperation with Elderhostel offers adults opportunities to witness legislative proceedings on the House floor, meet with Washington leaders and decision makers, attend Capitol Hill committee hearings, and tour national landmarks. Another program, The Smithsonian Institution Close Up: An Intergenerational Adventure, is a week-long program created for grandparents and grandchildren to explore the nation's capital and share the legacy of America's greatest citizens displayed in Smithsonian museums.

Usually 20 participants from across the nation participate as a group in the program. Experienced instructors lead the groups, and sessions are informal to promote the exchange of ideas. During this Washington learning adventure, older adults explore critical issues with policy analysts, media representatives, members of the administration, and other Washington experts. They examine topics covering the presidency, domestic issues, international relations, and the media. Included in the program are tours of historical sites and opportunities for cultural activities, such as an evening at the theater. A sample offering for a week could include a study visit to Mount Vernon, home of George Washington; a seminar on the media; a foreign policy seminar; a diplomatic visit to a foreign embassy; attendance at a legislative committee hearing; and a twilight tour of the Washington monuments.

The Close Up Foundation programs are for citizens from all areas of the nation and from all walks of life. The program cost provides for a generous package of services including accommodations and meals. Program funding is derived primarily from registration fees paid by participants; community, corporate, and philanthropic contributions; and an appropriation from Congress.

For more information, contact Program for Older Americans, Close Up Foundation, 44 Canal Center Plaza, Alexandria, VA 22314, phone: 800-256-7387; www.closeup.org.

Although people may think of community-based education as occurring primarily in a classroom setting, outdoor programs also present older adults with learning opportunities. For example, Camp Cheerio, nestled in the Blue Ridge Mountains of North Carolina, offers adults aged 50 and older the opportunity to enjoy camping experiences similar to those traditionally offered to youth and teens. During the five-day camp sessions, participants stay in cabins, and have the option to participate in activities such as fishing, guided morning walks, arts and crafts, ping-pong, archery, riflery, skeet shooting, table/card games, bingo, and tennis. During these programs, older adults learn the importance of good physical and mental health and develop new skills such as camping, canoeing, and working in a group situation. Visit the Camp Cheerio website at www.campcheerio.org/sac/index.php.

At-Home Educational Experiences

With the advance of technology, both well and frail older adults can take part in new educational ventures from the convenience of their own homes. These programs reduce structural barriers (e.g., inconvenient timing and hard-to-reach locations) that often discourage older adults from attending university or community-based courses and programs.

For many years, special programs from public and state libraries have provided educational services to older adults via bookmobiles, cable television, and books by mail (Manheimer et al., 1995). In addition, librarians and volunteers provide reading programs and materials to persons who are homebound and residents of nursing homes and other institutional settings.

SeniorNet, a nonprofit membership organization based in San Francisco that began in 1986, offers computer training and networking capabilities to adults 50 years of age and older. Community organizations (e.g., banks, senior health organizations, financial service companies, and private foundations) sponsor local SeniorNets by furnishing computer equipment, scanners, and digital cameras, and contributing to the cost of establishing and maintaining the sites. Using a "seniors teaching seniors" model, over 5,000 seniors serve as mentors, instructors, and learning center administrators to teach members how to use computers at the sites. In 2006, more than 200 corporate learning centers and affiliates were located throughout the United States and Canada, housed in a variety of settings, including senior centers, community centers, public libraries, schools and colleges, and clinics and hospitals. A typical center contains 6 to 10 computers. In addition to providing basic and advanced computer instruction, most centers offer open lab time where students can use computers to practice their skills or to work on individual projects. In addition to computer technology–related activities and support, SeniorNet offers semester-length online classes on literature appreciation, Latin, and Greek. A nationwide online "electronic community" also fosters long-distance information sharing among the program's 25,000 members through a variety of online discussion boards called SeniorNet Round Tables. Members, particularly those not living near a site, have the opportunity to interact with one another, participate in network forums, and seek and give information through databases and special-interest groups. Members also receive newsletters and discounts on computer-related and other products and services. SeniorNet holds regional and national conferences and participates in research on older adults and technology. The cost of individual membership in the SeniorNet organization is $40 (SeniorNet, 2006).

Some older adults find self-directed learning opportunities such as correspondence study and telecourses appealing. These courses, offered through the continuing education division of many colleges and universities, were among the early innovations in long-distance learning. Today, older adults have the option of enrolling in a rapidly growing number of internet courses. Although these distance education programs are not marketed specifically for older adults, their independent structure may be attractive to some older adults (Brubaker & Roberto, 1993). In particular, older individuals who are self-disciplined and internally motivated to learn, who live in rural or more remote areas, and/or who have limited mobility or transportation can participate in courses of personal interest without leaving their homes.

The goal of *Seniors Surf the Net,* is to provide older adults living in central Pennsylvania access to reliable information about local services, medical care, and community events from a single web portal. Multiple local human service agencies joined with the Dauphin County Area on Aging and Comcast Cable to create the website. To help seniors become more comfortable and proficient in accessing internet sites, hands-on training sessions are provided throughout the year by a Comcast representative, at a local computer lab. In 2006, over 40 older adults received instruction on how to surf the net. More information can be obtained at www.dauphininfo.com.

For Your Files: Computer Learning Through SeniorNet

SeniorNet provides adults aged 50 and older with information and instruction on computer technologies so they can use their new skills for their own benefit and to benefit society. More than 80,000 older adults have been introduced to computers at SeniorNet learning centers. All centers share common goals and objectives, but each has its own activities. Here are some examples:

- The center in Bakersfield, California, has joined with the Senior Aid Program at the Mexican-American Opportunity Foundation to prepare Spanish speakers to go back into the workforce.
- In Honolulu, a group of members produced a 10-minute video about Hawaii, the college (Honolulu Community College), and SeniorNet, using both video and computer technology.
- The Chicago Department of Aging established a learning center on the South Side to serve its predominantly African American population. It is open seven days a week and has about 20 seniors stopping by daily.
- The instructors of the Peoria, Illinois, center helped set up computers in nursing homes and retirement homes and now go online with the residents.

Visit the SeniorNet website at www.seniornet.org.

CHALLENGES FOR EDUCATIONAL PROGRAMS

As we previously noted, future cohorts of older adults will have higher levels of formal education, so participation by older adults in formal and informal learning situations is likely to continue to increase. The demand for increased opportunities for lifelong learning will no doubt challenge people to rethink the role of education as well as where and how such educational experiences are delivered. We end this chapter by addressing several current and future challenges facing education programs for older adults.

Increasing Participation of Older Adults

The growth in the number of older learners is not necessarily reflected in increasing enrollments within most traditional postsecondary institutions. The main focus of higher education has always been on collegiate and postcollegiate students. The pedagogical norm at most colleges and universities does not suit the unique needs of older adults (Manheimer, 2002; Yankelovich, 2005). Most older adults are not attracted to lengthy course commitments or to lecture halls in which traditional college-age students listen passively. Thus, to attract more older adults, institutions of higher education may need to rethink their curricula, course content, and didactic delivery style (Novak, 2001).

For older adults who do choose to enroll in educational programs and courses at colleges and universities, the cost of attending usually is not a primary concern. The problems concern access. Older adults are far more dependent on a skillfully and sensitively planned environment than are younger students, who can overcome barriers (Regnier, 1988). Inconvenient parking facilities, lack of concern for physical safety of those walking to and from the classroom (e.g., poor lighting), and lack of physical comfort (e.g., uncomfortable chairs, lack of climate control, and unpleasant and unattractive classrooms) discourage them from enrolling in classes (Moore & Piland, 1994). Moore and Piland suggest that colleges conduct a "physical environment audit" (1994, p. 316), with active involvement from older adults, to illustrate appropriate areas of the campus for older adult learner activities and to suggest realistic alterations in others that could house senior educational services. In addition, colleges and universities may need to make several significant administrative changes to meet the needs of older students. For example, they must consider the schedule/time of course offerings, the support services available to the older students, and the relevance of the learning to real-world issues facing older adults (Bass, 1992).

In addition to physical barriers, older adults face psychological and social barriers when contemplating entering the higher education arena (Dickerson, Myers, Seelbach, & Johnson-Dietz, 1990). A pervasive obstacle to participation in lifelong education by today's older adults is that they have a lower level of educational experiences than younger adults. Older adults often hold negative self-images about their ability to learn that make them apprehensive about mixing with younger students. Although society expects adults to fulfill many roles in their later years (e.g., retiree and grandparent), the role of student is not commonly encouraged.

Institutions of higher education sponsoring senior educational courses and programs must address the inclusion of participants from all races, cultures, and socioeconomic groups. Today, the majority of the older learners attending traditional classroom courses or participating in nontraditional programs (i.e., LLI programs and Elderhostel) are those with the highest levels of education, income, and employment. Although LLI programs and Elderhostel provide "scholarships" or "hostelships" to encourage attendance by individuals from all economic strata, their attempts to recruit a more diverse group of older individuals have not been very successful.

Expanding the Content of Education Programs

In addition to efforts to make formal educational opportunities more accessible to older adults, attention must be directed toward the content of educational experiences. According to Fischer (1992), colleges and universities have at least four major responsibilities to older adult learners. First, they need to help them understand the values, culture, and technology of today. Second, higher education must act as a catalyst for mobilizing young-old adults for productive roles in society for the 20 to 30 years of life after retirement. Third, colleges and universities have a responsibility to foster diversity in intellectual, cultural, and social life by educating students of all ages about aging and ageism. Finally, higher education has the responsibility of enhancing the effective use of society's limited resources by reducing older adults' needs for health and social services.

Ensuring the Quality of Educational Programs

Quality control is an issue of concern for all educational programs. Community-based educational offerings for older people have diverse sponsors, program types, audiences, and content. There is no central system of support for monitoring of these activities, so their patterns depend on the preferences of administrators and the needs of local communities. This often makes them responsive to the wishes of the older learner but does not facilitate development of easily described categories of programs, nor does it provide much assistance in predicting a program's success with other sites and sponsors (Peterson, 1990).

Financing Education Programs

A concern for institutions of higher education is the method of financing educational activities for older people. Federal and foundation funds are not nearly sufficient for the number of programs currently operating or planned. Peterson (1990) suggests that long-range funding must come from the states or from the sponsoring institutions themselves. Public institutions will need state support in revising program priorities to meet the needs of the aging population. Typically, state support is primarily for credit students, with noncredit enrollees paying most of their program costs. Because older people generally are not willing to pay high tuition for noncredit courses, colleges and universities must either find new support mechanisms or pursue new definitions of credit courses.

Yet another concern is the limited funding that directly supports the availability of educational opportunities. With decreases in federal dollars for educational programs, community-based programs will need to further develop private sponsorships. Although many foundations have given local awards, only a few have devoted large amounts of money to this area and have continued support of educational programs through several years (Peterson, 1990).

Addressing the Future of Senior Education Programs

The role and purpose of education for future cohorts of older adults will no doubt be as varied as the older population itself. Educational opportunities for older adults will need to address their different needs. According to McClusky (1974), older adults have five needs that educational programs can address. Education programs can help older adults address *coping needs*—those that help individuals deal with the social, psychological, and physiological changes brought about by aging. Courses on health, physical exercise, adjustment to retirement, and learning how to live with losses are examples of education that addresses coping needs. *Expressive needs* are activities in which older adults derive satisfaction, pleasure, or meaning. Given that much of learning during the life course is related to skill acquisition, there may be a greater demand for these types of educational opportunities by future cohorts of older adults. *Contribution needs* of feeling wanted and needed, and fulfilling a useful role, can be addressed through educational opportunities that allow older adults to act as mentors or peer counselors. Educational programs that empower older adults so they can have influence and control over their quality of life deal with *influence needs.* Courses that address these needs teach older adults about their legal rights or how they can assume leadership roles within their communities. Finally, individuals' needs to feel better off in later life compared with an earlier time in life are *transcendence needs.* Any educational experience that allows older adults to advance artistically, occupationally, educationally, or physically has the potential of addressing transcendence needs (Crandall, 1991).

In summary, future educational opportunities will need to be available at every stage of the life course and will need to offer content that fulfills the varied social and emotional needs of older adults. Several of the top 50 resolutions made by delegates to the 2005 White House Conference on Aging make reference to the importance of lifelong education. For example, delegates voted to

- educate Americans on end-of-life issues;
- prevent disease and promote healthier lifestyles through educating providers and consumers on consumer health care; and
- improve health decision making through promotion of health education, health literacy, and cultural competency.

Strategies for implementing these resolutions included the development of

- innovative and educational models on prevention and health throughout the lifespan using e-learning; and
- web technologies and educational programs that are culturally and linguistically appropriate and relevant for health decision making.

CASE STUDY

Can Further Education Help a Downsized Worker?

Martin, 45, entered the workforce shortly after graduation from high school. His first job was with a state highway department, in which he worked as a construction supervisor for seven years. He was caught up in a reorganization and was laid off from that job. For the past 21 years, he has been employed with a major private sector highway construction firm for which he has performed many duties, including work as a materials tester, safety officer, office manager, and highway construction supervisor. Martin and his wife, Nancy, who is an administrative assistant with the U.S. Forest Service, have been earning excellent wages and benefits for more than 20 years. They have two children: a daughter in her second year of college and a son employed in a successful position with a major insurance company.

Two months ago, Martin was officially informed by his company that his job would be eliminated by the new owners. Once again, Martin found himself in a downsizing situation in which the higher salaried positions were being eliminated to cut the operating expenses of the company. As a dislocated worker, Martin thought that this time around he would have considerably more difficulty finding a job, especially without the benefit of more education.

Martin had always wanted to pursue educational opportunities beyond high school, so he and Nancy had stressed the benefits of higher education with their children. Fortunately, Martin and Nancy have been careful with their finances. Even with a daughter in college, they were not panicked about Martin losing his job. Their finances were such that Martin was thinking that this might be a good time for him to reevaluate his educational opportunities.

Case Study Questions

1. This chapter discusses three philosophical perspectives about lifelong learning. Which of those perspectives most closely pertains to Martin's situation? Why?

2. What statistics and studies described in the chapter could you cite to Martin that would reassure him that a decision to return to a higher education learning environment need not be threatening because of his age?

3. What differences in attitudes might Martin encounter as a middle-aged learner in the 1950s and the 1990s?

4. If you were counseling Martin on his options, which options described in the chapter might best meet Martin's educational goals? Which generic educational programs and services might not meet Martin's needs at this time in his life?

5. If Martin decides to enroll at a local college, what problems, barriers, and frustrations might he have to overcome as an older learner? Cite chapter discussion to support your answer.

Learning Activities

1. Investigate what educational opportunities are available to older adults in your community, at your college, or at other institutions. Find out about the older adults who are involved in these classes.

2. Interview an older participant in Elderhostel or other educational programs about the experience. What did the participant gain from it, what did he or she like and dislike, and why is he or she involved?

3. Sit in on a class that is geared toward older adults. How is it similar to or different from classes you attend? Interview students or the teacher of the course. What type of experiences have they had? What do they like, and what would they change? Is this something they do or plan to do on a continuing basis?

4. Interview someone involved in arranging Elderhostel or other types of educational opportunities for older adults. How did he or she decide what to offer? To whom are the classes marketed? How successful has the program been?

5. Check local newspapers, television ads, and magazines to see how education opportunities are marketed to older adults. Check the web to see what information is provided on Elderhostel and other education programs.

6. Interview people in their 40s and 50s, and those 60 and older. What types of educational opportunities interest them, if any? What are their reasons for being interested in taking these classes?

For More Information

National Resources

1. American Library Association (ALA), Adult Services Division, 50 Huron Street, Chicago, IL 60611; phone: 800-545-2433; www.ala.org.

    The ALA's activities are focused in many areas, including developing innovative programs that support libraries in acquiring new information technology and training people in its use and supporting libraries as centers for culture, literacy, and lifetime learning.

2. Elderhostel, 11 de Lafayette, Boston, MA 02110; phone: 800-454-5768; www.elderhostel.org.

    Elderhostel is a nonprofit educational organization that offers academic programs hosted by educational institutions in the United States and around the world. Individuals 55 years of age and older are eligible, and a spouse or an adult companion may attend with an age-eligible participant. Students live on college and university campuses and in marine biology field stations and environmental study centers and enjoy the cultural and recreational resources that host institutions and communities have to offer. We can hardly wait!

3. *Gerontology and Geriatrics Education.* The Haworth Press Inc., 10 Alice St. Binghamton, NY 13904; phone: 800-429-6784; www.haworthpress.com/store/product.asp?sku = J021.

    Articles published in this journal focus on the exchange of information related to research, curriculum development, course and program evaluation, classroom and practice innovation, and other topics with educational implications for gerontology and geriatrics. It is designed to appeal to a broad range of students, teachers, practitioners, administrators, and policy makers.

Web Resources

1. National Institute for Literacy: http://novel.nifl.gov.

    The home page of the National Institute for Literacy offers information about literacy forums and listservs (email discussion groups), regional and state literacy resources, and links to other internet resources.

2. SeniorNet, 1 Kearny Street, Third Floor, San Francisco, CA 94108; phone: 415-352-1210; www.seniornet.org/php/default.php.

    Don't forget to drop by the SeniorNet site. Find out more about the program, the members, and the activities at various sites.

3. Lifelong Learning Survey: http://research.aarp.org/research/reference/publicopinions/aresearch-import-490.html.

    This website contains an AARP study entitled "AARP Survey on Lifelong Learning." The results from this study showed that younger retirees, age 50 and older, prefer a more "hands-on" approach and are more interested in learning about personal development, health care, and finances than older retirees. Of the 1,019 retirees surveyed, 90% prefer learning by watching, listening, and then thinking.

4.   Generations on Line: www.generationsonline.com.

This organization provides both a service for access and a product for learning aimed at older adults who cannot afford or choose not to enroll in computer training or Internet training. The specially programmed self-training software introduces older adults to the internet and provides four basic functions: electronic mail, discussion, research, and a gateway to popular sites. The software is provided at a minimal cost to senior centers, libraries, retirement homes, and other locations where older adults might congregate.

NOTE

1.   Unless otherwise noted, the background information about Elderhostel comes from Mills (1993). Current statistical data about the program came from Elderhostel's website (www. elderhostel.org) and national office.

7

Senior Centers and Recreation

Last fall, a distraught daughter called the San Francisco Senior Center (SFSC) and asked the Social Services Director for advice to help her 85-year-old Italian-American mother, Jane, who had suddenly stopped talking. After an extensive discussion with the daughter, the Social Services Director suspected that Jane had been suffering from isolation and depression, which are documented as common and sometimes deadly in the elder population. The Social Services Director suggested that both Jane and her daughter visit SFSC to observe the activities and meet senior participants. Coming from a large city back East where she walked frequently, Jane was naturally attracted to the Aquatic Park location's Gardening and Walking Group, whose members walk from the center to the Fort Mason Community Garden each Wednesday. As Jane continued to come to SFSC, she found many walking companions who enjoyed walking and visiting this San Francisco garden while sharing their concerns about the challenges of aging. Jane has since become known as "fast Jane" for her ability to out-walk even the youngest participants in the group. In addition, Jane participates in the healing class each Monday, and almost every day she visits the center where her new friends look forward to her company. (San Francisco Senior Center Website, 2004: www.sfsenior.com/inspiring_stories.htm)

Stop for a moment and think about the activities in which you participate during your free time away from work or school. Do you read a good book? Garden or fix things around the house? Exercise? Jump in the car and take a short day trip? Play golf or tennis? Go fishing? Attend a concert or a movie? Gather with friends for a coffee? According to researchers, most of our leisure patterns are highly individualized and stable across our life course until very late in life. So the chances are that you will be enjoying the same leisure activities in later life until an intervening variable, such as health status or functional ability, forces a change (Janke, Davey, & Kleiber 2006; Kelly, Steinkamp, & Kelly, 1986; Stanley & Freysinger, 1995). Now think about why you participate in your favorite leisure activity. Does it help you unwind? Make you feel connected with others? Do you gain a sense of accomplishment? Feel productive? Improve your mood?

Researchers have identified numerous benefits associated with participation in leisure and recreational activities. Involvement in formal leisure activities has been positively associated with increased happiness (Menec, 2003) and decreased depressive symptoms (Musick & Wilson, 2003). Engagement in physical leisure activity has been associated with maintenance or prevention of negative physical health declines (DiPietro, 2001) and improvements in psychological wellbeing (Menec, 2003). According to Dumazadier (1967), leisure has three main functions—relaxation, entertainment, and personal development—and thus acts as a buffer against major life stresses. Although these functions are important at each stage of the life course, engaging in leisure and recreational activities provides a number of benefits for older adults. Leisure activities can replace a work role, expand on preretirement skills and interests, assist in maintaining a positive self-concept, and enhance mental wellbeing (Hooyman & Kiyak, 1996; Kelly, Steinkamp, & Kelly, 1987; Lawton, Moss, & Fulcomer, 1982; Riddick & Stewart, 1994). In addition, participating in leisure activities can help older adults such as Jane deal more effectively with stressful life events through shared companionship, can reduce feelings of loneliness, and can increase the ability to cope with significant life changes such as widowhood and retirement (Atchley, 1997; Coleman & Iso-Ahola, 1993).

Some researchers who have examined how patterns of leisure participation changes over time have found stability in time spent in leisure activities (Lee & King, 2003; Singleton, Forbes, & Agwani, 1993), whereas others have found a gradual reduction in leisure participation and diversity of leisure activities (Armstrong & Morgan, 1998; Verbrugge et al., 1996). One of the few longitudinal studies conducted on changing patterns of leisure activities among people over the age of 50 was conducted by Janke et al. (2006). They examined leisure participation patterns over an eight-year period in three subdomains of leisure activities: informal leisure activities, which include socializing with friends and family, visits with others, and telephone conversations; formal leisure activities, which include participation in clubs and organizations; and physical leisure activities, which include participation in sports or exercise of both low and high intensity. Results indicated that participation in informal leisure activities remained consistent until late in life (mid-80s and older) when participation declined markedly. Over time, two factors influenced informal leisure participation rates. Retirement was associated with an increase in informal leisure activities and an increase in the number of functional limitations was associated with a decline in informal leisure participation rates. Older adults' participation in formal leisure activities declined at a faster rate later in life (early to mid-80s) and, as the severity of functional limitations increased over time, participation rates declined. Participation in physical leisure activities remained fairly consistent until the eighth decade of life when rates of participation declined significantly. However, physical and mental health was found to be related to rates of participation in physical leisure activities. As physical health declined and the severity of depressive symptoms increased, rates of participation in physical activities decreased. Janke and colleagues (2006) concluded that, overall, leisure activities remain fairly stable over time, and that participation is positively associated with a number of physical and psychological factors. The changes that do occur in patterns of leisure activity are influenced more by health status, not age *per se.*

One source of leisure activities for older adults is the senior center. According to Krout (1989b), a senior center is a designated place with a broad array of services and activities targeted to older people. It offers opportunities for social interaction, development of strong friendships, and promotion of feelings of self-worth and community belonging. In this chapter, we begin by reviewing the federal policies that have contributed to the growth of senior centers. This is followed by a discussion of who attends senior centers, the various models of senior centers, and the types of programs offered. In the final section, we present the challenges that lie ahead for senior centers.

POLICY BACKGROUND

The first senior center was established in 1943 in New York City (Leanse, Tiven, & Robb, 1977). The founders established the William Hodson Community Center to help alleviate loneliness among older adults observed by social workers in the city's Welfare Department. According to the center's first director, the center needed to offer older adults a meeting place but, more importantly, needed to offer services that would help participants remain in the community (Perspective on Aging, 1993). California was the location of the next two senior centers, which offered a variety of recreational and educational services (Kent, 1978; Maxwell, 1962). By 1966, there were 340 centers; today, between 12,000 and 15,000 senior centers are located across the country, serving 10 million older adults annually (Administration on Aging [AoA], 2002a; Wagner, 1995a).

According to the National Institute of Senior Centers (1978), senior centers are based on the philosophy that aging is a normal developmental process, that human beings need peers with whom they can interact and who are available as a source of encouragement and support, and that adults have the right to have a voice in determining matters in which they have a vital interest. As such, the center is a major community institution that is geared to maintain good mental health and to prevent breakdown and deterioration of mental, emotional, and social functioning of the older person (1978, p. 5).

The NISC (National Council on Aging, 2005, para. 3) defines a senior center as a place where older adults come together for services and activities that reflect their experience and skills, respond to their diverse needs and interests, enhance their dignity, support their independence, and encourage their involvement in and with the center and community.

As senior centers emerged as a significant community resource for older adults, the Older Americans Act (OAA) played an important role in the creation and support of more facilities. In the original Act (1965), funds were available for senior center operations under Title IV, and dollars under Title III supported many of the programs offered at these sites.[1] The 1973 amendments of the OAA created a new Title V under which senior centers became the focal point of providing services to older adults. These amendments introduced the term "multipurpose senior center" and provided funding for renovation or acquisition of facilities to be used as multipurpose centers—community organizations designed to be the center for developing and delivering a range of services. Amendments in 1978 eliminated Title V and placed support for senior centers under Title III. In addition, the amendments required that, when feasible, Area Agencies on Aging (AAAs) designate a central point for the delivery of services and give special consideration to senior centers. In part because of this increased support for senior centers under the OAA, the number of senior centers increased dramatically. By the end of the 1970s, there were an estimated 6,000 to 7,000 centers. As funding for OAA programs in the 1980s flattened and declined, few additional legislative changes affected senior centers. In Title III under the OAA 2000 amendments, a multipurpose center was defined as "a community facility for the organization and provision of a broad spectrum of services, which shall include, but are not limited to provision of health (including mental health), social, nutritional and educational services and the provision of facilities for recreational activities for older persons" (§ 102 [33]). The OAA reauthorization in 2006 did not contain language that would affect senior center operations. Although Title III monies fund senior centers, those dollars must also support the other programs designated under Title III. Krout

(1990) notes that the average percentage of federal contributions to senior centers fell from 29% in 1982 to 19% in 1989. Currently, approximately half of all senior centers ($n = 6,614$) receive some funding from OAA monies (AoA, 2002a). Thus most centers are funded entirely or in part by local nonprofit organizations, local, state, and federal governments, and charitable organizations such as the YMCA, United Way, and Catholic Charities.

USERS AND PROGRAMS

Most of the research on senior centers during the past 25 years has focused on identifying organizational characteristics of senior centers, characteristics of participants, and types of programs and services offered. As Wagner (1995a) and Strain (2001) point out, much of the research on demographic characteristics of senior center participants and the role these characteristics play in predicting senior center participation paints a somewhat contradictory picture. This is no doubt reflective of the diverse communities in which centers are located and the differences in the type of programs and activities provided by centers. In addition, it is estimated that only 15% of older adults participate in senior center activities annually (National Council on Aging, 2005).

Characteristics of Senior Center Participants

Early studies of senior center participants reported equal percentages of female and male participants (Silvey, 1962; Storey, 1962), whereas more recent studies reveal that the majority of participants are women (Krout, 1983b; Krout, Cutler, & Coward, 1990; Strain, 2001). Early studies of senior center participants found that senior center participants were primarily in their 60s (Harris & Associates, 1975; Storey, 1962). More recently, researchers have found that senior center participants are older than non-participants (Calsyn, Burger, & Roades, 1996) but Strain (2001) found in a Canadian sample of older adults that the young-old were more likely to become participants than those in other age groups. However, others have found a curvilinear relationship between age and senior center attendance, as those least likely to participate are the young-old and the old-old (Aday, 2003; Krout, Cutler, & Coward, 1990; Turner, 2004). When examining frequency of attendance and age, the results have been inconsistent. Strain (2001) found that, over a four-year period, there was no relationship between frequency of attendance and age (Strain, 2001). However, Miner, Logan, and Spitz (1993) found that frequency of attendance was related to age. Older participants were more likely to report that they attended the senior center frequently than were their younger counterparts, who were more likely to report rarely attending. There was no discernible pattern between age and attending senior centers "sometimes." Miner, Logan, & Spitz, (1993) concluded that observations by senior center directors that younger participants were interested only in occasional trips and special events appear to be supported by these findings. Indeed, the results on both attendance and frequency support the notion that senior center participants are aging in place and that younger cohorts are not frequent users of senior center activities. This suggests that the young-old adults who attended in the 1960s and 1970s are "aging in place" and that a new cohort of younger participants are not being recruited into senior centers (Krout, 1989a; Krout et al., 1990; Miner et al., 1993).

Are older adults of color less likely to be senior center participants? Calsyn and Winter (1999) found that race was not a predictor of senior center participation. Other studies have found race to predict participation. Some researchers have found that older adults of color were less likely than their White counterparts to attend senior centers (Aday, 2003; Harris & Associates, 1975; Krout, 1987b, 1988; Leanse & Wagner, 1975), but Ralston (1985) reported that older Blacks were more likely than Whites to indicate a willingness to attend a senior center. A national sample of recreation and senior center directors were asked to estimate the percentage of their participants by ethnic group (Wacker & Blanding, 1994). Overall, older Blacks constituted an average of 8% of the participants, older Hispanics 5%, and Asian and Native Americans 2% each. The percentage of minority participants, however, varied across programs. For example, the percentages of older Black and Hispanic participants ranged from 0% to 95% and from 0% to 98%, respectively. Similar percentages were noted for older Asian Americans and Native Americans. These variations in participant characteristics may reflect the location of the center: senior centers located in neighborhoods having high numbers of older adults of color probably report higher percentages of minority users. Overall, older adults of color are underrepresented at most senior centers, except for those centers primarily serving them.

For Your Files: The New Leaf Outreach to Elders

The New Leaf Outreach to Elders (formerly Gay and Lesbian Outreach to Elders or GLOE) serves lesbian, gay, bisexual, and transgender elders aged 60 and over. The New Leaf Outreach to Elders program provides a range of senior social services promoting independent living and improving quality of life. The program offers information and referrals, support services, friendly visits for the homebound, educational and cultural activities, holiday events, group outings, and women's and men's social/recreational activities and groups. Outreach to Elders has a Geriatric Mental Health component that offers in-home, senior-specific counseling services and medication management.

For more information, contact The New Leaf Outreach to Elders Program at 1390 Market St., Suite 800, San Francisco, CA 94102, 415-626-7000; www.newleafservices.org.

Health and functional status appear to differentiate users of senior centers from nonusers. Early studies by Hanssen et al. (1978) and Harris and Associates (1975) found that those with poor functional ability and poor health were less likely to attend. More recent studies report similar findings. In their study of 282 senior centers in New York, Cox and Monk (1990) found that only 10% of participants were classified by directors as frail, and Aday (2003) found that only 2.6% and 20.9% of senior center participants in seven states had self-rated health as poor or fair, respectively. Similarly, in another study, only a small percentage of participants had a disability that required special programming accommodations (Wacker & Blanding, 1994). For example, an average of less than 9% of participants had physical disabilities or hearing impairments, 6% had visual impairments, and only 3% had cognitive impairments. Krout et al. (1990) also reported that older adults with fewer problems with activities of daily living were more likely to attend a senior center than were their less well counterparts. Strain (2001) also found that those who had attended a senior center in the past six months had fewer Instrumental Activity of Daily Living (IADL) limitations than did non-participants. One exception to these findings was a study by Miner et al. (1993). The authors found that frequency of attendance did not differ by functional ability; seniors with disabilities who had ever attended a senior center participated as frequently as did their healthier counterparts. They concluded that, although functional disability may make a difference in whether older adults ever attend a senior center, it does not influence how often they attend. Strain (2001) also found that changes in participation patterns of senior center participants over time were not related to the changes in IADL limitations.

Socioeconomic status measures of education and income have been found in some studies to be predictors of senior center attendance. Attendees are more likely than nonattendees to have lower incomes (Calsyn, Burger, & Roades, 1996; Krout, 1990; Strain, 2001). When examining the relationship between education and senior center participation, Krout et al. (1990) found participation was highest among those with mid-levels of education, whereas other studies found no relationship between education and attendance (Krout, 1991; Strain, 2001). However, Miner et al. (1993) found that those with more economic resources and higher levels of education were more likely to report "rarely" attending senior centers. They concluded that those with higher incomes and education levels had other, more expensive, alternatives for leisure activities and supportive services. Data suggest that senior centers serve neither the very rich nor very poor but are attracting older adults whose incomes are lower than those of the older adult population in general (Wagner, 1995a). Other participant characteristics associated with senior center attendance have been higher levels of social interaction (Krout et al., 1990), having a desire to have more contact with friends and family, size of family networks (Di & Berman 2000), living alone (Aday, 2003; Strain, 2001), and being unmarried (Calsyn et al., 1996; Di & Berman, 2000; Turner, 2004). Finally, lack of attendance may also reflect lifelong patterns of participation in voluntary or community associations (Krout, 1989b).

In summary, although findings from national and local data are somewhat contradictory, we can make some generalizations about the typical senior center participant, who is generally a woman in her middle 70s, of lower to middle economic status, living alone, White, in good physical health, and with slightly less than a high school education.

BARRIERS TO SENIOR CENTER PARTICIPATION

What factors prevent older adults from attending senior centers? Some evidence suggests that many older adults living in the community are simply unaware of the different activities and services offered at senior centers (Walker Bisbee, Porter, & Flanders, 2004). Indeed, Krout (1981, 1982, 1984) found that, although a high percentage of respondents were aware of the existence of senior centers, non-participants knew little about senior center programming.

Transportation problems and lack of transportation services to and from senior centers act as a hindrance to senior center attendance (Harris & Associates, 1975; Jirovec, Erich, & Sanders, 1989; Ralston, 1982; Walker et al., 2004). However, other studies found that availability of transportation was not significantly related to attendance (Hanssen et al., 1978; Krout, 1983a; Leanse & Wagner, 1975).

Researchers have identified other personal perceptions that inhibit senior center participation. Non-users often report that they believe senior centers are for those who are "old and frail," or say they are reluctant to attend because they do not want to be labeled as a "senior citizen" (Leanse & Wagner, 1975; Walker et al., 2004). Other non-users perceive that participants are cliquish and unwelcoming, or they are uncomfortable because the groups attending the center are either too small or too large (Walker et al., 2004).

For Your Files: Manzano Mesa Multigenerational Center

The Center for all Ages Manzano Mesa Multigenerational Center in Albuquerque, first opened in 2002, is for seniors, youth, and the entire community. Membership is almost equally divided among participants over age of 55 (3,094) and those under the age of 55 (4,582). Activities are especially designed for seniors and youth, and include everything you can find at a senior center as well as activities for youth aged 6 and up. Programs for older adults include health screening and promotion, senior fitness programs, legal services, estate planning, and many other classes and activities. The Manzano Multigenerational Center provides both breakfast and lunch for seniors. Services for youth include both before- and after-school care for children, as well as many recreational and cultural programs. For more information, contact the center at (505) 275–8731; www.cabq.gov/seniors/Manzano.html.

MODELS OF SENIOR CENTERS

As senior centers sprang up across the nation in different social contexts and locations, they developed different organizational structures. Taietz (1976) was the first to identify the different models of senior centers. On the basis of his study of senior centers across the country, he suggested that centers could be categorized as based on either a social agency model or a voluntary organizational model. Senior centers based on a social agency model have programs designed to meet the needs of older adults, with those who are poor and disengaged being the likely participants. In contrast, the voluntary organization model assumes that older adults who are more active in voluntary organizations and who have strong attachments to the community are the ones who will participate in senior centers. Krout (1989b), however, argued that such a dichotomous distinction might not accurately reflect the wide variation of senior centers and their participants. For example, although some participants attend senior centers for recreational and educational opportunities, they may have other unmet nutritional and health needs.

Moreover, the model that a senior center adopts may be linked to its geographical location. For example, rural senior centers differ from urban centers in several organizational characteristics: they are likely to have smaller budgets, fewer paid staff, and fewer resources (Krout, 1987a). Thus community size makes a significant difference in program planning activities, interagency networking, and the types of services and activities that senior centers offer. Centers located in smaller communities are less likely to create new programs, work with other aging and nonaging organizations in joint projects, and make referrals to other agencies (Wacker & Blanding, 1994). Not surprisingly, programs in larger communities are able to offer a wider range of services, including support groups, outreach, and job and employment counseling. The same pattern holds true with activities: Rural centers are less likely than centers located in urban areas to offer many cultural, educational, social, recreational, and outdoor activities.

Best Practice: Serving Rural Seniors

Weld County covers 4,004 square miles in north-central Colorado—an area larger than Rhode Island, Delaware, and the District of Columbia combined. The challenge was how to set up and support senior programs in the county's 28 smaller communities, which range from 150 to 10,000 in population. The solution began in March 1975 after a VISTA volunteer had spent three months assessing both the needs of the rural Weld seniors and the barriers to providing services to them. Without exception, the response from the agencies was the same: "Weld County is so large we simply do not have the staff to do outreach work in the rural communities. Everything is concentrated in Greeley; we have nothing in the small towns."

With this information in hand, a plan was developed and approved by the county commissioners to bring the services and the seniors in the rural areas together. Small-town governments were encouraged to hire a senior aide for 20 hours per week with the promise that the county would pay the aide's salary through an employment and training program for the first year. At the end of the first year, 11 senior aide sites were in place. Today, 21 sites are active, most fully supported by their towns.

Through the years, the senior aide program has grown not only in terms of numbers of sites in place but also in its program offerings. Originally, most senior aides worked out of their homes, offering simple information and referral activities. Today, nearly all the aides work in viable senior centers; some aides have become full-time town employees; and all use volunteers in their centers. Many have new, modern centers and offer a respectable range of recreational outings, educational classes, regular senior meals, and intergenerational programs.

A unique and successful aspect of this program is the monthly day-long training meetings that provide a forum for training and information exchange. The meetings continue to this day and rotate among the participating towns, giving each aide a better understanding of the similarities and differences among the communities. A technical advisor, provided by the Area Agency on Aging, helps the senior aides develop their monthly agendas. These meetings include a wide range of informative programs designed to help the aides provide up-to-date information and quality senior services to their communities. The senior aging network uses the monthly meetings to get the word out about their services and how to access them. The advisor also travels to each town to provide one-on-one technical assistance when needed. In 1980, the senior aides incorporated under the name WELDCOS, Inc. They applied for general fund dollars from the county commissioners and have received a yearly allocation that they divide among themselves. Aides use the funds to help pay utilities, buy craft materials, pay for a fundraising event, purchase equipment, and take seniors on outings. Records show that the program generates more than 50,000 volunteer hours annually for the senior centers and their communities. Community volunteers, coordinated by the aides, also assist with the overwhelming transportation needs generated in this large, rural county. The program continues to grow and thrive, providing valuable assistance and opportunities for seniors in small towns.

For more information, contact Weld County Area Agency on Aging, P.O. Box 1805, Greeley, CO 80632; phone: 970-353-3800, ext. 3323; www.co.weld.co.us/departments/agencyonaging.html.

PROGRAMS OFFERED AT SENIOR CENTERS

The variety of services and activities offered by senior centers can be classified in several ways. The National Institute of Senior Centers classified senior center activities on the basis of participant characteristics. For example, senior centers can provide services to community institutions, group services such as education and group social work, and individual services such as health maintenance and counseling (Lowy & Doolin, 1985). In contrast, Krout (1985a) distinguished between activities and services offered through senior centers. Activities are programs offered by the center for personal enrichment and enjoyment, whereas services are designed to relieve or prevent problems for at-risk older adults. Although the type and number of services and activities offered by senior centers have expanded through the years, centers have always offered creative activities such as arts and crafts; recreational activities such as cards, bingo, parties, and dances; and services such as information, referral, and meals (Krout, 1985a; Leanse & Wagner, 1975; Wacker & Blanding, 1994). Although the availability of services and activities offered at senior centers will vary by the location and size of the center, the services and activities likely to be available at most local centers are listed in Exhibit 7.1.

EXHIBIT 7.1 Types of Services/Programs and Activities Offered at Senior Centers

Recreational opportunities
Health and wellness
Educational opportunities
Meals and nutritional education
Transportation
Arts and humanities
Employment assistance
Intergenerational programming
Information and referral
Support groups and counseling
Social and community action opportunities
Employment assistance
Volunteer activities

Source: Adapted from Wagner (1995a).

Krout's (1985a) national survey of senior centers reported that more than 75% of centers offered information and referral, outreach and transportation services, meals, health education, and screening. More than half of the centers offered home-delivered meals, friendly visiting, telephone reassurance, consumer information, crime prevention, financial/tax services, housing information, legal assistance, and assistance with Social Security and Medicare. Less than one-quarter offered adult day care services, job training and placement, protective services, and peer counseling.

A comparison of Krout's (1985a) data with an early study conducted in 1975 by Leanse and Wagner revealed that the types of services offered by senior centers have diversified and grown, especially services such as home-delivered meals, classes and lectures, and active recreational activities (Krout, 1989b). Findings from a national sample of both senior centers and recreation programs serving older adults were similar to Krout's (1985a) findings in that the majority of senior centers offered health services such as fitness classes, blood pressure checks, vision and hearing tests, and health education, and provided meals, transportation, and outreach (Wacker & Blanding, 1994). Fewer than half offered housing support/assistance, employment counseling, crisis counseling, or adult day care. Although senior centers were providing the usual craft and social activities, few were providing outdoor recreation activities or more physical activities such as swimming, golf, and tennis.

This study also revealed a more recent trend in the type of activities offered at senior centers: the inclusion of intergenerational programs. Seventy percent of senior centers offered some type of intergenerational activity. Examples of intergenerational programming included lunch buddies, whereby older adults are paired with schoolchildren to eat lunch together twice a month, pen-pal programs, and a gift shop for kids at the senior center.

Wacker and Blanding (1994) also examined programmatic characteristics by age of participant. Centers with a higher percentage of adults over 70 years of age compared with the percentage of participants under age 70 offered significantly different types of programs. For example, programs with older participants were significantly more likely to offer the 22 services listed in Exhibit 7.2 than were programs with younger participants. Programs with older participants were likely to offer more health-related services (e.g., health education, blood pressure checks, and vision and hearing tests) and support services (e.g., nutrition, outreach, transportation, and legal aid) than were programs with a younger clientele. More research is needed to determine whether the participant profile influenced programmatic differences or whether the programs offered drew a particular type of participant.

Not surprisingly, differences in programming exist among centers with varying budgets and locations. Centers with larger budgets and more staff are likely to offer a higher number of services and activities (Krout, 1987a; Wacker & Blanding, 1994), and there appears to be a relationship between budget size and location. Two studies by Krout (1984, 1987a) found that budgets of senior centers in rural communities were smaller than budgets of centers located in more urban areas.

Senior centers also serve as a focal point for services and, in many cases, as a source of information and referral for participants. A handful of studies reported that those attending senior centers believed that their center was a source of information about other community services and played an important intermediary role between themselves and other service providers (Delisle, Boucher, & Roy, cited in West, Delisle, Simard, & Drouin, 1996).

EXHIBIT 7.2	Percentage of Services Provided by Senior Centers and Recreation Programs by Age of Participants		

Agency/Organization	Programs With Older Participants (n = 218)	Programs With Younger Participants (n = 336)	X^2
Fitness class/opportunities	95.0	91.0	NS
Information and referral	93.3	73.3	.00
Health education	91.2	71.4	.00
Blood pressure check	90.0	73.4	.00
Vision-hearing tests	81.9	61.8	.00
Nutrition site	81.0	58.2	.00
Transportation	80.0	61.4	.00
Financial education	79.4	56.9	.00
Leisure education	78.4	68.7	.02
Intergenerational activities	78.2	58.9	.00
Outreach	76.3	47.4	.00
Adult education	73.3	54.4	.00
Legal aid	70.1	48.3	.00
Cholesterol testing	56.9	52.7	NS
Support groups	56.4	45.1	.01
Recycling	52.0	50.0	NS
Housing support/assistance	49.0	31.0	.00
Job/employment counseling	41.1	30.0	.01
Government commodities	37.2	31.0	NS
Gift shop or store	33.3	22.9	.00
Hotline crisis counseling	17.0	19.0	NS
Adult day care	16.4	11.1	NS

Source: Wacker and Blanding (1994). Reprinted with permission from the National Recreation and Park Association.

Best Practice: Rural Adult Day Program in a Senior Center—Bozeman, Montana

The National Institute of Senior Centers, in collaboration with the National Council on Aging, identified 10 outstanding caregiving programs for inclusion in a best-practice publication entitled *Together We Care—Exemplary Caregiving Programs in Senior Centers*. One of the programs selected was The Bozeman Senior Center, whose service area extends beyond the city to rural south-central Montana. The Bozeman Senior

Center established an adult day service in 1997 in recognition of the intensifying demand on family caregivers. Inclusion of the day center within a senior center gives the program important links to other services, including meal programs and gives continuity to senior center participants who have become frail over time by creating an opportunity to continue participating in an activity they highly value—going to the center. Just as importantly, the center can become a place of activity and respite for the caregiver. Services provided by this adult day service center include meals and other nutritional support, case management (made possible by a Medicaid waiver), socialization, exercises, games, other activities, a free medical equipment loan program, and transportation to medical appointments. This adult day service center can serve up to 12 persons per day on weekdays and is closed on weekends. Center vehicles may travel 30 to 40 miles one-way outside of Bozeman city limits to pick up clients. Family caregivers find support through annual training and frequent information updates, some through radio talk shows that help them remain up to date on ways to deal with illnesses or disabilities. Depending on the nature of the family member's illness, respite may be for provided for several hours on one day or may extend over the better part of a week. Weekly visits to the senior center by occupational or speech therapists, even a podiatrist, eliminate the need for caregivers to take family members on separate visits to such specialists. Staff may refer caregivers to support groups and maintain telephone contact with long-distance caregivers. For eligible participants, a Medicaid waiver makes case management service possible at no cost, and some participants have private health insurance that contributes towards costs. Other sources include a county allotment, United Way, and personal and business donations. All day care clients pay fees determined through a preliminary interview to determine level of payment, and scholarships are available for those unable to pay. For more information, contact the Bozeman Senior Center, 807 N. Tracy, Bozeman, MT, 59715, 406-586-2421.

Source: National Council on Aging (2002, p. 9).

For Your Files: National Recreation and Park Association

The National Recreation and Park Association (NRPA) is a national nonprofit service organization dedicated to promoting the importance of recreation and parks and to ensuring that all people have an opportunity to make the best and most satisfying use of their leisure time. The Leisure and Aging Section of the NRPA represents and assists professionals who are involved with helping older adults remain healthy and active through participation in recreational pursuits. It also provides leadership and advocacy to ensure the availability of leisure and recreation opportunities for older adults. NRPA has a number of publications available, such as *Active Aging in Vital Communities: Innovative Programs for Older Adults*, *Best Practice Programs in Leisure and Aging*, *Leisure and Aging: A Selected, Annotated Bibliography*, and *Dynamic Leisure Programming With Older Adults*. For more information, contact NRPA at 22377 Belmont Ridge Road, Ashburn, VA 20148-4501; phone: 703-858-0784; www.nrpa.org.

EXHIBIT 7.3   Percentage of Referrals Made to Selected Agencies by Senior Center and Recreation Programs by Age of Participant

Agency/Organization	Programs With Older Participants (n = 218)	Programs With Younger Participants (n = 336)	X^2
Other seniors centers	86.1	69.8	.00
Area Agency on Aging	86.1	68.3	.00
Nutrition sites	84.7	63.3	.00
City/county Social Service Dept.	83.1	58.1	.00
Local Health Dept.	76.0	56.2	.00
Home Health	73.4	42.7	.00
Legal Aid	73.1	47.2	.00
Local Social Security Office	69.3	41.0	.00
Human service organizations (Salvation Army, etc.)	69.0	46.6	.00
Special disability groups	67.0	50.9	.00
Adult day care facility	66.6	43.4	.00
Recreation centers	66.5	70.4	NS
Case management	66.2	37.1	.00
Libraries	66.1	56.8	NS
Service clubs	60.0	52.6	NS
Schools/universities	59.4	50.8	NS
Nursing homes	57.9	40.5	.00
Local hospitals	53.1	37.8	.00
Travel agencies	49.3	43.2	NS
Religious organizations	42.2	36.2	NS
Private physicians	40.0	23.3	.00
State Office on Aging	39.1	33.0	NS
Financial Planning Services	37.0	31.2	NS
Youth groups	36.3	33.9	NS
YMCA/YWCA/Jewish Community Centers	35.0	34.0	NS
Health Maintenance Organizations	32.0	26.4	NS
Outdoor organizations	30.0	28.4	NS

Source: Wacker and Blanding (1994). Reprinted with permission from the National Recreation and Park Association.

As shown in Exhibit 7.3, programs with predominantly older participants referred their participants to support services and long-term care services more often than did programs with predominantly younger participants. For example, more referrals were made to legal aid and nutrition programs, as well as to case management services, nursing homes, home health agencies, and adult day care programs. Thus, as a source of information and referral, senior centers must be aware of a wide range of community services and must respond to changing needs as participants age in place in their programs.

In an attempt to promote formal, national quality control standards for senior centers, the National Institute of Senior Centers (NISC) instituted an accreditation process in 1998. The accreditation process is based on a peer review process, an onsite visit, adherence to standards issued by NISC, and a recommendation to accredit by the National Senior Center Accreditation Board (National Council on Aging, 1998). As of 2006, 126 senior centers have met the accreditation self-assessment requirements and peer review process (National Council on Aging, 2006a). In addition, some states have also instituted a certification process. For example, North Carolina has developed a certification process that designates senior centers as Centers of Merit or Centers of Excellence based on the scope and quality of outreach and access to services, programs and activities, planning, evaluation, input from older adults, staffing, operations, and the physical plant (North Carolina Division of Aging, 2001).

ADDRESSING DIVERSITY

As discussed in Chapter 1, the percentage of older adults of color has been rising steadily and is expected to increase from 18.1% of the older adult population over age 65 to 38.7% in 2050 (Federal Interagency Forum on Aging-Related Statistics, 2006). In addition, gay/lesbian elderly are becoming more "visible" and it is estimated that between 3% and 8% of elders are gay, lesbian, bisexual, or transgender (GLBT) (Cahill, South, & Spade, 2000).

As discussed previously, senior center attendance by non-majority older adults remains low. Barriers to participation can be attributed to system or community barriers such as lack of transportation or geographical segregation. In many communities, both large and small, neighborhoods are often segregated by socioeconomic class and race, thus making attending senior centers in other neighborhoods difficult. Indeed, senior centers located in urban neighborhoods tend to have elders from specific ethnic or racial backgrounds, whereas participant diversity among suburban centers is more difficult to achieve.

Organizational characteristics such as lack of culturally aware programming or culturally competent staff (Kim, Kleiber, & Kropf, 2001; Pardasani, n.d., 2004) or individual barriers such as a perceived lack of a welcoming environment by a majority of participants can act as barriers to participation. A history of discrimination no doubt makes it difficult for many older persons to feel comfortable attending senior centers when they are in the minority. To address the issue of increasing diversity among senior center participants and to provide programs that appeal to and support the unique needs of these subpopulations, two approaches or models of centers have emerged. As shown in the model in Exhibit 7.4, one approach to addressing diversity has been the Open + Targeted Model where the older adults targeted for participation represent the entire senior community. Increasing diversity among members is addressed via outreach efforts to specific subpopulations within the senior community or to incorporate the unique elements of ethnic diversity within the center's programming. An example of this approach is the San Francisco Senior Center, which has a mission to serve seniors who are economically and ethnically diverse, who are well or frail, and who live alone, with family, or with caregivers. Although the senior center targets the entire senior population in San Francisco, there are programs targeting specific groups such as the Deaf Senior Group, the Chinese Outreach Program, and the Senior Literacy Project. Another example of the Open + Targeted Model is the Pimmitt Hills Senior Center in Falls Church, Virginia, that identifies itself as a multicultural center whose participants include elders from China, Taiwan, Iran, and South America. In addition to offering exercise, leisure, educational, and arts activities, Pimmitt Hills incorporates other programming such as English as a second language classes, Persian calligraphy, Iranian cultural music and dance, Chinese calligraphy, and an American cultural seminar.

The second model or approach to addressing the diversity among elders in a community is the Targeted Model, where senior centers serve a specific subpopulation of elders and provide programming and services that address the unique needs of that group. Examples of the Targeted Model are the Yu-Ai Kai Japanese American Community Senior Service in San Jose, California; the Hispanic Senior Center in Cleveland, Ohio; and the Korean American Senior Center in Chicago. The programming offered to participants is more specific to the needs of the subgroup the center is targeting. For example, the Korean American Senior Center in Chicago provides culturally and linguistically isolated Korean American seniors with support and assistance, culturally familiar meals, adult literacy and translation assistance, cultural arts, and citizenship classes, and delivers home care and counseling services through culturally sensitive staff. Over 100 Korean elders partake in the noontime meal every day. Another example is the GLBT Senior Center in Cleveland that convenes twice a week at the Lesbian and Gay Community Center in Cleveland and offers social events, fitness programs, and lunch, or the Gay & Lesbian Center Village at Ed Gould Plaza in Hollywood, California, which offers support and counseling as well as social and educational events. As our older adult population becomes increasingly diverse, senior centers will have to determine the approach or model that best serves all the elders in their communities.

CHALLENGES FOR SENIOR CENTERS

Senior centers provide older adults with a place to pursue leisure activities, to socialize with others, and to receive important health, social, and educational services and information. As the United States experiences social and demographic changes, senior centers will face a number of challenges.

Who Will Senior Centers Serve in the Future?

The "greatest generation" born in the 1920s and 1930s currently comprises the majority of senior center participants; the first wave of "new" older adults—the baby boomers— have now entered their sixth decade and represent the future of senior center participants. However, there is evidence to suggest that attracting this new cohort of seniors to senior centers may be challenging. Recent work by Putnam (1993, 2000) has brought to our attention the fact that membership and participation in a variety of local and civic organizations has been declining at an accelerated rate during the past 25 years. Between 1970 and 1990, average attendance by Americans at some type of monthly club meeting has fallen off by almost 60% (Putnam, 2000). The fact that many senior participants are "aging in place" at senior centers established in the mid-1970s is reflective of a generation with a long history of civic

EXHIBIT 7.4 Two Models of Serving Diverse Older Adults in Senior Centers

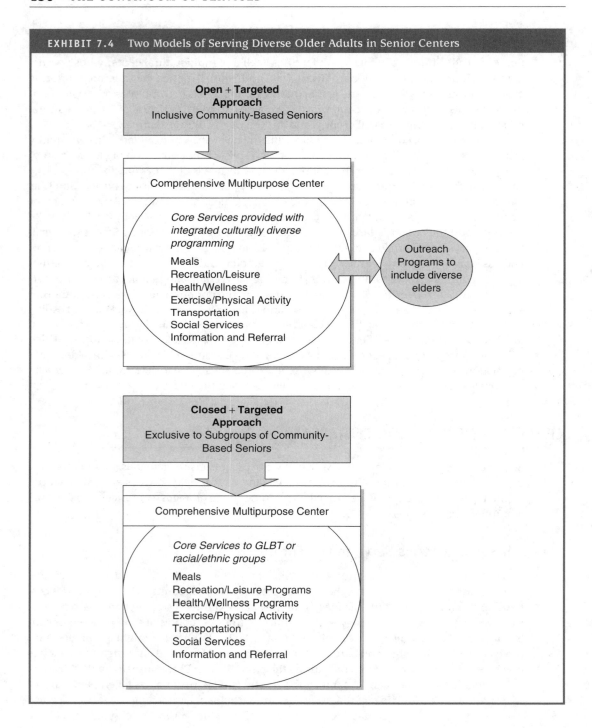

involvement, whereas their children and grandchildren are much less engaged in most forms of community life. In contrast, baby boomers and gen-Xers participate in more individualized leisure activities. The difference can be summed up this way: Fewer baby boomers belong to a bowling league compared with their parents; however, there is an increase in number of boomers bowling in a non-league setting (Putnam, 2000). Thus senior centers will have to look to ways to re-engage and connect with baby boomers who have grown up with a different concept of group association and membership. Senior centers must be aware of what interests baby boomers and adjust programmatic offerings to match their recreation and leisure interests. Younger cohorts who will be recruited to attend senior center activities will carry with them leisure and recreation interests that will no doubt differ from those of the current cohort of older participants. Some possible programmatic changes might include incorporating the latest computer technology for information and entertainment, acting as brokers for arranging individual leisure pursuits, including adventure leisure activities and eco-tourism, and changing food programs to accommodate a wider variety of discerning tastes and extending hours of operation to include evenings and weekends. To attract a more active, more health-conscious cohort of older adults, senior centers must become "vital aging" centers that foster self-development and intellectually challenging opportunities (e.g., language courses, cooking, financial management, lectures, exhibits) and health education and wellness (including personal trainers and public health and nutrition consultants) (MacNeil, 2001; Marken, 2005). Others suggest that providing opportunities to engage in altruistic activities, civic engagement, and intergenerational activities will also be attractive to a new generation of older adults (Eaton & Salari, 2005; Marken, 2005; Williams, Haber, Weaver, & Freeman, 1998; Wagner, 1995b).

Although senior centers are working to attract younger participants, they will also have to determine how to serve their oldest-old participants who are more frail. Unfortunately, there is a dearth of information about how senior centers currently serve at-risk older adults, the impact of involving at-risk older persons with well participants, and how at-risk older adults can successfully be recruited in senior center activities (Krout, 1993b). Cox and Monk (1990) found that senior center directors perceived that the well participants would be resistant to including impaired older persons into their programs. Several directors in their study reported being concerned about becoming "babysitters" for nursing home residents, and felt that they did not have the staff to meet the needs of impaired older adults. Cox and Monk also pointed out that if senior centers are going to include frail elders in their programs, they must receive assistance from other agencies in obtaining diagnostic, program, and service resources. As Krout (1995) observed, senior centers must carefully examine the advantages and disadvantages that serving older adults who are frail will have on their operational, programmatic, and budgetary functions.

Do Senior Centers Need a Name Change?

The senior center of the future may not be called a "senior center." Evidence suggests that some older adults and baby boomers do not attend a senior center because of the stigma associated with being identified as an older adult (Walker et. al., 2004). In a survey of 244 senior center directors, 63% were in favor of changing the name "senior center"

(Kelley, 2005, cited in National Council on Aging, 2006b). Some communities have already made the name change. Senior centers in Lincoln, Nebraska, are now called ActivAge Centers (Lincoln Area Agency on Aging, 2006). It is likely that this trend will increase in the coming years as senior centers move to "reinvent" their images. Of course, not everyone is in favor of moving away from using the term "senior center." Using "senior center" in the name clearly identifies it as a place for older adults, and thus increases the likelihood that community members will recognize the purpose of the organization.

How Will Senior Centers Respond to Diversity Among Seniors?

How will senior centers respond to the increasingly diverse elderly population in their communities? Which model should communities embrace to accommodate this growing diversity—the Open + Targeted Model or the Targeted Model? Clearly, research is needed that measures the individual and organizational benefits of each type of model. However, one way we can begin to think about how senior centers are organized to address diversity is to employ the social capital framework (Putnam, 2000), which refers to understanding the social connections that are created within our communities and organizations. Two concepts of social capital that are germane to our discussion are the dimensions of bonding and bridging. Bonding refers to networks that are, by choice or necessity, inward looking, and reinforces exclusive social identities among homogenous groups. Senior centers that can be characterized as Targeted Models, such as those which serve exclusive subgroups of minority or GLBT elders, have a high degree of bonding among their members and provide those within this social network with an environment in which they feel welcome and where they receive both practical and emotional support. Bridging characterizes social networks that are outward looking and encompass people across diverse social divides such as race and social class, yet who share broadly similar demographic characteristics (Woolcock, 2001). Senior centers that fit the Open + Targeted Model could be considered to have a high degree of social bridging. Bridging outcomes include increased levels of trust and reciprocity, and serve to build connections between diverse heterogeneous groups. As Halpren (2005) notes, both bridging and bonding have different types of benefits, but a social network based too much on one or the other is likely to be a disadvantage to individuals and to communities. According to Halpren, a healthy and effective community needs a blend of both forms of social capital. Interestingly, there is some evidence to suggest that if particular social and ethnic groups have protected enclaves where bonding can occur, they will be more likely to form bridges with people who are very different from themselves (Halpren, 2005). If senior centers can organize themselves around the concepts of bonding and bridging, they may be able to more effectively address the cultural diversity that exists within their communities. Senior centers must consider offering culturally diverse meals and activities, increasing staff sensitivity, and dealing with issues of inclusion by the majority group (Ralston, 1991). Just as U.S. society continues to struggle with racial segregation and racism within many of its cities, senior centers will no doubt be confronted with these same issues as they strive to be more inclusive of minority elders.

Supporting the Senior Centers of the Future

Among the top 50 resolutions put forth by delegates of the 2005 White House Conference on Aging, one gave specific attention to senior centers. The resolution—to encourage the redesign of senior centers for broad appeal and community participation— is to be implemented through the following strategies:

- Support an expanded role for senior centers as focal points for community-based services and civic engagement for senior centers as independent service through (a) combined service for all economic levels, cultural competence, and diversified populations and generations (volunteer opportunities, transportation, nutrition, etc.) and mental health services; and (b) NISC accreditation.
- Support efforts to modernize and upgrade facilities and programming that will attract and serve existing and new generations through (a) healthy aging— physical, emotional, and mental health services; (b) civic engagement to provide community support; and (c) design for all economic levels and capabilities.
- Impose a federal requirement that all 50 states, territories, and tribes establish statutes defining "multipurpose senior centers" as *the* community-based focal point for planning and coordination for the organization and provision for a broad spectrum of services suited to the diverse needs and interests of self-determining older persons.
- Create a separate and distinct title in OAA for multipurpose senior centers which are a system serving older adults, caregivers, and their families.
- Support policies and encourage efforts to create and expand opportunities and partnerships that integrate senior centers, health care systems, service providers, communities, business, and public and private organizations to serve culturally diverse populations across all social and economic lines.

The Senior Center of the Future

So what will senior centers look like in the future? In addition to the programmatic changes mentioned above, Schoeffler (1995) argues that, at a minimum, every senior center must provide information and referral services and be used as an intake location for delivering other community services. It is hard to know for certain what form or function senior centers will embrace in the coming years. But what is certain is that if senior centers wish to continue to be effective places, they must be flexible and adapt to the changing natures of our communities and elderly population. Conducting frequent needs assessments and hiring staff trained in gerontology will be critical to maintaining the viability and relevancy of senior centers in the coming years and to meeting the challenges that lie ahead. In the near future, senior centers will be challenged to respond to the needs and demands of a new generation of older adults. Perhaps, as a result, senior centers of the future will bear little resemblance to the senior centers that currently exist.

CASE STUDY

Loneliness of a Caregiver

Alex, 77, laid down the natural science journal he was reading and thought for a moment about the turn of events in his life since his wife, Susan, had been diagnosed with Alzheimer's disease five years earlier. When he retired from the university and she from public school teaching, they had literally catapulted into a new life of worldwide travel and volunteer work with the local Friends of the Library and several conservation groups. Their life contained all the excitement and stimulation they had hoped it would when they began planning for their retirement. Hardly a day passed when they were not socializing with friends and other volunteers. Even Alex's lifelong lapses into depression had virtually disappeared.

At first, after Susan's diagnosis, they kept up a good front. Few of their social contacts realized what was happening to Susan. Now, he thought, everything has changed. Susan needed constant supervision. Other than their two daughters, who visited once a month, a couple of neighbors who dropped in to say hello, and the home health aide, Alex had few contacts with the outside world. It embarrassed him to think that twice in the last year he had checked into emergency care at the hospital on orders from his doctor to have a psychiatric evaluation. Once he was released; the other time he was admitted for three days of psychiatric tests and counseling.

On his worst days, Alex wonders why he is alive. On better days, he's gratified that he is still able to take care of his wife. At the same time, he also wonders how much longer he can tolerate the isolation and loneliness. His psychiatrist and the home health aide are advising him to hire a respite worker to come in and sit with Susan a couple of afternoons a week so that he can visit the downtown senior center.

Case Study Questions

1. Why do you believe Alex's psychiatrist and his wife's home health aide are recommending that he connect with the local senior center? Cite research in this chapter that supports your response.
2. On the basis of what you know about Alex, what the literature says about the typical senior center participant, and theories of service use, what are the chances that Alex will follow the advice of his psychiatrist?
3. Describe a typical senior center offering of activities and services. Which of these offerings might be most beneficial to Alex? Why?
4. What barriers to becoming involved in the senior center do caregivers like Alex face? What other community support services could be helpful at this time?
5. Why do you think Alex and his wife did not join the senior center at the time of their retirement? What research supports your answer?
6. Describe a senior center program that would be most appealing to Alex.
7. What are the benefits to Alex, Susan, and society in helping Alex reconnect with his community?

Learning Activities

1. Interview two or more people who are in their 50s about their leisure and recreational activities. Do they participate in passive, social, or physical activities? How do they think the pattern of their leisure activity will change as they become older or retire? Would they be interested in joining a senior center when they get older? Why or why not? What type of activities do they think senior centers should provide to people in their generation? If possible, interview a group with diversity based on gender, income, and race.

2. Visit the local senior center. What activities are available there? What percentage of program offerings are for recreation? What percentage are social support services? On the basis of your review, do you think this center acts as a focal point for older adults in your community?

3. Interview the director of a local senior center. What percentage of the participants are aging in place? What strategies has the center used to attract younger participants? What, in the director's opinion, is the most innovative program the center offers? If money were no object, what program or service would the center provide?

FOR MORE INFORMATION

National Resources

1. National Institute on Senior Centers, 409 Third Street S.W., Suite 200, Washington, DC 20024; phone: 202-479-1200; www.ncoa.org/content.cfm?sectionid = 44.

   The National Institute on Senior Centers is funded under a cooperative agreement between the Administration on Aging (AoA) and the National Council on the Aging. The institute is a resource for older Americans through multipurpose senior centers and community focal points. The institute offers training, technical assistance, and materials, and sponsors research initiatives.

2. National Senior Games Association, P. O. Box 82059, Baton Rouge, Louisiana 70884-2059; phone: 225-766-6800; www.nsga.com/about.html.

   The mission of the National Senior Games Association is to motivate senior men and women to lead a healthy lifestyle through the senior games movement. The NSCA governs the Summer National Senior Games, better known as the Senior Olympics, which is the largest multisport event in the world for seniors. It supports and sanctions member state organizations that promote the year-round participation of older adults in events such as archery, badminton, basketball, shuffleboard, table tennis, horseshoes, volleyball, cycling, swimming, softball, tennis, triathlon, and golf.

3. National Recreation and Park Association (NRPA), 22377 Belmont Ridge Road, Ashburn, VA 20148-4501; phone: 703-858-0784; www.nrpa.org.

   The Leisure and Aging Section of the NRPA represents and assists professionals who are involved with helping older adults remain healthy and active through participation in recreational pursuits. NRPA's publications include *Best Practice Programs in Leisure and Aging*, *Leisure and Aging: A Selected, Annotated Bibliography*, and *Dynamic Leisure Programming With Older Adults*.

Web Resources

1. Council on Aging Senior Center, Shelby, NC: www.seniorcenter-coa.org.
   This is an excellent example of a senior center website. It is the home page for the senior center in Shelby, NC, and lists activities, events, and services for and about seniors in Shelby. Visitors can access information about recreation and leisure programs and activities, volunteer opportunities, community news, and other community services for older adults.

2. Seniors' Center, Boulder, CO: http://bcn.boulder.co.us/community/senior-citizens/center.html.
   This site is a "senior center" on the web. Visitors will find information about all types of services and programs for older adults, from a list of local grocers and senior discounts to information about health matters and travel.

3. Shepherd's Centers of America: www.shepherdcenters.org.
   Shepherd's Centers of America is an interfaith, nonprofit organization whose primary purpose is to enrich the lives of older adults. The home page explains the philosophy behind the centers and provides a list of centers across the country.

4. Northshore Senior Center, Bothell, WA: http://northshoreseniorcenter.org.
   The home page of the Northshore Senior Center provides information about how to join the center, volunteer opportunities, and the computer learning center. Visitors can access the center's newsletter and catalog.

NOTE

1. Unless noted otherwise, the history of senior centers comes from Krout (1989b).

8

Employment Programs

At 57 years of age, John suddenly found himself unemployed when his company was sold. He had worked in almost every area of the lumber business and had expected to work for the same company until he retired. The new owners offered him a position at half the salary he had been earning. With at least eight years until retirement and his youngest child still in college, John simply could not accept the offer. He was frightened about his financial future. Through a friend, he heard that the local employment service operated a federally funded program for adults aged 55 and older. John qualified for the program as a displaced worker and because of his age. His employment specialist helped him regain his self-confidence and set new employment goals. The program enrolled him in a correspondence course and an on-the-job training program with a local appraisal company. After successfully completing his training, the employment counselor helped John establish himself as a self-employed appraiser.

In 1986, the first of the baby boomers turned 40 and became "older workers." By 2006, many of these individuals were seriously contemplating the date of their retirement. In the interim, some individuals, like John, found that their age worked against them in maintaining their current positions, seeking new jobs, or requesting training—although most employers rate older workers highly on such traits as loyalty, dependability, and attitude toward work. For a variety of reasons, including industry's need for workers and the economic needs of some older adults, employers can no longer ignore this growing segment of the workforce.

We begin this chapter by examining work-related policies that protect older workers. We then profile older workers and their employers, with particular focus on federally supported employment training programs designed specifically for older adults. We conclude the chapter with a discussion of the challenges facing older worker and employment programs.

POLICY BACKGROUND

The Age Discrimination in Employment Act (ADEA), first passed in 1967, is the single most important law protecting the rights of older workers. It provides that workers over the age of 40 cannot arbitrarily be discriminated against because of age in any employment decision, including hiring, discharges, layoffs, promotion, wages, and health care coverage (Brown,

1989). The 1986 amendments to the ADEA prohibit most employers from setting a mandatory retirement age. There are, however, a few exceptions to the ADEA. For example, the ADEA does not protect workers who are employed by companies that have fewer than 20 employees, and the ADEA permits the mandatory retirement of "executives or persons in high policy-making positions" (p. 186) at age 65 if their annual retirement pension benefits equal or exceed $44,000. In addition to the ADEA, more than 40 states have their own laws against age discrimination in employment that often provide greater protection than the federal law.

Congress also enacted the Older Workers Benefit Protection Act in 1990 to make clear that discrimination based on age in virtually all forms of employee benefits is unlawful. Specifically, it applies to employee benefits and benefit plans established or modified on or after its enactment (October 16, 1990; April 14, 1991 for private employers). The major goal of the Act is to establish regulations prohibiting age discrimination for most employee fringe benefits (Wiencek, 1991). It provides statutory recognition of early retirement programs and enacts into law the "equal benefit" or "equal cost" principle, requiring employers to provide older workers with benefits at least equal to those provided for younger workers, unless the employers can prove that the cost of providing an equal benefit is greater for an older worker than for a younger worker.

The Americans With Disabilities Act (ADA) of 1990 also provides additional protection for older workers. Although disabilities are not a result of normal aging, the ADA classifies many ailments associated with older adults as disabilities. Older adults who have been unemployed because of disability will have substantially improved opportunities to re-enter the workforce. Under the law, individuals must be considered for employment if they can perform the essential functions of the position with reasonable accommodations.

The federal government has also been instrumental in creating employment programs for older workers. These include the Experience Works, the Senior Community Service Employment Program (formally known as the Green Thumb Program), the Community Service Employment for Older Americans under Title V of the Older Americans Act (OAA), and the Senior Employment Program. Each of these will be explained in greater detail later in this chapter.

In 2000, then-President Bill Clinton signed into law the Senior Citizens' Freedom to Work Act, eliminating the earnings limitation for Social Security for those adults older than normal retirement age. The passing of this law was heralded by some members of Congress as the "dawn of a new age for older Americans." The goals of the act are twofold: to allow those older adults already working to receive more wages and to encourage more older adults to get into the labor force. Critics point out that the overwhelming majority of older adult retirees are not advantaged by the Freedom to Work Act because only about one in five taxpayers older than age 65 reports wages or earned income from employment. A review of labor statistics in 2002 indicated that little has changed for older adults, yet evidence suggests that, over time, benefits will be seen (Song, 2003–04).

USERS AND PROGRAMS

Characteristics of Older Workers

The proportion of older people working decreases with age. In 2005, 75% of men between the ages of 55 and 61 and 52% of men aged 62 to 64 were in the civilian labor force

(Federal Interagency Forum on Aging-Related Statistics, 2006) (see Exhibit 8.1). Only 34% of men between the ages of 65 and 69, and 13% of men over age 70 and older were in the labor force. Labor force participation rates of older women show a similar decline with age.

Approximately 63% of all women aged 55 to 61 were working, yet only 24% of women between the ages of 65 and 69, and 7% of women aged 70 and older, were employed. In all age groups 55 years and older, men are more likely than women to be employed (He et al., 2005). Some 10.82 million men aged 55 and older and 5.25 million women over age 55 work in nonagricultural industries (He et al., 2005).

Rates of labor force participation also vary between members of various ethnic groups. As shown in Exhibit 8.2, in 2003 non-Hispanic White and Hispanic men had higher rates of participation than did older Black men. Among men aged 60 to 64, 58% of non-Hispanic White men, 58% of Hispanic men, and 47% of Black men were employed. For men aged 70 to 74, a higher percentage of non-Hispanic White men were employed (20%) than either Blacks (16.2) or Hispanics (15%). A lower percentage of women than men were employed at every age and in each ethnic group. Among older women, a higher percentage of non-Hispanic White women and Black women than Hispanic women were employed. At age 60 to 64, 47% of non-Hispanic White women, 42% of Black women, and 36% of Hispanic women were employed (He et al., 2005).

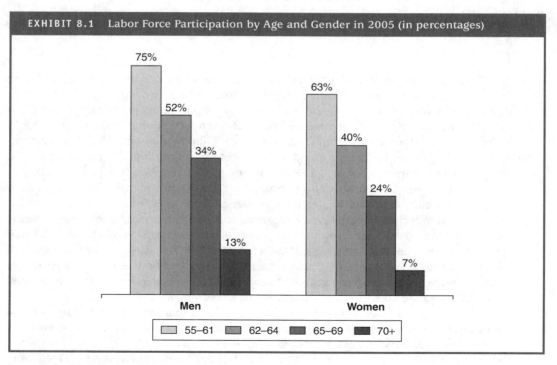

EXHIBIT 8.1   Labor Force Participation by Age and Gender in 2005 (in percentages)

Source: Federal Interagency Forum on Aging Related Statistics, 2006

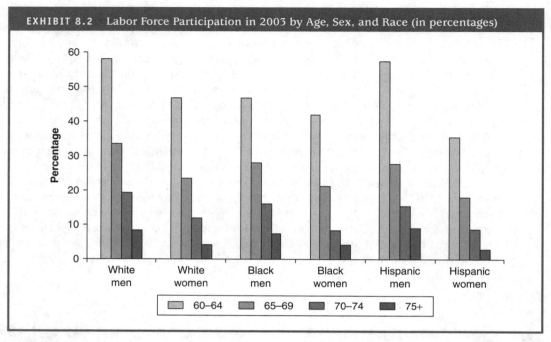

EXHIBIT 8.2 Labor Force Participation in 2003 by Age, Sex, and Race (in percentages)

Source: He et al. (2005).

There are two exceptions to the decline of older workers gainfully employed with advancing years. There is a shift among married couples from two-worker to single-worker units, with wives assuming a greater share of work responsibility outside the home when their husbands leave the labor force for health-related reasons (Johnson & Favreault, 2001). The second exception is the slight increase at age 73 in the numbers of male pensioners employed in full-time jobs year round. This is most likely a result of the elimination of the Social Security earnings test at age 72 for this cohort (Benitez-Silva & Heiland, 2006).

According to the U.S. Bureau of the Census (2001), the majority of male workers aged 65 or older are in administrative and management, professional, and sales occupations. Administrative support jobs (principally clerical jobs) and service occupations account for the largest share of older women workers. Further examination reveals that the occupations held by adults aged 65 or more are the ones that workers aged 30–39 are least likely to hold (e.g., sales, administrative support, farming, transportation, and service-oriented jobs). Only in blue-collar, non-executive jobs is the percentage of older adults (62.4%) approximately the same as those for workers aged 55–64 (61.7%) and 40–54 (63.4%) (Hedge, Borman, & Lammlein, 2006).

Of the 5 million older adults in the labor force, fewer than half are on full-time schedules (Administration on Aging [AoA], 2005a). About 68% of the baby boomers work full time; 12% work part time. Workers aged 50 and older are more likely than younger workers to be self-employed (17% vs. 12%) or small business owners (9% vs. 5%) (Sloan Work and Family Research Network, 2006). Of adults over age 65 who were employed in 2002, 19.3% were self-employed (Karoly & Zissimopoulos, 2004).

The availability of unearned income, particularly the availability of pension income, is a key factor in determining whether older individuals continue working after receipt of Social Security benefits. Only about 10 to 12% of older men and 6 to 8% of older women who receive income from a private pension or retirement savings plan remain in the workforce (Purcell, 2000). According to the 2006 Metlife National Survey of Aging Workers, 72% of retirees say they continue working because they need the income to live, 54% want to stay active and engaged, 43% want to engage in meaningful work, 43% desire to maintain their lifestyle, and 41% want to build up retirement savings. Seventy-five percent of older adults aged 66 to 70 work because they want to stay actively engaged (DeLong & Associates, 2006).

Workers aged 55 and older have a lower unemployment rate than younger age groups. The unemployment rate for workers aged 35 to 54 is 4.8% compared with 3.9% for workers aged 55 to 64 and 3.6% for workers 65 and older (Whittaker, 2005). Once older workers become unemployed, however, they experience a longer period of unemployment than do other workers. For example, individuals 55 to 64 years old report being unemployed an average of 22.8 weeks, and those 65 and older report being unemployed an average of 20.3 weeks, compared with 15.9 weeks for all workers aged 16 and older (U.S. Bureau of Labor Statistics, 2006a). Approximately 2% of older persons not in the labor force in 2005 indicated that they would like to be working (U.S. Department of Labor, 2006a). The most common reasons for not looking for work were discouragement over job prospects, facing lower levels of replaced earnings, illness or disability, and family responsibilities.

Employers of Older Workers

Federal Employment and Training Programs

Government programs provide the majority of employment and training programs for older persons. Experience Works (formerly known as Green Thumb) is the oldest and largest operator of employment and training programs for older Americans. It was founded in 1965 by the National Farmers Union, as part of President Johnson's War on Poverty. Originally designed to put older, rural Americans to work to beautify the nation's parks and highways, the program began with 280 participants in four states. Since 1994, it has provided employment, training, and service opportunities to more than 55,600 older Americans in 50 states and territories (Experience Works, 2006).

Participants in the Experience Works program must be 55 years of age or older; have annual family income of not more than 125% of the established federal poverty income guidelines; establish residency in the state in which they enroll in the program; and be eligible to work in the United States. Through Experience Works, participants receive training experience at an approved government or private nonprofit agency (i.e., the host agency), educational opportunities, counseling, and information to help them find and keep a job. Participants average 20 hours per week of community service work at their host agencies and may not work more than 1,300 hours per year. They receive either the federal or state minimum wage, whichever is higher in the state in which they live. Employers of Experience Works workers include schools, hospitals, housing facilities, public works and transportation, social services, and nutrition programs.

In 1969, Congress funded a demonstration project to promote useful part-time opportunities in community-service activities for unemployed low-income older adults.

The success of this project resulted in statutory financing in 1973 for the Senior Community Service Employment Program (SCSEP). In 1978, this program became Title V of the Older Americans Act. Although the Department of Labor manages the SCSEP, it allocates the majority of funds to 10 national organizations: AARP; the Asociacion Nacional Pro Personas Mayores; Experience Works; the National Caucus and Center on Black Aged; the National Council of Senior Citizens; the National Council on the Aging; the National Indian Council on Aging; the National Asian Pacific Center on Aging; the National Urban League; and the U.S. Department of Agriculture, Forest Service. The governors of each state receive the remaining funds to operate the SCSEP. The governors decide which state agency in government has the authority for program management and oversight. In most states, the State Unit on Aging (SUA) has this responsibility (U.S. Department of Labor, 2006b).

SCSEP programs provide subsidized minimum-wage jobs in community service positions in public and nonprofit organizational settings for persons aged 55 and older whose incomes are no more than 125% of the poverty level. Senior participants work 20 hours a week for the minimum wage and minimal benefits. The goal is to ultimately place these individuals in unsubsidized employment. Nationally, the unsubsidized placement rate is about 26%; this figure, however, varies widely by sponsor (U.S. Department of Labor, 2006b).

Although regulations allow contractors to provide training to participants, they devote few financial resources to this activity. Most of the efforts go into creating community jobs for participants and matching participants with existing jobs (Schultz, 2001). SCSEP workers provide whatever services are needed locally. Programs deliver two-thirds of their services to the general community; the remaining services assist the older population in the community. The largest service categories are social services and education. Most participants are female (71%) and White (58%) (U.S. Department of Labor, 2006b).

For Your Files: Job-Seeking Online

Older workers wanting to re-enter the workforce can now find job openings as well as online support for their search and interview process through internet employment services such as Retired Brains (www.retiredbrains.com), Too Young to Retire (www.2young2retire.com), and Senior Job Bank (www.seniorjobbank.com). The internet sites are supported by employer ads and do not charge the prospective worker a fee. Sites often have web links to free documents with titles like *How to Start Your Own Business after 50* and *Creating Your Resume* that can be downloaded.

A smaller workforce program authorized under Title V is the Section 502(e) experimental projects. The purpose of these projects is to ensure second-career training and the placement of eligible Title V participants in jobs in the private business sector. In contrast to the SCSEP program, 502(e) programs can pay participants more than federal minimum wage, can subsidize a greater number of hours per week, and offer greater flexibility in the income eligibility requirements for program participants. Enrollees may have incomes of up to 150–165% of the poverty level, compared with 125% for SCSEP. Unfortunately, there is no separate appropriation for 502(e) programs. Sponsors must divert part of their Title V funding to run these training-oriented programs. The only in-depth examination of the 502(e) project estimates that the number of experimental project participants was about 3% of the total SCSEP enrollment (Centaur Associates, 1986). Women constituted about 70% of program enrollees. Most of these 502(e) placements were in the health, clerical, and services occupations.

The Job Training Partnership Act (JTPA) of 1982 is a comprehensive workforce development program with several programs that provide employment and training activities. In general, JTPA IIA programs provide basic educational and occupational skills training to persons who are economically disadvantaged and other persons with multiple barriers to employment (e.g., age discrimination) to prepare them for employment and economic self-sufficiency (Hale, 1990). Although all adults, regardless of age, can use JTPA services, participation by older adults is low. In 1995, some 176,000 adults participated in JTPA IIA programs beyond initial assessment; of these, only 3,513 (2%) were 55 years of age or older (Gross, 1998). Title II-A, the 5% Set-Aside program, was designed to provide funding specifically for older adults (age 55 +) with low income (i.e., no more than 100% of the poverty guidelines or 70% of the lower living standard income level). These programs provided training for placement of older individuals in employment opportunities with private business concerns. Approximately 66% of the states administered Title II-A 5% Set-Aside program through the state JTPA office. In 20% of the states, the SUA administered the program. This program was discontinued under the Workforce Investment Act of 1998, which became fully effective on July 1, 2000. Under the new legislation, older workers are served under the adult training component of JTPA IIA, leaving SCSEP as the only program specifically providing training to low-income older workers.

Older adults also may receive training through Title III of JTPA, which provides monies for training, placement, and other assistance to dislocated workers. The law extends eligibility to individuals who meet other criteria, including long-term unemployed persons who have limited opportunities for employment or reemployment in the area in which they reside. This category includes older individuals who may have substantial barriers to employment because of age (Alegria, 1992).

Another federally funded program is the Senior Employment Program (SEP). Founded in 1965, more than 92,000 older adults currently participate in employment activities through SEP programs nationwide. Participants receive over 1 million hours of skilled training and provide more than 45 million hours of service to the community. To be eligible, workers must be aged 55 and older and have a family income of no more than 25% above the federal poverty line. Enrollment priority is given to persons over age 60, veterans, and qualified spouses of veterans. Wages are equivalent to the highest of federal minimum wage, state minimum wage, or prevailing wage allowable. Participants work an average of 20 hours per week. Employment opportunities include a wide variety of facilities, including day care centers, senior centers, schools, hospitals, and government agencies (U.S. Department of Labor, 2006b).

Private Sector Employers

Most employers view older workers as mature and stable contributors to their organization. Older workers are perceived as having lower absenteeism rates than younger workers and as possessing good work ethics (Tourigny & Pulich, 2006). However, the same employers tend to believe that older workers cannot learn new things, take on new responsibilities, and be productive beyond the scope of work they have traditionally completed. Employers also do not view older workers as needing to build their careers. Thus they are reluctant to invest too much time, energy, and money in older workers because they do not see it as a good return on their investment.

The belief that older workers cannot learn new things and are unable to utilize computer technology in the workplace is held by many employers. However, research indicates that older workers are not afraid of using computers; they just haven't had as much opportunity to use them as younger workers (Rizzuto & Mohammed, 2005). Most older adults agree that they would be happy to learn if offered the opportunity. Their success is based on their willingness to learn and the employers' commitment to their achievement.

Some companies view workers over the age of 50 as an asset rather than a liability. One such company, USB Financial Services in Winston-Salem, NC, purposefully employs more financial advisors who are aged 50 or older than not. USB management recognized that clientele were more receptive to the advice of older advisors than younger advisors. In a business move that runs counter to current management thinking that younger workers are more cost-effective, USB management sought and trained older workers who were successful in their previous careers as financial advisors (Craver, 2007).

Best Practice: Mature Services

Mature Services, Inc. provides workers aged 40 and older in northeastern Ohio who want to enter or re-enter the workforce a number of employment services. A senior employment center provides job search services, job fairs, meetings with employers, and a computer resource room. It also provides a full-service staffing agency that works to match job seekers aged 40 and older with employers.

For more information about this employment program, contact Mature Services, 415 S. Portage Path, Akron, OH 44320; phone: 330-762-8666; www.matureservices.org.

CHALLENGES FOR OLDER WORKER AND EMPLOYMENT PROGRAMS

Society is redefining the meaning of work and retirement. It is not uncommon for today's workers to pursue multiple careers throughout their lifetimes. Frequently, workers who pursued one lifelong career retire from it only to continue working in another field or in their primary field while receiving some retirement income (Hirshorn & Hoyer, 1994). In addition, given the changing demographics of society, there will be increasing numbers of older workers, as well as a greater need for them. We end this chapter by examining several challenges facing older worker and employment programs as they address the changing needs and values of an aging workforce.

Increasing Enrollments in Job Training Programs

Eligibility requirements limit the number of midlife and older persons who take part in SCSEP and JTPA programs. The inclusion of Social Security benefits and/or Title V income in calculating income eligibility for JTPA enrollment leads to the ineligibility of many older worker applicants. Beginning in 1995, states could request a waiver that allows for excluding 25% of Social Security when making eligibility calculations. Program administrators at the state and local levels need to start a more aggressive awareness campaign to increase the number of older adults enrolled in this program.

Providing Opportunities for Older Workers

In both the public and private sectors, training is a key element in the successful integration of older workers in the labor force. The rapid introduction of new technologies and productive innovations requires a reorientation by employers and workers of all ages toward the concept of lifelong learning and skills upgrading (DeLong & Associates, 2006). In addition, business must look beyond the "McJobs" opportunities for older workers (Hushbeck, 1990) and support the use of older workers to their full potential (Hedge, Borman, & Lammlein, 2006).

In rural areas, the agricultural economic base, low population density, and relative isolation from larger urban areas often limit the employment opportunities for older workers. The aging network needs to become more involved in offering and facilitating training programs that prepare older workers for the more limited employment opportunities in rural areas as well as helping them prepare for their retirement years.

Entry or re-entry into the labor force may be difficult for some older women without recent job experience. Upon finding a job, older women typically receive less pay and fewer benefits than older men. Older women earn 55 cents for every dollar that older men earn, and only 80% have access to health insurance through their employer (Sloan Work and Family Research Network, 2006). These women may benefit from special programs designed to better integrate them into the labor force to gain better positioning. One such program, formed in 1981 to empower all displaced homemakers and help them in achieving economic self-sufficiency, is the National Displaced Homemakers Network. In 1993 it reorganized and changed its name to Women Work! The National Network for Women's Employment, in recognition of the range of economic transitions women face throughout their lives. Today, Women Work! is one of the leading organizations advocating for women to train and qualify for jobs in the information technology field and nontraditional occupations. Recognized as experts on employment and training issues, Women Work! and its nationwide network affect policy by working with lawmakers, business leaders, nonprofit organizations, and labor unions to create and strengthen programs and policies for women.

Educating Employers

Stereotypes of aging still hold fast in the workplace. Older workers confront more restricted job opportunities than do otherwise identical younger workers. With the changes in demographics, greater awareness and understanding of older workers as resources are needed. Furthermore, employers need accurate information about the myths and realities of older workers. Many would probably be surprised to know that older workers have lower rates of absenteeism, experience less stress on the job, and remain productive workers.

Increasing Self-Employment

Many baby boomers reaching retirement age want to continue working. For those not willing or able to remain in their current position, the most flexible way to remain in the workforce is through self-employment. In a 2003 MetLife study of retirees, 36% of 60–65-year-olds and 42% of 66–70-year-olds identified themselves as being self-employed. Increasing rates of self-employment also suggests that limited employment options exist for older adults in the workplace. Some workers reported feeling forced into self-employment due to age discrimination at their workplace, and considered self-employment their best option (DeLong & Associates, 2006).

Preparing for Retirement

Regardless of how, at what age, or why older adults leave the workforce, they are often ill-prepared for life as a retirees. Teaching men and women about finances and other retirement issues should begin early in their work careers. This introduction to retirement issues serves two purposes: consciousness-raising and information dissemination (Shagrin, 2000). Personnel offices, training offices, and employee-counseling services within organizations should provide workers with adequate information concerning financial options for retirement because many individuals are unaware of, or do not fully understand, their retirement benefits. This may be a particular concern for women and low-income individuals who, because of financial concerns, may not even consider retirement as an option or have exacerbated fears about retirement (Daily, 1998).

Several private organizations are testing models of flexible retirement options. These programs help upcoming retirees make an easier transition from work to retirement; companies view such programs as a cost-effective means for solving their labor shortages. For example, the National Rural Electric Cooperative Association has a "phased retirement" option for its older workers. When employees reach retirement age under their pension plan, the pension may start even if they continue working on a full- or part-time basis. Other benefits, like health insurance, continue to be available during the phased retirement period (U.S. Department of Labor, 2000b). Other companies offer cafeteria-like options for older workers on a preretirement basis, such as part-time work, flextime, and vacation-work combinations. Another approach used by some companies is internal job redesign that allows for work-schedule adjustments based on demographic and lifestyle changes as employees age (Bond, Thompson, Galinsky, & Prottas, 2002; Clark & Quinn, 2002). Both preretirement planning and flexible retirement plans stand to benefit both the employer and the employee by providing adequate time to prepare for the transition from work to retirement.

Promoting Older Worker Programs in the Future

The 2005 White House Conference on Aging gave specific support for employment programs. Two of its top 50 resolutions focused on older workers:

- Promote incentives for older workers to continue working and improve employment training and retraining programs to better serve older workers.
- Remove barriers to the retention and hiring of older workers, including age discrimination.

Suggested strategies for implementing these resolutions include:

- Provide greater access to education and training for older worker via education grants, tuition waivers, and new financing mechanisms like a training education 401K.
- Require local workforce investment boards to set aside a minimum amount of funds to support the training of older workers.
- Remove barriers to the retention and hiring of older workers, including age discrimination.
- Retain and increase funding for Title V programs to allow people to enroll sooner and serve older workers who are economically disadvantaged.
- Implement phased retirement options to encourage flexible work options for older workers' businesses.
- Encourage the development of technologies so that, after people retire, they can return to work from home or near their communities in less manual jobs to perform more meaningful work.

CASE STUDY

Beginning the Journey to Financial Independence at Midlife

Sally, a 58-year-old widow, has had no income for the last six months. She is unable to pay her rent, and has had to move in with her sister. Before medical problems forced her to quit her job, Sally had been employed for three years at the local university, clerking in the student bookstore. Her supervisor was complimentary about her organizational skills and how well she worked with the students and faculty. It was a pleasant job, although far from her original career goals. As a young woman, she had aspirations of becoming a chaplain or working in some aspect of the ministry, or at least in some type of helping profession. Marriage and family interrupted this dream. She left school one semester and a thesis shy of a Master of Divinity degree. During the past 30 years, a series of unfortunate events has left Sally with few resources. Other than her three uninterrupted years working in the student bookstore, her work history is patchy. Mostly, Sally fulfilled a traditional role as homemaker until her husband died four years ago. To keep in touch with her love of helping people, she volunteers at least five hours per week in the social ministries of her large church.

Sally and her husband had no children, and her sister is her only living relative. Although Sally appreciates her sister's kindness, she desperately wants to be independent. When she finally rebounded from her recent medical problems, she began looking for work. She has been searching for a job for four months with no promise of employment—at least employment that can support her. Sally is angry and frustrated. She is sure she is being discriminated against. She suspects that her age and being overweight are contributing to her lack of success. Overall, Sally's self-esteem at this point in her life is low, and she is running desperately short on financial resources.

Case Study Questions

1. What protection does Sally have against discrimination? How realistic is it that these protections will alleviate her present situation?

2. On the basis of statistics on older workers, in what fields is Sally most likely to find employment? How do these jobs relate to her employment goals?

3. Sally could continue her job search on her own. Eventually, she might be successful. What other employment assistance might she explore? Do you believe she would qualify for these employment programs? Why?

4. Although Sally is classified as an older worker, how does her situation differ from that of a worker 65 or 70 years of age? What impact does being female have on her situation, if any?

5. Which of the special employment programs for older workers described in the chapter would be most appropriate for Sally? Why? If you were the older worker employment specialist working with Sally, what would be your goals for her?

Learning Activities

1. At what age would you like to retire? From what job do you see yourself retiring? How far up the career ladder will you have climbed? What will be your ending salary? What steps do you need to take throughout your adult life to achieve these goals?

2. Interview an employee counselor who deals with retirement planning. What information and training does the counselor provide? What types of employees (e.g., women, men, age, position) seek or attend retirement planning? When does the counselor recommend that employees start to plan for retirement? How much savings/pension should the average employee try to secure for retirement?

3. Plan your retirement. Will you take on a second career, travel, take classes—or do it all? If planning a second career, describe what it would be, and look in your local newspaper, employment agency, and senior job line to check on availability, pay, and requirements (experience and skills).

4. Interview someone who has retired from one career and has now embarked on another. How did the individual decide on the second career? How did the person find the position, learn skills, and so on? How is the second career different from the previous one?

5. Interview an advocate, attorney, or someone who deals with age discrimination in employment. What type of cases has the person handled? How successful are people in fighting age discrimination? What types of positions or older adults seem more prone to age discrimination?

For More Information

National Resources

1. Experience Works, 2200 Clarendon Blvd, Suite 1000, Arlington, VA 22201; phone (toll free): 1-866-EXP-WEKS; www.experienceworks.org.

   Experience Works empowers low-income older Americans aged 55 and older to remain productive and independent by providing them with employment and training opportunities.

2. U.S. Department of Labor, Office of Public Affairs, 200 Constitution Avenue N.W., Room S1032, Washington, DC 20210; phone: 202-639-4650; www.dol.gov/opa/media/press/opa.

   The Department of Labor is responsible for the Senior Community Service Employment Program for low-income older adults over age 55.

3. AARP, 601 E Street N.W., Washington, DC 20049; phone: 1-888-OUR-AARP; www.aarp.org.

   AARP is a nonprofit organization helping older adults maintain independence, dignity, and purpose. AARP has a number of publications about older workers and preretirement planning.

4. Equal Employment Opportunity Commission, 1801 L Street N.W., Washington, DC 20507; phone: 1-800-669-4000; www.eeoc.gov.

   The Equal Employment Opportunity Commission enforces the Age Discrimination in Employment Act and investigates age discrimination complaints.

Web Resources

1. America's Job Bank, U.S. Department of Labor: www.ajb.dni.us.

   This online listing links visitors to computerized network of 1,800 state employment offices and their active job listings. There are approximately 250,000 listed in America's Job Bank files. There is no cost to employers for posting their vacancies or to job seekers.

2. National Council on the Aging's MaturityWorks: www.maturityworks.org.

   MaturityWorks is devoted to employment and training issues affecting middle-aged and older workers. Website visitors can link to the National Council on the Aging's workforce resources, other workforce-related sites, and the Senior Community Service Employment Program sites.

3. Urban Institute: www.urban.org.

   The Urban Institute, a nonprofit policy research organization located in Washington, D.C., investigates the social and economic problems confronting the nation, including those facing older workers.

4. National Older Worker Career Center (NOWCC): www.nowcc.org.

   NOWCC is a nonprofit organization that expands employment and training opportunities for America's fast-growing population of workers aged 40 and over. This website also provides information on the Senior Environmental Employment Program (SEE), which offers nationwide opportunities for individuals aged 55 and over to apply skills and experience ranging from clerical to scientific and assists the U.S. Environmental Protection Agency in pollution prevention and control projects.

5. The SPRY (Setting Priorities for Retirement Years) Foundation: www.spry.org.

    SPRY is an independent, nonprofit 501(c)(3) research and education organization that helps people prepare for successful aging. SPRY emphasizes planning and prevention-oriented strategies in four key areas: Health & Wellness; Mental Health; Financial Security; and Life Engagement. The SPRY Foundation's report, entitled *Redefining Retirement: Research Directions for Successful Aging Among America's Diverse Seniors*, suggests that minority seniors do not share the traditional idea of age-related retirement and retirement planning. Visit the Foundation's website to read this and other SPRY reports.

9

Income Programs

Scott and Stacy are somewhat anxious as they wait for their appointment with a retirement planner. Like many couples in their mid-40s, they have not given serious thought to retirement. Most of their financial planning has centered on preparation for sending their two children to college. After hearing so much in the media lately about whether Social Security will be there for them when they retire, they are wondering whether they are making the best plans for their own future. Unanswered questions for them at this time include the following: Will Social Security be a retirement resource for them? Are they saving enough money and in the right way to supplement their Social Security? How do their work pensions fit into all this? What level of income will they need in retirement for quality of life? What sources of help could they turn to if something terrible and unforeseen happened to their income security?

The economic circumstances of older Americans have improved substantially during the past three decades, with average incomes and assets for persons over 65 rising dramatically. Median incomes for older adults have risen, whereas the share of older adults in poverty has dropped. As shown in Exhibit 9.1, the percentage of older adults living in poverty declined from 24.6% in 1970 to 9.8% in 2004 (Federal Interagency Forum on Aging-Related Statistics, 2006). The decrease in the percentage of older adults living in poverty coincides with the passage of public programs for income security (Moon & Ruggles, 1994). The percentage of older adults living in poverty, however, varies significantly by age, gender, race, and ethnicity. In 2002–2004, the poverty rate for persons age 65 to 74 was 9.4% compared with 9.7% for persons between the ages of 75 and 84, and 12.6% for persons 85 years of age and older. Almost 12.5% of older women live in poverty compared with 7.7% of older men. In contrast to the 8.3% of White older adults living in poverty, 23.8% of non-Hispanic Black older adults, 8.4% of non-Hispanic Asian older adults, and 21.4% of Hispanic older adults live in poverty (Federal Interagency Forum on Aging-Related Statistics, 2004, 2006).

In 2003, the median income for older married-couple households was $36,006 (He, Sengupta, Velkoff, & DeBarros, 2005), which is substantially higher than for older male and female householders living alone ($17,359 and $13,775, respectively). Here, too, there are variations in income between subgroups of elders. For example, in 2003 the median income of married persons aged 65 to 69 was $45,305 compared with $29,280 for married persons aged 75 and older (He et al., 2005). Older women living alone, regardless of age, had

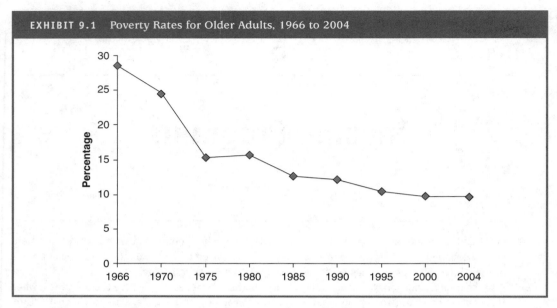

EXHIBIT 9.1 Poverty Rates for Older Adults, 1966 to 2004

Source: Federal Interagency Forum (2000); U.S. Bureau of the Census (2006a).

a lower median income than their male counterparts. On average, the median income of older non-Hispanic White men ($35,187) is nearly twice as much as older Hispanic men ($18,990), more than double that of older Black women ($14,371), and three times greater than older Native Hawaiian/Pacific Islander women ($9,693) and older Hispanic women ($11,157). Moreover, older men in all minority groups have higher median incomes than their female counterparts (U.S. Bureau of Census, 2006c).

Thus the differential income distributions between older women and older men and between older Whites and non-Whites result in a greater reliance on income support programs by older women and by older non-Whites. In this chapter, we provide the policy background for three primary income programs: Social Security, pensions, and Supplemental Security Income. We then describe the users of these programs and conclude with challenges facing income programs as the next century approaches.

POLICY BACKGROUND

Social Security

The Social Security Act of 1935 established the basic Old Age Benefits program and a federal–state system of unemployment insurance. In 1939, Congress added survivors' and dependents' benefits, and in 1956 it expanded Social Security to include disability insurance

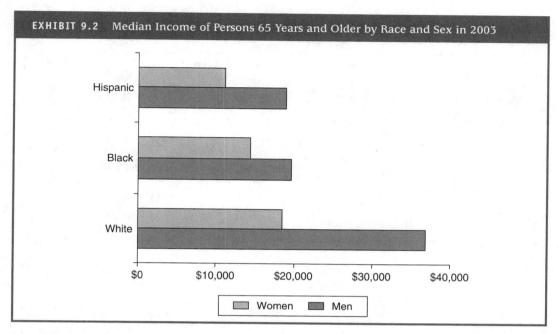

EXHIBIT 9.2 Median Income of Persons 65 Years and Older by Race and Sex in 2003

Source: U.S. Bureau of the Census (2006c).

to protect workers with severe disabilities. Although numerous adjustments have been made to the Social Security system since its inception, there have been few major programmatic changes (see Chapter 2 for details).

Exhibit 9.3 summarizes the various programs available under Social Security. To be eligible for retirement benefits under the Old Age, Survivor, and Disability Insurance (OASDI) program, a worker must have worked in covered employment for the required number of calendar quarters. Coverage is nearly universal for work done in the United States; it covers about 95% of all jobs. In 2006, about 197.1 million persons worked in employment or self-employment covered under the OASDI program. Older adults comprise 15% of current beneficiaries: 9.5 million aged 65–69, 7.1 million aged 70–74, and 13.9 million aged 75 + (Social Security Administration, 2006a).

The three basic categories of benefits under Social Security are (a) retirement benefits, (b) disability benefits, and (c) dependents' and survivors' benefits. Once a worker qualifies for retirement benefits, he or she (together with the survivors) first becomes eligible to claim early retirement benefits at age 62. To receive disability benefits, a worker must have a physical or mental impairment that prevents any substantial gainful work, and the disability must be expected to last, or to have lasted, 12 months or to be expected to result in death (Matthews, 1992). To be eligible for dependents' and survivors' benefits, the worker has to have had enough credits to qualify for his or her own retirement or disability benefits.

EXHIBIT 9.3 Benefits Provided Under Social Security in 2006

Type of Benefit	Who Qualifies	Average Amount of Benefits Paid to Recipient	Number of Beneficiaries
Survivor's benefits	Children under 18 A child who is under 19 but still in high school A child who is 18 or older but who becomes disabled before age 22 A widow(er) who is caring for children under age 16 or disabled A widow(er) age 60 or older, or a widow(er) age 50 or older, who is disabled	About $2,098 per month for a widow(er) and two children	Social security pays monthly survivor benefits to 6.9 million Americans.
Disability	Workers are considered disabled if they have a severe physical or mental condition that prevents them from working. The condition must be expected to last for at least 12 months or to result in death. Once benefits begin, they continue for as long as the worker is disabled.	The average monthly payment to a disabled worker is $947; for a disabled worker with a spouse and two children, the average pay is about $1,593. The disabled worker and eligible family members receive checks each month. A worker who receives disability payments for two years becomes eligible for Medicare.	More than 5 million disabled workers under 65 and 1.6 million dependents receive Social Security.

EXHIBIT 9.3   (Continued)

Type of Benefit	Who Qualifies	Average Amount of Benefits Paid to Recipient	Number of Beneficiaries
Retirement	Full retirement benefits are now payable at age 65, with reduced benefits available as early as age 62. The age for full benefits will gradually rise in the next century until it reaches age 67 in 2027 for people born in 1960 or later. Reduced benefits are still available at age 62.	Social Security pays monthly retirement benefits to more than 31 million retired workers and their families. Average: wage earner $1,011 High: wage earner $2,116	More than 9 out of 10 Americans who are age 65 or older get Social Security benefits.

Source: Social Security Administration (2006a).

Pension Benefits

The Civil Service Retirement Act was enacted in 1920, providing pension coverage for the first time to federal civilian employees (Schultz, 2001). A year later, the implementation of private, employer-sponsored pension plans was encouraged by the passage of the Revenue Act of 1921. This legislation exempted both the income of pension and profit-sharing trusts and the employer contributions to these plans from income taxation.

Through the years, serious problems (e.g., inadequate funds and misuse of funds) have undermined the worker protection provided under employer-sponsored programs. In response to abuse and mismanagement in the private pension system, Congress enacted the Employee Retirement Income Security Act (ERISA) of 1974. It was the first comprehensive effort to regulate private pensions. The major objectives of this Act are to (a) ensure that workers and beneficiaries receive adequate information about their employee benefit plans, (b) set standards of conduct for those managing employment benefit plans and plan funds, (c) determine that adequate funds are being set aside to pay promised pension benefits, (d) ensure that workers receive pension benefits after they have satisfied certain minimum requirements, and (e) safeguard pension benefits for workers whose employers end their pension plans (Coleman, 1989).

A major shift in the type of pension programs provided by employers began in the 1980s. In the mid- to late 1980s, plans established by single employers dominated the labor market. By 2005, many plans were insolvent or were absorbed by multi-employer plans (Pension Benefit Guaranty Corporation, 2006). Regardless of the origin of the plan, types available include defined benefit and defined contribution plans.

Defined benefit pension plans promise to pay a yearly pension benefit to workers who qualify on the basis of age and service. These plans provide retirees with a steady income stream that commences with retirement and continues until that person's, or in some cases the spouse's, death. In almost every defined benefit plan, the employer assumes the risk of making sure that adequate money is available to pay the promised benefit (Barocas, 1994). When an employer offers a defined benefit plan, participation is generally automatic, as it does not require the employee to make any contributions (Costo, 2006).

Defined contribution plans specify employer and employee contributions but do not guarantee future benefits. Funds accumulate in an account, and the returns to the accumulated funds determine the retirement benefits. The employee is responsible for investing the contributions. The most common and frequently employed defined contribution arrangements are 401(k) plans (Burman, 2004).

In 2005, 60% of private sector employees were covered by retirement benefits; 22% participated in a defined benefit plan; 42% were in a defined contribution plan; and 9% were enrolled in both (Costo, 2006). Fewer Blacks, Hispanics, and women participate in retirement benefits plans than do Whites and males at all ages (Herz, Meisenheimer, & Weinstein, 2000).

Supplemental Security Income

Administered by the Social Security Administration, the SSI program provides income support to persons aged 65 and older and to children and adults who are blind or have a disability. Established in 1972, SSI replaced the federally aided state programs that had prevailed for several decades. Distribution of the first SSI payments occurred in January 1974. The program has not experienced any significant changes since its original legislation.

SSI acts as an important safety net for older adults receiving few or no Social Security benefits. Under this program, each eligible person living in his or her own household, having limited or no other income and few assets, receives a monthly cash payment. Eligibility and federal payment standards are nationally uniform and strict. To receive SSI, a person must be aged 65 or older, blind, or have a disability, and must have assets (excluding a home, car, and personal belongings) of no more than $2,000 for an individual and $3,000 for a couple (Social Security Administration, 1996). In addition, the recipient's monthly income (e.g., Social Security, pensions, bank account interest, and stock dividends) must not exceed the guidelines established by each state. Many recipients receive only partial SSI benefits because benefit levels are reduced by one dollar for each dollar of countable income. In 2005, the maximum federal SSI benefit amounts to approximately 73% of the official poverty guideline for single older adults and 81% for older couples (Social Security Administration, 2006a).

For Your Files:	Financial Abuse, Undue Influence, Scams, Frauds, and Protection of Assets

According to the Clearinghouse on Abuse and Neglect of the Elderly (CANE), older individuals may be more susceptible to financial exploitation and fraud simply because many have assets in the forms of savings, stocks, insurance policies, and property. Seniors with dementia or mental health concerns may be particularly vulnerable to financial abuse by friends and family members or court-appointed guardians who exert undue influence. They may also be targeted for identity theft or become victimized by predatory lending practices. In 2003, CANE posted an annotated bibliography containing citations for references that address these and other aspects of elder financial exploitation. Included are a number of articles that address the need for protection of assets and other consumer issues. To review the bibliography, visit the CANE website at www.elderabusecenter.org/default.cfm? p = cane_finabuse.cfm.

USERS AND PROGRAMS

Social Security is an important source of income for many families and is the primary source of money income for older adults. As shown in Exhibit 9.4 (Social Security Administration, 2006a), retired workers (63%), survivors of deceased workers (13%), disabled workers (14%), and spouses and children of retired and disabled workers (10%) receive Social Security benefits under one of its programs. Nine of every 10 older adults receive income from Social Security. Moreover, for 20% of older adults, Social Security is their only source of income; 13% of older adults depend on Social Security for 90% or more of their income (He et al., 2005). Among older adults, White (92%) and Black (88%) elders are somewhat more likely than Hispanic elders (76%) to receive Social Security (U.S. Bureau of the Census, 2000b).

The monthly Social Security benefit amount a retired worker will receive depends on the worker's age and earning record. Nearly one-half of all new retired worker benefits are awarded at age 62, and more than two-thirds are awarded before age 65. According to the Social Security Administration (2006a), the average monthly benefit for retired workers in 2006 was $1,011. Older male retirees received an average monthly benefit of $1,189 compared with $829 received by older female retirees. At least 72% of couples and individuals aged 65 and older receive pension income, including both private and government

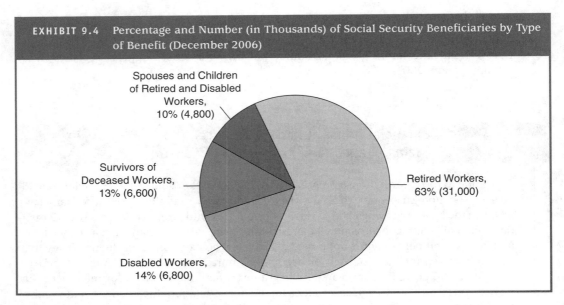

EXHIBIT 9.4   Percentage and Number (in Thousands) of Social Security Beneficiaries by Type of Benefit (December 2006)

Spouses and Children of Retired and Disabled Workers, 10% (4,800)

Survivors of Deceased Workers, 13% (6,600)

Retired Workers, 63% (31,000)

Disabled Workers, 14% (6,800)

Source: Social Security Administration (2006a).

employee pensions (Wu, 2006). The proportion of retirees receiving pension income is greater in the middle and higher income brackets than in the low to moderate income brackets.

Since the 1970s, approximately 50% of private industry has offered pension plans to its workforce. Yet only 52% of retirees are receiving benefits (He et al., 2005). In 2004, 11 million retirees—approximately 30% of the older population—had pension income. The median income from private pensions for men 65 years of age and older was $12,000 compared with $6,141 for women. Although older women's pension coverage has increased, it still remains below that of men: 22% of retired women compared with 43.5% of retired men receive a pension (Wu, 2006). A greater percentage of White older adults (45%), compared with Black (28%) or Hispanic (21%) older adults, received pensions (Social Security Administration, 2000a).

In 2002, approximately 113,000 beneficiaries aged 55–61, 305,000 aged 62–64, and 3.2 million aged 65 + received federal, state, local, or military pensions, and survivor and disability benefits (Social Security Administration, 2002). The median benefit paid to retirees aged 65 + by federal, state, and local pension plans was $13,680. In addition, approximately 1.8 million retirees and survivors received military retirement benefits (Schultz, 2001). The military retirement program, touted as the best pension in the United States, provides full benefits that begin immediately on retirement, requires no financial contribution from military personnel, pays at least 50% of basic pay to those with 20 years' service and 75% after 30 years of service, and does not subject benefits to an earnings test.

In 2005, approximately 2 million older adults received SSI benefits. The average monthly amount for an older beneficiary was $321; the maximum federal monthly SSI check was

$579 for one person and $869 for a couple (Social Security Administration, 2006a). Older women were more likely than older men to receive SSI benefits. Black (9%) and Hispanic (11%) older adults were more likely to receive SSI than were their White (2%) counterparts (Wu, 2006).

For Your Files: **Tax Counseling for the Elderly (TCE) Program**

The Tax Counseling for the Elderly (TCE) Program offers free tax help to individuals who are aged 60 or older. Trained volunteers from nonprofit organizations provide free tax counseling and basic income tax return preparation for senior citizens. Volunteers who provide tax counseling are often retired individuals associated with nonprofit organizations that receive grants from the IRS. As part of this IRS-sponsored TCE Program, AARP offers the Tax-Aide counseling program at nearly 8,000 sites nationwide during the filing season. Trained and certified AARP Tax-Aide volunteer counselors help people of low- to middle income with special attention to those aged 60 and older.

For more information on TCE call 1-800-829-1040 or see www.aarp.org/money/taxaide/volunteertaxaide/a2004-01-22-volunteerwithtaxaide.html.

CHALLENGES FOR INCOME PROGRAMS

There is growing consensus among business, government, and academic experts that most Americans do not realize how much it costs to retire (Armstrong, 2005; Eschtruth, 2006; Nijssen, 2004). Younger workers think they have plenty of time to prepare for their retirement years and often do not take advantage of company-sponsored retirement plans or savings initiatives. Midlife employees recognize the need to plan proactively for retirement but often view themselves as unable to save more. As a group, they appear conservative and do not understand much about such topics as budgeting, types of investments, risk, and the time value of money. Older employees tend to fall into one of two groups: those who have planned well and those who have not. Environmental, personal, and social circumstances prevent many older adults from having a financially secure retirement. We end this chapter by discussing some challenges facing income programs as the number and proportion of persons entering the retirement years grow.

Maintaining a Person's Standard of Living

Despite increased benefit levels, there is still a large gap for most workers between their Social Security benefits and the income needed to maintain living standards in retirement (Munnell, Webb, & Delorme, 2006; Schultz, 2001). Experts often promote a "three-legged stool" model for financial preparation for retirement. Personal savings, Social Security, and pension income represent the three components or "legs" of the retirement income stool (Barocas, 1994). As previously mentioned, Social Security benefits are a significant source of retirement income for many older adults; however, for millions of older adults, Social Security represents the only leg on their retirement stool. The challenge is to encourage broader pension coverage for low-wage workers and to encourage financial planning for retirement.

Financial planning for retirement is a difficult and complex task. Both individuals and companies must invest more in preretirement planning as a means of helping employees take greater responsibility for their retirement income. The challenge for both the public and private sector is to (a) increase the availability of preretirement education for all individuals; (b) improve the quality of available programs by ensuring that programs assist employees in evaluating their current financial state, defining their personal goals, and identifying a financial game plan to make certain that the resources are available to achieve their personal goals; and (c) encourage people to begin preparing for retirement at an early age (Barocas, 1994; Schultz, 2001).

Enhancing the Income of Older Women

Studies have shown that women make substantially less than men in the labor market. This discriminatory pattern influences women's pensions, Social Security benefits, annuities, and bank savings. In addition, women who divorce or separate from their husbands may lose any resources developed during a marriage (e.g., rights to an ex-husband's pension and other financial assets). These women also may have discontinuous work careers that decrease their ability to achieve pension vesting rights and lower the wages on which retirement income is calculated (U.S. Dept of Labor, 2006c). To improve the income adequacy for women, policy makers must address the inequities of Social Security, particularly for working women, as well as inequities in private pension systems.

Increasing Participation in Income Programs

The federal government estimates that about 37% of older adults eligible for SSI do not participate in the program (Social Security Administration, 2001/02). Two key reasons appear to be lack of knowledge about it and the stigma associated with being involved with a means-tested program (Schultz, 2001). In recent years, the Social Security Administration has undertaken activities to increase awareness and participation in the program (e.g., public service announcements) but with little success. Another factor that may contribute to incentives to seek SSI payments is the income and resource test. SSI limits the amount of assets, earned income, and unearned income the individual may have and still qualify for benefits. The asset limit ($2,000) has not been increased since 1984, and the disregards for earned and unearned income ($65 and $20 per month, respectively) have not been changed since the program began (Social Security Administration, 2005).

Ensuring the Long-Term Financing of Social Security

As people are living longer and receiving Social Security benefits for longer periods of time, the total benefits paid annually by Social Security are increasing. Some economists predict that the cost of benefits will exceed the amount of payroll taxes collected within the next decade. In the past, efforts to deal with Social Security's financial difficulties have generally featured cutting benefits and raising tax rates on a pay-as-you-go basis. The pay-as-you-go approach means that taxes collected by workers in a given year are spent to pay benefits in the same year. The Social Security Trust Fund, which holds the money, is more of a money-transfer system, not a savings program. Therefore, the collection of Social Security tax is sensitive to the ratio of the number of current workers and those receiving benefits (Brown, Hassett, & Smetters, 2005). In 1950, the ratio was 16:1; by 2001, it had dropped to 3.4:1. It is projected that there will be two workers for each beneficiary in 2040. Under current program policies and regulations, individual tax will need to be increased 45% to cover retirement benefits. Government officials and Congress agree that the current approach needs to change, but are unable to agree on a single plan for dealing with the predicted financial difficulties.

In May 2001, President George W. Bush established a bipartisan, 16-member commission to study and report specific recommendations to preserve Social Security for older adults. The commission recommended that, to remain solvent, the current Social Security program should introduce up to three proposed voluntary personal account models. In each model the worker has the opportunity to invest a small percentage of their taxable wages however they see fit (i.e., stocks, bonds, and mutual funds) rather than pay it directly into the Social Security fund. The higher rates of return that would be achieved by investing funds in the stock market (or other private investments) would produce future benefits greater than or equal to the existing level of scheduled benefits. While this approach may appear fiscally sound and benefit the individual, the need to reduce current long-tem expenditures and increase long-term funding streams remains. Hence, adoption of these recommendations remains elusive. Economists continue to work with the Social Security Administration, Congress, and the President to develop strategies that will benefit everyone. The commission's final report can be accessed online at www.csss.gov/reports/Final_report.pdf. For additional information on the challenges facing Social Security reform, go to the Center for Retirement Research at Boston College website at www.bc.edu/centers/crr.

Maintaining and Enhancing Income Programs in the Future

The delegates to the 2005 White House Conference on Aging passed four resolutions specifically related to retirement income:

- Establish principles to strengthen Social Security.
- Provide financial and other economic incentives and policy changes to encourage and facilitate increased retirement savings.
- Modernize the Supplemental Security Income (SSI) Program.
- Strengthen the Social Security Disability Insurance Program.

The delegates proposed numerous strategies for strengthening the Social Security Program, including

- maintaining the entire Social Security (SS) system without privatization, including survivor benefits, disability program, and current cost of living adjustment (COLA) formula;
- investing a portion of SS Trust Fund in equity and bond markets and dedicating the inheritance tax for estates to the SS Trust Fund; and
- retaining the progressive defined benefit structure by removing caps on earnings for SS contributions.

To encourage Americans to save for retirement, the delegates suggested strategies such as establishing financial education as a high school and college graduation requirement and providing incentives for annuities or appropriate installment savings programs to support lifetime income. The strategies proposed for modernizing SSI and strengthening SSDI focused primarily on simplifying the application process and improving benefits.

In closing, obtaining financial security in later life will require that employment opportunities exist for older workers who wish to remain or re-enter the workforce, that public and private pensions expand the number of workers covered, and that Social Security benefits continue to act as the third leg of the financial retirement stool. Perhaps the increase in the number of older adults who will be faced with retirement decisions in the next decade will facilitate a change in policy about work, retirement, and income security in retirement.

CASE STUDY

When the System Fails

Sonny, who is 66 years old, and his wife, Magdalena, who just had her 63rd birthday, never expected to find themselves in such a financially precarious position and so frustrated with their own government at this point in their lives. When they were married 45 years ago, they had made so many plans. They were proud that their hard work had realized a modest retirement savings and that their three children were responsible, hardworking young adults. Sonny was especially proud of his service to his country during World War II.

Sonny retired at age 65 with a Social Security benefit of $1,000 per month and a union retirement benefit of $400 per month. Magdalena had never worked outside the home. She had no credits toward Social Security, and at age 63 was not eligible to draw an early Social Security retirement benefit on Sonny's credits of work or apply for Medicare. Nevertheless, their income had been adequate because their home and vehicles were paid for and they had no other outstanding debts.

Their retirement dreams began to fade as Magdalena's health deteriorated. Side-effects from diabetes, diagnosed when Magdalena was 15 years old, have caused kidney failure. Magdalena is now receiving dialysis twice a month and spends part of her time in a wheelchair. She is also considered legally blind. The predicament for Sonny and Magdalena now is that the health plan that covered Magdalena's medical expenses expired because it had limited time coverage from Sonny's former employer, that Magdalena is not eligible for SSI because their income of $1,400 per month is too much to qualify, and that she cannot qualify for private insurance because of her pre-existing condition. Although a Social Security regulation permits persons with dialysis to qualify for benefits including Medicare before age 65, Magdalena has twice been denied this benefit on the grounds that she is not disabled. Their savings have been completely depleted to pay for Magdalena's dialysis and other medical expenses. To their anger, shame, and frustration, Magdalena is receiving a six-month limited health benefit from their state's medically indigent uninsurable program. At the end of the six months, they will still have another year of uncovered medical expenses before Magdalena can qualify for Social Security unless they can find some help to turn this situation around.

One day at the dialysis center, Magdalena was talking with the receptionist about not understanding why Social Security would refuse her application for early disability under the special dialysis rule. Why would Social Security not consider Magdalena disabled?

Case Study Questions

1. Are Sonny and Magdalena justified in their frustration? Do they have the right to expect a source of income maintenance and health insurance coverage, given their situation?

2. Name as many help source agencies or programs that you can think of that Sonny and Magdalena might have contacted regarding this situation.

3. It is obvious that money is tight for this couple at this time. One human services professional might see the best course of help as being to put Sonny and Magdalena in touch with a variety of charity programs that could help them with food, clothing, utilities, and free medical service. Another professional might see the best course as being to appeal their case to Social Security. Which professional would you be and why?

4. In what type of community human service environment does a dialysis center receptionist care and know where to refer a patient for help in a matter such as Magdalena's?

5. Often, in working with older adults, professionals speak of clients who "fall through the cracks." What do you think this expression means? Do you think Sonny and Magdalena fit this description? Why or why not?

6. What could have been a worst-case scenario for this couple? How typical do you think their situation is? What does it show about the importance of income-maintenance programs for many older adults?

Learning Activities

1. Put together a monthly budget that includes expenses such as rent or mortgage, food, utilities, medical expenses, entertainment, insurance, and other items that you believe are necessary for a comfortable and satisfying lifestyle. What would you need currently to support yourself? Project your income needs to maintain that lifestyle at age 70. What

changes may occur in your income needs? What is your plan to ensure that your income is sufficient?

2. Interview someone from your local Social Security office. With what issues does the office primarily deal in relation to income and benefits? Whom do the office staff see more—women or men? What is the clients' typical level of income? Do many of the recipients have alternative income sources? Does the office offer information on income planning for retirement? What counseling and information services does the office provide, and for what are beneficiaries most likely to ask?

3. Investigate retirement-income plans. How accessible is the information (both to obtain and to understand)? What places carry the information, and to whom is it targeted? Are there specific brochures for women, men, minorities, and income levels, and in languages other than English?

4. Talk to two older family members to find out what plans they have made for their income needs in their old age. Do they feel that their income is adequate? If you could, what suggestions would you make to them about how they can plan for their income for retirement?

For More Information

National Resources

1. Social Security Administration, 6401 Security Blvd., Baltimore, MD 21235; phone: 800-772-1213; www.ssa.gov.

    The Social Security Administration is responsible for the administration of the Social Security and the SSI programs. Free publications are available.

2. Pension Rights Center, 1350 Connecticut Avenue, N.W., Suite 206, Washington, DC 20036-1739; phone: 202-296-3776; www.pensionrights.org.

    The Pension Rights Center works to protect the pension rights of workers, retirees, and their families. The center publishes handbooks and packets on pension law and retirement systems.

Web Resources

1. Social Security Online: www.ssa.gov.

    The Social Security website is one of the most comprehensive sites in the aging network. Visitors can request a copy of their earning record, browse information about the history and legislation on Social Security, access publications online, and review statistical information about benefits and beneficiaries.

2. Canada Pension Plan: www.hrdc-drhc.gc.ca/isp/common/cpptoc_e.shtml.

    Check out Canada's retirement pension program and compare it with the U.S. Social Security program.

3. Benefits Link: www.benefitslink.com/index.html.

    Benefits Link is a free nationwide link to information and services for employers sponsoring employee benefit plans, companies providing products and services for plans, and participating employees. There are links to new benefits information, public discussions of benefits design, internet resources, and online benefits newsletters.

4. U.S. Department of Labor: www.dol.gov.

   The U.S. Department of Labor's site has a number of resources, including a link that provides pension information.

5. Social Security Administration (SSA) for Women: www.ssa.gov/pressoffice/forwomen.htm.

   The Social Security Administration has launched this website to provide basic Social Security information on retirement, survivors, disability, and SSI benefits that pertain to women.

6. BenefitsCheckUp: www.benefitscheckup.org.

   The National Council on the Aging created BenefitsCheckUp to help older adults quickly identify federal and state assistance programs that may improve the quality of their lives. Family and friends can also obtain facts about benefits for which their loved ones may qualify.

7. The National Council of La Raza (NCLR): www.nclr.org.

   NCLR is a private, nonprofit, nonpartisan organization established to reduce poverty and discrimination and to improve life opportunities for Hispanic Americans. On the website is a policy report entitled, "Social Security Reform: Issues for Hispanic Americans."

8. President's Commission to Strengthen Social Security (CSSS): http://csss.gov.

   CSSS was created to evaluate and recommend ways to keep the Social Security program fiscally sound. The website will provide information about the commission's meetings, minutes from the meetings, and the final report issued by the commission. People can use the website to contact the commission with any comments or ideas.

10

Nutrition and Meal Programs

The door opens, and Alice beams with pride as she ushers you into her apartment. She prepares lunch, but you notice that there's nothing in the fridge. It's empty. That's the first sign. She offers you coffee, and you get Nescafé. That's the second sign. You know that she's giving you the last food she has until she visits a food pantry later in the week, a wonderful, welcoming agency that receives its food from The Greater Boston Food Bank. You have no choice but to eat Alice's food. Refusing to do so would hurt her more than the hunger that hurts her most every day. Alice relies on emergency food assistance to survive. She lives on her small Social Security income to pay her rent and utility bills and to buy clothes and food. "I have lived through the depression, and know how to stretch a dollar," she explains. "But it's just not enough."[1]

The consumption of food is not only a biological necessity for health and vitality but also a social activity that is rich with symbolism. It is often an integral part of holiday gatherings and celebrations of all types. Although most of us are aware of the social nature of food consumption, we are only vaguely aware of the necessity of good nutritional habits. Good nutritional habits are important in all stages of life, but in later life, as individuals grow older, age-related changes in various body systems as well as in social relationships can place them at risk of inadequate nutritional intake. In this chapter, we review the extent of malnutrition and hunger among older adults, the physical and psychosocial factors that influence nutritional status in later life, the policies that support nutrition programs of older adults, the types of nutrition programs available, and the characteristics of those who use such programs.

FOOD INSECURITY AND HUNGER AMONG OLDER ADULTS

Evidence supports the notion that many older adults are at risk of poor nutritional intake, malnourishment, food insecurity, or hunger (see Exhibit 10.1 for a definition of these terms). A study conducted by the U.S. Bureau of the Census found that approximately 1.4 million (55%) of adults aged 65 and older experienced food insecurity and 1.5% of elderly households experienced hunger (Nord, Andrews, & Carlson, 2002). The Urban Institute (1993) conducted a national study that examined food deprivation among older adults. Researchers asked respondents whether (a) they got enough food and enough of what they wanted to eat,

(b) food was always available and whether they had the resources to purchase food, (c) they skipped meals because they had no food, (d) they resorted to alternative action such as borrowing money to buy food, and (e) they had to choose between purchasing food and other necessities. The latter four questions were used to measure food insecurity. Researchers found that, overall, almost 400,000 older adults reported that they sometimes or often did not have enough food to eat in the month prior to the survey. Older adults with low incomes were twice as likely as those with high incomes to indicate that they did not get what they wanted to eat. With regard to food insecurity, 1.5 million older adults reported that they had experienced at least one of four indicators of food deprivation in the six months prior to the survey. Slightly less than half a million had skipped meals in the past month because of lack of food or food resources. In addition, more than 600,000 had had days in the six months prior to the survey on which they had had no food or resources to purchase food. Older adults who reported that they had had days with no food or food resources were asked what strategies they used to stretch their food supplies. Most reported that they bought or served less-expensive meals (44%), served smaller meals (37%), borrowed money (30%), took money from savings (30%), or got food from a food bank or food pantry (20%). Many respondents had to make a decision between eating and paying for other necessities. Almost 800,000 had had to make the choice between buying medicine and buying food in the six months prior to the survey. In a more recent attempt to measure the extent of food insecurity, America's Second Harvest conducted a study of 31,342 agencies operating food programs and 52,878 clients of emergency food programs. Results indicated that 17% of the clients served by America's Second Harvest food program sites have elderly adults as members of the household. Thirty-six percent of households with older adults reported being food insecure without hunger; 16.2% reporting being food insecure with hunger. In addition, many of the clients who received food from food banks relied on other food programs, such as senior nutrition sites (18.3%), home-delivered meals (5.7%), and senior brown bag programs (11.7%) (America's Second Harvest, 2001). Finally, research collected by mayors across the country reported that requests for emergency food assistance by older adults in major U.S. cities increased by an average of 19% during 2002 (U.S. Conference of Mayors, 2002).

Older adults who do not have adequate nutritional intake are at risk of negative physical outcomes. Researchers have found a link between food insecurity and increased risk of additional health problems, reduced muscle mass, a compromised immune system, and mortality (Arora & Rochester, 1982; Chandra, 1992; Choi, 1999; Wolfe, Olson, Kendall, & Frongillo, 1998). Furthermore, inappropriate diets may induce diseases such as coronary heart disease and a reduction in general wellbeing (Hamburg, Elliot, & Parron, 1982; Kannel, 1986).

PHYSICAL AND PSYCHOSOCIAL FACTORS
THAT INFLUENCE NUTRITIONAL STATUS

A number of physical and psychosocial factors are thought to influence nutritional status (see Exhibit 10.2). For example, changes that older adults experience in taste, smell, and vision may inhibit their ability to enjoy food (Saxton & Etten, 1994). In addition, changes in the digestive system and the ability to chew may impair the digestion of food and make eating less enjoyable. Chronic conditions such as arthritis, orthopedic impairments,

---

EXHIBIT 10.1   Definitions of Nutritional Status

- *Food insecurity* occurs whenever the availability of nutritionally adequate and safe food or the ability to acquire foods in socially acceptable ways is limited or uncertain.
- *Hunger* is the uneasy or painful sensation caused by a recurrent or involuntary lack of food and is a potential, although not a necessary, consequence of food insecurity. Over time, hunger may result in malnutrition.
- *Food insufficiency* means an inadequate amount of food intake due to lack of resources.

Source: Anderson (1990).

EXHIBIT 10.2   Factors Affecting Nutritional Status in Older Adults

Physical
Cognitive status
Chronic and acute illness
Oral/dental health status
Chronic medication use
Dependence and disability

Psychosocial
Social support and isolation
Economic status
Ethnic status
Accessibility and availability of food programs
Advanced age

Source: Adapted from Goodwin (1989); White, Ham, & Lipschitz. (1991).

---

cataracts, and hypertension have been found to be negatively associated with poor nutritional intake (Dwyer, 1991). For example, impairments that affect mobility, such as arthritis, can make shopping, preparing, and eating difficult. Individuals with cognitive impairments are at obvious risk of poor nutrition. Loss of memory, disorientation, and impaired judgment can reduce food intake (White, Ham, & Lipschitz, 1991). Because the use of medications—either over-the-counter or prescribed—is high among older adults, they are at risk of experiencing adverse drug-nutrient interactions. White et al. (1991) suggest that many drugs have adverse effects on appetite and cause the depletion of certain minerals.

Not only do physical changes make the task of eating more difficult, but changes in the social environment can have a detrimental effect on dietary patterns. Throughout our lives, eating is an activity that we rarely do in isolation. It is a social activity associated with various rituals in our culture. Think about the food rituals in your family. Do you have a special place you like to go to eat when celebrating a birthday? Do you look forward to eating or cooking certain meals during the holidays? Are there special restaurants you enjoy? Chances are that these rituals are enjoyed with friends and family. And on those occasions when you are alone, you are probably less likely to cook and more likely to eat something of questionable nutritional value from a fast-food restaurant. Because eating is such a social activity, social isolation can result in negative changes in eating patterns. Indeed, researchers have found that living alone is associated with a lack of interest in preparing and consuming food and a less favorable dietary pattern (Davis, Randall, Forthofer, Lee, & Margen, 1985; Ryan & Bower, 1989; U.S. Census Bureau, 2004). For example, in a national study of 4,402 adults aged 55 or older, Davis, Murphy, Neuhaus, and Lein (1990) found significant variations in living arrangement and dietary quality. Men living alone had poor-quality diets compared with men who were living with a spouse, and the percentage of men living alone with poor-quality diets increased with age. Among women aged 55 to 64, 22% of those living alone had poor-quality diets, compared with 14% of those living with a spouse. There was no significant difference in dietary quality and living arrangements for women aged 65 to 74 and 75 or more years. Overall, a higher percentage of women, regardless of their living arrangement or age, had poor-quality diets compared with men.

Included among those living alone are widowed older adults. Older adults who are widowed may be at risk of poor nutritional habits because of changes in income and social interaction patterns. Moreover, being responsible for new roles associated with meal preparation (e.g., shopping or cooking) for which they were not previously responsible can have negative dietary consequences. Although some evidence supports the relationship between living arrangement and dietary intake, other studies have found no relationship (Green et al., 1993; Schafer & Keith, 1982). Such variations may suggest that simply measuring whether one lives alone does not adequately capture other factors that may be influencing nutritional intake, such as loneliness and number of social contacts. For example, Walker and Beauchene (1991) found a moderate relationship between loneliness and poor nutrient intake. Moreover, it may be appropriate to consider the length of time respondents have lived alone, which may reflect the degree of adjustment to altered eating patterns.

Income has an obvious effect on the quality and amount of nutritional intake. Posner (1979) points out that older adults with low incomes have less money to spend on food, thus reducing chances of an adequate diet. The U.S. General Accounting Office reported in 1992 that poor elderly persons compared to nonpoor elders consumed less of some essential nutrients and that as many as half of poor elders consumed less than two-thirds the recommended daily allowance of vitamin C, calcium, and other nutrients. More recently, the USDA reported that the rate of food insecurity among elderly households with incomes below the poverty level was 22.6%, which was more than 12 times that of elderly households with incomes above 185% of the poverty rate (Nord, 2002). Seven percent of elderly households with incomes below the poverty rate reported hunger from food insecurity. In addition, those living in poverty may not have accessibility to health care services needed to diagnose and treat diseases linked to poor nutritional status. Rural older adults are also at risk of inadequate nutritional intake (Sharkey & Haines, 2002). This may partly be because rural older adults have more risk factors associated with increased food insecurity. Rural elders are more likely than their urban counterparts to have incomes below the poverty level, to have more health problems, to have fewer social and health services, and to be socially isolated (Quandt & Rao, 1999; Rogers, 1991; Schwenk, 1992). Rural elders who are older, male, and Black and have low incomes are more likely to have inadequate nutritional intake (Fischer, Crockett, Heller, & Skauge, 1991; Ralston & Cohen, 1994).

Older minority and ethnic adults are also at risk of experiencing nutritional problems. A national study found that Black and Hispanic elders had higher levels of food insecurity than did White elders (18.9% and 15.4% vs. 3.7%, respectively; Nord, 2002). Although tremendous variations exist among and between ethnic groups in their history and cultural characteristics, they share some sociodemographic characteristics that make them susceptible to poor nutritional intake. In general, Black, Hispanic, and Native American older adults are more likely than their White counterparts to have incomes below the poverty line, are likely to have lower levels of education and poorer health status, and to need assistance with everyday activities than do older Whites (U.S. Bureau of the Census, 1996a). These increased levels of functional impairment, low income, and education put older adults of color at an increased risk of malnutrition and unbalanced diets (Saxton & Etten, 1994). Moreover, language difficulties that exist among some older adults such as first-generation Asian Americans and Hispanics can act to isolate them from nutrition education and programs. Finally, Dwyer (1994) notes that nutrition education and programs that are insensitive to the cultural variations in diet may act as an obstacle to participation by older adults of various racial and ethnic backgrounds.

In response to the nutritional needs of older adults, a network of nutrition services and programs has been created. We describe these efforts in the following section.

POLICY BACKGROUND

Congress initiated nutrition programs for older adults with the passage of research and demonstration projects in 1968 under Title IV of the Older Americans Act (OAA). Four years later, Congress authorized the Nutrition Program for Older Americans as Title VII; however, the program was not implemented until 1973 (U.S. Senate Special Committee on Aging, 1993). Congress reorganized the nutrition program in 1978 by placing it under Title III in the OAA.

The purpose of the nutrition program for older adults under the OAA is to provide nutritionally balanced meals and nutrition education, opportunities for social interaction, and other support services (U.S. Senate Special Committee on Aging, 1993). Specific goals for the program identified in the 2006 amendments of the OAA are

- to reduce hunger and food insecurity;
- to promote socialization of older individuals; and
- to promote the health and wellbeing of older individuals by assisting such individuals to gain access to nutrition and other disease prevention and health promotion services to delay the onset of adverse health conditions resulting from poor nutritional health or sedentary behavior.

Under current OAA legislation, congregate meal programs are required to provide at least one hot meal five or more days a week in a congregate setting, adult day program, or multigenerational site (except in rural areas and where it is deemed unfeasible); such programs may include nutrition education services. The act also authorizes home-delivered meal programs that deliver at least one hot, cold, frozen, dried, or supplement meal at least five days a week (except in rural areas and where it is not feasible). Each meal must provide a minimum of one-third of the recommended daily allowances and be prepared with the advice of dietitians. The 2006 amendments also provides for nutrition screening, nutrition education, nutrition assessment, and counseling. Finally, the OAA legislation authorizes an evaluation of the effect of the nutrition projects on improvement of the health status, including nutritional status, of participants; prevention of hunger and food insecurity of the participants; and continuation of the ability of the participants to live independently. Research will also examine the cost-benefit analysis of nutrition projects, including the potential to affect costs of the Medicaid program, and an analysis of how nutrition projects may be modified to improve the nutritional outcomes of the participants.

Funding for nutrition services has increased slightly and then declined over the past 10 years. In fiscal year 1998, total funding for the Title III congregate and home-delivered meal programs was $486.4 million, and by 2001 it rose to $530.4 million, which represented 53% of the Title III budget (Administration on Aging [AoA], 2001e). In 2005, the total budget was $570,100 ($387,274 for congregate meal programs and $182,826 for home-delivered meal programs), but by 2006 the budget declined to $567,223, ($385,319 for congregate meal programs and $181,904 for home-delivered meals) (AoA, 2006c). The congregate meal and home-delivered meals programs use funds from other sources to supplement the costs of providing meals, as only 43% of the cost of a congregate meal and 26% of the cost of home-delivered meals comes from Title III funds. The remainder comes from participant contributions, state, local, and private funds, and the Nutrition Services Incentive Program which provides cash or commodities to support the meal program (Ponza, Ohls, & Millen, 1996). The Nutrition Services Incentive Program, formally administered by the U.S. Department of Agriculture until it was transferred to the OAA in 2000, provides nutrition programs with high-protein foods, meat, and meat alternative commodities. Programs can opt to receive a cash payment in place of donated food (AoA, 2003a). Funding for the Nutrition Services Incentive Program in 2006 was $147,846 (AoA, 2006c). Funding for nutrition services is also provided under Title VI, which is a grant program for tribal organizations to help them deliver social and nutrition services to older American Indians, Alaskan Natives, and Native Hawaiians. In 1994, Title VI grantees received nearly $17 million in Title VI funds for nutrition and supportive services and served 1.3 million meals to 41,000 congregate participants and 1.5 million meals to 47,500 home-delivered participants (AoA, 2004b).

Food Stamp Program

The first U.S. food assistance programs were developed in the 1930s during the Depression, when the government purchased surplus agricultural commodities and distributed them to the poor (Kuhn et al., 1996). In 1964, Congress established the Food Stamp Program using coupons, and in 1971 it enacted national eligibility standards, although the states still had a choice of food assistance programs. By 1974, however, the Food Stamp Program became a nationwide mandatory program (Lipsky & Thibodeau, 1990). The goal of the Food Stamp Program is to alleviate malnutrition among low-income families and individuals of all ages by providing food coupons or a debit card that participants can use to buy a nutritionally adequate diet (Kuhn et al., 1996; Sing, Cody, Sinclair, Cohen, & Ohls, 2005). To be eligible for food stamps, participants must meet income and asset guidelines. Older adults who receive SSI automatically meet the eligibility requirements for food stamps; however,

SSI recipients in California are not eligible for food stamps because the state includes extra money in the amount it adds to the federal SSI payment instead of issuing food stamps (Social Security Administration, 2001). Although the average amount of food stamp benefit is $70 per month, 40% of recipients receive $50 or less each month in food stamps (Barrett, 2006). In 2005, the Food Stamp Program served approximately 1.9 million older adults aged 60 and over, representing 17% of all food stamp participants, up from 15% in 1992 (Barrett, 2006; U.S. Department of Agriculture, 2001a). The participation rate for food stamp–eligible elderly adults is significantly lower than for any other age group. In 1999, 5.3 million elderly individuals were estimated to be eligible for food stamps; however, only 32% of these individuals participated in the food stamp program, leaving 3.6 million eligible elders without benefits (Castner, 2000). Reasons for non-participation include perceived lack of need, lack of information about the program, low expected benefits, and stigma associated with applying for assistance (McConnell & Ponza, 1999; Sing et al., 2005).

Nutrition Screening Initiative

In response to the Surgeon General's report *Healthy People 2000* (U.S. Department of Health and Human Services, 1990), which called for increased nutrition screening of older adults, the Nutrition Screening Initiative was conceived (Wellman, 1994). The goal of the Nutrition Screening Initiative is to promote routine nutritional screening and better nutrition care, especially among older adults.

The cornerstone of the Nutrition Screening Initiative project was the creation of a nutrition screening tool to be used by various professionals working with older adults. The screening tool, called DETERMINE, is designed to identify older adults who are at risk of poor nutritional health (see Exhibit 10.3). The screening tool asks simple questions about eating habits, illness and medication use, financial hardship, health status, and social contact. The checklist is the initial step in preventing, identifying, and correcting poor nutritional status of older adults. More than a million checklists have been distributed to laypersons and health care professionals nationwide in the hope that more older adults will be screened for nutritional deficiencies (Wellman, 1994). Nutrition programs are encouraged to use the DETERMINE screening tool as a means of providing nutrition screening to identify participants at high nutritional risk (AoA, 2001b).

In the next section, we discuss the various nutrition programs that have emerged from both the public and private sectors and provide a profile of nutrition program participants. We end this chapter with a discussion of the challenges facing nutrition programs.

USERS AND PROGRAMS

Nutrition programs for older adults, much like the continuum-of-care model discussed in Chapter 1, exist on a continuum based on functional status and socioeconomic need. Balsam and Osteraas (1987) developed the continuum of community nutrition services. As shown in Exhibit 10.4, older adult nutrition programs exist within a continuum of community nutrition programs and serve both independent and frail older adults. We explain the different nutrition programs that serve older adults in more detail below.

EXHIBIT 10.3 DETERMINE Nutritional Screening Tool

The Warning Signs of poor nutritional health are often overlooked. Use this checklist to find out if you or someone you know is at nutritional risk.

Read the statements below. Circle the number in the yes column for those that apply to you or someone you know. For each yes answer, score the number in the box. Total your nutritional score.

DETERMINE YOUR NUTRITIONAL HEALTH

	YES
I have an illness or condition that made me change the kind and/or amount of food I eat	2
I eat fewer than 2 meals per day.	3
I eat few fruits or vegetables, or milk products.	2
I have 3 or more drinks of beer, liquor or wine almost every day.	2
I have tooth or mouth problems that make it hard for me to eat.	2
I don't always have enough money to buy the food I need.	4
I eat alone most of the time.	1
I take 3 or more different prescribed or over-the-counter drugs a day.	1
Without wanting to, I have lost or gained 10 pounds in the last 6 months.	2
I am not always physically able to shop, cook and/or feed myself.	2
TOTAL	

Total Your Nutritional Score. If it's —

0-2   **Good!** Recheck your nutritional score in 6 months.

3-5   **You are at moderate nutritional risk.** See what can be done to improve your eating habits and lifestyle. Your office on aging, senior nutrition program, senior citizens center or health department can help. Recheck your nutritional score in 3 months.

6 or more   **You are at high nutritional risk.** Bring this checklist the next time you see your doctor, dietitian or other qualified health or social service professional. Talk with them about any problems you may have. Ask for help to improve your nutritional health.

These materials developed and distributed by the Nutrition Screening Initiative, a project of:

 AMERICAN ACADEMY OF FAMILY PHYSICIANS

 THE AMERICAN DIETETIC ASSOCIATION

 NATIONAL COUNCIL ON THE AGING, INC.

Remember that warning signs suggest risk, but do not represent diagnosis of any condition. Turn the page to learn more about the Warning Signs of poor nutritional health.

Source: Reprinted with permission of the Nutrition Screening Initiative, a project of the American Academy of Family Physicians, the American Dietetic Association, and the National Council on the Aging, Inc., and funded in part by a grant from Ross Products Division, Abbott Laboratories.

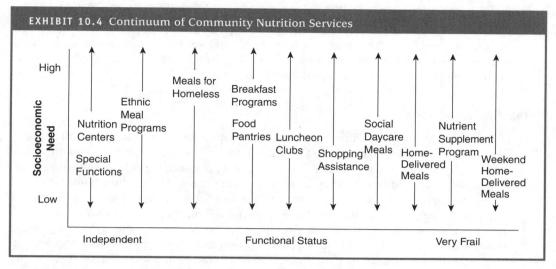

EXHIBIT 10.4 Continuum of Community Nutrition Services

Source: Adapted from Balsam and Osteraas (1987). Used with permission.

Congregate Meal Sites

As previously mentioned, the OAA nutrition program under Title III-C provides funds to support congregate meal programs. The program, funded by OAA dollars, reaches millions of older adults. In 2004, congregate meal sites funded under the OAA provided almost 106 million meals to 1.77 million older persons (AoA, n.d.). The goals of congregate meal programs are to (a) provide low-cost meals to older adults, (b) encourage wellbeing through social interaction and maintenance of good health, and (c) provide nutrition education, screening, counseling, and outreach (AoA, 1995c; Mullins, Cook, Mushel, Machin, & Georgas, 1993). Nutrition programs funded under the OAA are to target their services to isolated, low-income, and minority older persons. Individuals 60 years of age and older and their spouses can eat a nutritionally balanced hot meal for a suggested donation. Suggested donations range from $1 to $2; 94% of congregate meal participants and 73% of home-delivered meal participants make a contribution for their meal (Ponza, Ohls, & Millen, 1996). Congregate meal sites are located in a variety of places, including senior centers, schools, churches, and restaurants. Meals may be prepared on site or prepared at a central kitchen and delivered to sites. All congregate meal programs serve lunch. Approximately 13% have a supper option during the week, and 11% serve weekend congregate meals. Almost 75% of the programs offer modified meals (e.g., low-fat, low-cholesterol, or low-salt) to accommodate special diets.

Congregate meal programs also offer nutrition education programs, screening, and information about other community programs. Approximately 85% of congregate meal programs offer information and referral services to participants (Ponza et al., 1996). Providing participants with information and referral services makes congregate meal programs an important link in coordinating and delivering non-nutrition programs to older adults. Other congregate meal programs sponsored by nonprofit organizations such as the Salvation Army provide meals to low-income individuals and families of all ages. Unfortunately, the number of older adults who receive meals through these community congregate meal sites has not been documented.

Home-Delivered Meals

Home-delivered meals in most communities are provided by private nonprofit agencies and/or programs funded under the OAA. More than one home-delivered meal program may exist in any community and serve different target populations; Meals on Wheels is perhaps the most recognized home-delivered meal program in the country. Eligibility to receive home-delivered meals varies by program. In general, however, individuals must have difficulty attending a congregate meal site or preparing meals. Programs receiving Title III dollars must serve individuals 60 years of age or older. Most programs have a suggested donation amount or a sliding fee scale based on income. Programs deliver one or more hot, chilled, or frozen meals directly to the recipient's home each day during the week. Many programs offer frozen meals for recipients to use during the weekend.

More recently, nutrition programs have begun offering medical nutrition therapy for older adults who are nutritionally at risk or malnourished. According to the National Policy and Resource Center on Nutrition and Aging (1996), the medical nutrition therapy process is designed to help older adults who are at risk of malnutrition to obtain appropriate nutrition. On the basis of an assessment of the nutritional status of an at-risk older adult by a dietitian, a nutritional care plan is developed. The plan might recommend a change in daily diet or the incorporation of high-nutrient food into the diet. In addition, the food itself may need to be altered—for example, chopped or pureed to help those who have difficulty chewing or swallowing. Nutritional supplements or liquid meals might also be needed to meet an individual's nutritional needs. Because of the increased cost of providing medical nutrition therapy, the funding for such programs comes from client fees, contributions, and private payers.

In addition to the nutritional value that home-delivered meal programs offer their participants, volunteers play an important role in meeting clients' social needs. Volunteers who deliver the meals are often the only source of social contact for meal recipients, and in some cases they help clients with grocery shopping or other errands. Because of the increase in the number of frail older persons, many home-delivered meals have waiting lists. Forty-one percent of home-delivered meal programs have waiting lists of persons needing home-delivered meals and the mean length of time on a waiting list is between two and three months (Ponza et al., 1996). The total number of home-delivered meals has increased dramatically over the past 20 years. From 1980 to 1996, it increased by 227%, due in part to an increase in funding for home-delivered meals over the years (U.S. Senate Special Committee on Aging, 2000). In 1998, home-delivered meals funded under Title III-C of the OAA provided some 129.7 million meals to 896,153 older adults; in 2004, the number of home-delivered meals totaled 143 million to 968,062 older adults (AoA, n.d.; AoA, 2001c). One program, the San Francisco Meals on Wheels Program, delivers more than 1,500 meals to the homebound each day and has a waiting list of 275 individuals because of a shortage of volunteer drivers.

Best Practice: Two Coasts, Two Meals on Wheels Programs

San Francisco

In 1970, a group of civic-minded individuals living in San Francisco noticed a need among their elderly community. The people in need required nutritious meals delivered to their homes and friendly assistance with small tasks that they were unable to take care of themselves. To fill the need, this small group of dedicated volunteers started Meals on Wheels of San Francisco. They fixed the meals in their own neighborhood kitchens and then delivered them to their homebound neighbors. As the need for this service grew beyond anyone's expectations, Meals on Wheels volunteers, in their own cars, were supplemented with professional drivers and refrigerated delivery vehicles. Eventually, full-time social workers, nutritionists, and administrative staff were hired. In 1995, Meals on Wheels of San Francisco opened its own state-of-the-art kitchen.

In 1988, Meals on Wheels served 500 seniors per day. Today, more than 1,750 participants receive meals every day, either in their homes or at the organization's congregate nutrition site. In 2005, the program delivered 639,942 meals to homebound San Franciscan older adults. Meals on Wheels—San Francisco has 53 full-time staff, the majority of whom participate in delivering services. There is also a large volunteer force that provides additional services such as shopping, reading, and helping with pet care. For more information, contact Meals on Wheels of San Francisco, Inc., 1375 Fairfax Avenue, San Francisco, CA 94124, phone: 415-920-1111, www.mowsf.org.

New York City

In 1981, Gael Greene and James Beard founded Citymeals-on-Wheels by raising private funds to supplement the government-funded weekday meal delivery program. Citymeals now funds 102 community-based agencies that bring weekend, holiday, and/or emergency meals to homebound elderly New Yorkers who can no longer shop or cook for themselves. The program served 6,000 older adults in its first year. In 2006, Citymeals funded the preparation and delivery of more than 2.5 million weekday, weekend, holiday, or emergency meals to more than 17,500 homebound elderly New Yorkers.

For more information contact Citymeals-on-Wheels, 355 Lexington Avenue, New York, NY 10017, phone: 212-687-1234; www.citymeals.org; e-mail info@citymeals.org.

Sources: Meals on Wheels of San Francisco, www.mowsf.org/History.asp; and Citymeals-on-Wheels, www.citymeals.org.

Food Banks

Many communities have created food banks that serve families and individuals with low incomes. Food banks distribute to qualified individuals government commodities or food that has been donated by private citizens, farmers, food manufacturers, grocery stores, and restaurants. The Food and Nutrition Service, under the U.S. Department of Agriculture, supports two community food security programs: the Commodity Supplemental Food Program (CSFP); and the Emergency Food Assistance Program (TEFAP). The CSFP assists low-income older adults over 60 years of age in addition to low-income pregnant and breastfeeding women, new mothers up to one year postpartum, infants, and children up to age 6. To qualify for assistance, older adults must be residents and have incomes at or below 130% of the poverty income guidelines, and the program is not available in every state. Food packages include items such as cereal, rice, pasta, canned meat, fruits, and vegetables (U.S. Department of Agriculture, 2001b). The number of older adults enrolled in the CSFP has increased over the past 10 years from 219,000 persons in 1996 to 293,000 in 2000 to 459,000 in 2005 (U.S. Department of Agriculture, 2006b; U.S. Senate Special Committee on Aging, 2000). The TEFAP, administered by the U.S. Department of Agriculture, distributes to low-income individuals foods such as butter, flour, cornmeal, green beans, tomatoes, beef, and pork at no cost. In 2005, the program donated $154 million worth of surplus food. In 2006, Congress appropriated $140 million to purchase food under the TEFAP (U.S. Department of Agriculture, 2006c).

Food recovery and gleaning are programs that collect excess food for delivery to community food banks. Food recovery programs work with wholesale food markets or retail grocers to salvage edible but not sellable ripe fruits and vegetables. The program "From Wholesaler to the Hungry" is one organization that has helped more than 60 communities establish a food salvage program. In Portland, Oregon, a program called "Fork It Over" coordinates a Food rescue program where food banks and pantries pick up surplus restaurant food. Many fresh and prepared foods are donated, including unserved menu items, unserved buffet foods, produce, dairy items, deli items, catered foods, baked goods, meats, and seafood. This program recovered approximately 10,614 tons of food, much of which would have otherwise been landfilled had it not been donated (McGuire, 2002). Another way communities have gathered surplus food to distribute to low-income individuals is to harvest unusable produce left after a commercial harvest. These "gleaning projects" have played an important role in preventing hunger in their communities. For example, the Gleaning Project sponsored by the Washington State University Cooperative Extension Program trains volunteers from low-income families to harvest unusable produce left in farmers' fields. Families are able to keep what they need, and the rest is distributed to food banks and hot meal sites. In 1998, the Gleaning Project harvested 200,000 pounds of produce, with 80% of the produce given to food banks and meal sites and the remainder going to low-income gleaners' families.

Brown Bag Programs

Brown bag programs are also supplemental food programs for low-income seniors. Typically, low-income older adults can receive a grocery bag containing fresh or frozen produce, breads, and canned foods. Food for these programs comes from local grocery stores and private donations from food drives. Distribution sites, home delivery availability, frequency of distribution, and eligibility guidelines vary by community and by program. One example of a brown bag program is the Greater Boston Food Bank's "Let's Bag Hunger" program. The program has seven Elderly and Family Brown Bag programs in the Boston area, which serve more than 3,000 participants each month. This initiative provides a free 10- to 15-pound grocery bag filled with food once a month (Greater Boston Food Bank, 2001).

Shopping Assistance Programs

As noted above, many older adults have difficulty grocery shopping. Chronic conditions make traveling to grocery stores and selecting and carrying groceries home problematic. Lack of private transportation makes shopping burdensome as well. No doubt many of the participants who receive home-delivered meals are in need of assistance with grocery shopping. Communities have responded by offering shopping assistance services that escort older adults to food markets or deliver groceries to their homes. Volunteers, in conjunction with public transportation, often help with shopping assistance. Volunteers travel to the homes of older adults, escort older adults to the grocery store, assist them in shopping, and return home. Grocery delivery programs allow older adults to call in their grocery order to be filled and delivered by volunteers. A study that surveyed a random sample of nutrition programs across the country found that approximately 43% of meal programs for older adults provided escort shopping services and that 15% offered grocery delivery services (Balsam & Rogers, 1988).

For Your Files: **America's Second Harvest Food Bank**

America's Second Harvest—The Nation's Food Bank Network is the nation's largest charitable hunger-relief organization comprised of a network of more than 200 member food banks and food-rescue organizations. It serves all 50 states, the District of Columbia, and Puerto Rico. The America's Second Harvest Network secures and distributes nearly 2 billion pounds of donated food and grocery products annually and supports approximately 50,000 local charitable agencies operating more than 94,000 programs including food pantries, soup kitchens, emergency shelters, and after-school food programs. Last year, the America's Second Harvest Network provided food assistance to nearly 3 million seniors.

For more information, contact Second Harvest Food Bank at 35 E. Wacker Dr., #2000 Chicago, IL 60601, 800-771-2303; www.secondharvest.org.

Users of Congregate and Home-Delivered Meal Programs

Who attends meal programs? Who participates in the home-delivered meal program? Do these programs serve the most needy among the older population? To answer these questions, researchers have conducted studies to identify participant characteristics and benefits of attending meal programs on both the local and national levels. In the past 30 years, two national studies have investigated Title III nutrition program participants and outcomes. One of those studies was the longitudinal study of the OAA nutrition program outcomes initiated in 1978 (U.S. Department of Health, Education, and Welfare, 1979). The purpose of the evaluation was to assess program impacts on participants and to identify program characteristics and other factors that influence participant outcomes. Researchers collected information from a random sample of 91 meal sites and conducted interviews with program staff and representatives from related organizations. In addition, a sample of nutrition program participants was compared with a sample of non-participants. The evaluation gathered specific information about dietary and health status, isolation, life satisfaction, longevity, and independent living. Results revealed that the majority of participants had incomes below the poverty level and that one-quarter of the participants were minority group older adults. Participants had higher rates of social activity compared with the sample of non-participants. The majority attended once a week or more, and the more frequent attendees were long-term participants who were poor, more than 75 years of age, in poor health, living alone, and ethnic minorities. In the final report, Kirschner Associates (1983) concluded that the attendance did increase the nutrient intake of participants; participants also ranked the benefits of social interaction higher than the benefits of the meals.

Almost 15 years later, another comprehensive two-year evaluation of the Title III nutrition program was undertaken. The purposes of the study were to evaluate the program's effect on participants' nutrition and socialization compared with those of similar non-participants; to evaluate who used the program and how effectively the program served targeted groups in most need of its services; to assess how efficiently and effectively the program was administered and delivered services; and to clarify funding sources and allocation of funds among program components (Ponza et al., 1996). Data were collected from 55 state units on aging, 350 area agencies on aging, 100 Indian tribal organizations, a representative sample of 200 nutrition projects, a nationally representative sample of 1,200 congregate meal participants and 800 home-delivered meal participants, and personal interviews with a nationally representative sample of 600 non-participants eligible for the congregate meal program, and 400 non-participants eligible for the home-delivered meal program. The majority of congregate meal participants were women (69%); 45% had been participating in the congregate meal program for more than five years (Ponza et al., 1996). The average age of the participants was 76 years and 26% needed special transportation to get to the meal site.

Ponza and colleagues (1996) found that participants were more disadvantaged regarding income, living arrangements, and physical health than the older adult population in general. For example, between 80% and 90% of participants had incomes that were 200% below the poverty level—a rate that was two times higher than that of the overall U.S. older adult population. Moreover, more participants were living alone (60%) than the overall older population (25%). With regard to physical health, participants typically had two chronic health conditions, and almost a quarter reported difficulty in doing one or more everyday tasks. Racial and ethnic minorities accounted for 27% of congregate meal participants. The congregate meal participants were also found to be nutritionally at risk. Following the protocols under the Nutritional Screening Initiative, 64% of participants had characteristics associated with moderate to high nutritional risk and over 55% received half or more of their daily food intake from their congregate meal. Approximately two-thirds of participants were either over- or underweight, placing them at increased risk for nutritional and health problems.

Researchers also evaluated specific outcomes of improved nutritional status and increased social contacts. Researchers found that the nutrition program significantly influenced participants' overall nutritional intake. On a daily basis, participants had higher percentages of recommended daily allowances than did non-participants, and overall dietary intakes were better than those of non-participants as well. Results indicated that when compared with non-participants, participants had, on average, more social contacts per month. Overall, the results indicate that nutrition programs are accomplishing the mission of improving the dietary and social wellbeing of an at-risk population. Researchers conducting studies of local older adult nutrition programs report similar outcomes, with some variation of the ethnic makeup of participants. In a study of the Boston area congregate meal program participants ($n = 174$), Posner (1979) found that the majority of participants were White (93%), female (69%), and widowed (44%). The average age of participants was 73 years, and most participants were living alone. One-fifth had incomes below the poverty level; 44% had incomes that were at or below 125% of the poverty level. Respondents were asked to identify what they thought was the program's value for them. The opportunity for a nutritious meal and the opportunity for socialization were the two top reasons given by respondents for attending the meal program. Participants indicated that they realized financial as well as food-purchasing benefits (31% and 50%, respectively). That is, their participation in the nutrition program helped reduce the amount of food they bought. Significantly more older adults who lived alone realized these benefits. More than half the respondents indicated that attending the program had a positive impact on the social aspects of their lives. This included meeting more people and socializing more with peers (26%), reduced loneliness and improved morale (22%), and increased social activities outside their homes (22%). Finally, 47% of participants indicated that they engaged in social activities outside the meal program with peers whom they had first met at the site.

Similarly, in their study of 888 congregate meal participants, Mullins et al. (1993) found that the majority of participants were female (70%), White (65%), widowed (47%), and living alone (51%). A surprising number had relatively few associations with children, grandchildren, and siblings and had fewer close relationships than did respondents who received home-delivered meals. Moreover, more than one-quarter (26%) reported levels of loneliness greater than the median. Half the congregate meal participants rated their health as either fair or poor, and 66% indicated that they had a health problem which affected their daily activities. Many of the participants also indicated that their economic condition was problematic; more than half (54%) reported that not having enough money to live on was a somewhat or very serious problem. Respondents were also asked if they felt healthier because of their participation in the nutrition program. More than three-quarters of congregate meal participants indicated that attending the program was related to feeling healthier and making more friends.

Another study investigated the social and nutritional outcomes of a random sample of participants ($n = 140$) at 13 rural areas and eight urban congregate meal sites in Colorado (Wacker, 1992). The majority of respondents were female (83%), and 43% were widowed. Slightly more than half the respondents reported their health status was good (52%), and 31% indicated their health was fair. Most had a high school education (47%), whereas 29% reported having less than a high school education. Reflecting data from national studies showing that meal programs primarily serve those with low incomes, many of the study participants reported a similar financial picture. When asked about their financial wellbeing, 32% said they had just enough income to make ends meet; 47% indicated that they had enough to make ends meet, with a little extra left over sometimes. A significant majority of respondents had been attending the program for three or more years and attended at least once per week. When participants were asked why they attended the program, the most popular reasons given were socializing with others (84%), getting an affordable meal (75%), and liking the food being served (72%). In addition, 75% indicated that the meal program was an important part of their diet. Of those who indicated that they had changed their health habits (e.g., reduced amount of fat and sodium in their diets), 17% said that the nutrition education presented at the meal program influenced them to change.

Examinations of users of home-delivered meal programs have shown that recipients have more physical limitations, are more socially isolated, and have lower incomes than those who attend congregate meal programs (Ponza et al., 1996; AoA, 1983; Mullins et al., 1993). Home-delivered meal participants are a more frail and at-risk population than those who attend congregate meal programs. According to the national study of the OAA Title III meal program mentioned above, the average age of a home-delivered meal participant is 78 years; 70% are female, 60% live alone, and 95% receive five or more meals per week. One-quarter were minority and ethnic elders and almost half (48%) of participants had incomes below 100% of the DHHS poverty guidelines. When meal participants were asked how many times per month they saw relatives, friends, or neighbors, 38% reported never or less than once. Home-delivered meal participants have more than twice as many physical impairments as the overall elderly population. Over 75% report experiencing difficulty doing one or more everyday tasks, and 43% reported a recent stay in a hospital or nursing home. Approximately one-third also receive personal care and homemaker services from other agencies. These meal participants are also nutritionally at risk. Eighty-eight percent were determined to be at moderate or high nutritional risk and more than one-third saved part of the program meal to eat as a second meal or as part of a second meal or snack. Researchers also found that about one-half of home-delivered meal participants had incomes at or below poverty levels. The majority of homebound older adults have poor diets compared with persons who attend congregate meal programs (Ponza et al., 1996; Steele & Bryan, 1986; Stevens, Grivetti, & McDonald, 1992).

CHALLENGES FOR NUTRITION PROGRAMS

On the basis of empirical research during the past two decades evaluating the outcomes of nutrition programs, one can conclude that these programs are indeed successful. Programs funded under the OAA are serving older adults who are at risk of poor nutritional intake with meals that are critical to their daily food consumption. These programs also provide older individuals with social contacts that are beneficial for their psychological wellbeing. Despite these successes, meal programs for older adults face a number of critical issues.

Enhancing Awareness and Use of Nutrition Programs

Older adults who participate in nutrition programs derive nutritional and psychological benefits, yet many other older adults who also could benefit from attending do not participate. Peterson and Maiden (1991) explored the variables associated with awareness and use of congregate meal programs in a sample of 358 community-dwelling older adults. Those who were aware of the programs had more personal and social resources and less nutritional need. Those using nutrition programs, however, had fewer personal and social resources and greater nutritional need. Such research illustrates the need for more studies about the factors associated with awareness and use of programs to assist with outreach efforts. On the basis of their two-year evaluation of the senior nutrition program, Ponza and colleagues (1996) made the following recommendations for future directions of nutrition programs:

- As the percentage of persons in the oldest-old category increases, the need for home-delivered meals may increase.
- Programs must endeavor to better meet the specialized nutrition needs of their participants, including more choices in types of meals, and more options for meals available during the day and on weekends.
- Changes in the delivery of health care will also have an impact on nutrition programs. As individuals continue to be discharged more quickly from hospitals and nursing homes, nutrition programs will be serving an even more frail and functionally impaired population than in the past.
- There continue to be waiting lists at some nutrition sites for home-delivered and congregate meals, and high percentages of home-delivered and congregate meal participants continue to be nutritionally at risk. Programs will be challenged to serve the underserved population in an era of shrinking public and private dollars.

Serving a Diverse Older Population

Meal programs for older adults must be ever mindful of meeting the nutritional needs of an ethnically diverse population. Programs must ensure that the social atmosphere, as well as the meals, is welcoming to racial and ethnic elders by having culturally sensitive staff, preparing ethnic meals, offering culturally appropriate nutrition education materials, and obtaining input from minority participants (Briggs, 1992). Others have commented on the need to reach out to the most needy older persons. For example, Balsam and Rogers (1991) argue that outreach for nutrition programs must include older adults who are "socially impaired"—those who are socially isolated, homeless, live in single-room occupancy dwellings, suffer from substance abuse, or are deinstitutionalized. Because such persons might not be readily welcomed at congregate meal sites, programs targeted to older adults at the margins of society might be created (Doolin, 1985). Adding to and customizing meals will also mean that more dieticians knowledgeable in working with older adults will be needed to help guide and advise expanding nutrition programs (Wellman, Rosenzweig, & Lloyd, 2002).

Funding Nutrition Programs

As always, the reliance on public money to fund nutrition programs runs the risk of cutbacks and perhaps elimination when fiscal budgets become tight. Alternative funding from businesses, civic organizations, and foundations will be sources of financial support that programs must tap to maintain and expand services (Balsam & Rogers, 1991).

Implementing Meal Programs for a New Generation of Older Adults

Finally, nutrition programs will have to change as the population ages and as cohorts with different needs and preferences replace the current participants. Because evidence indicates that nutrition and eating habits vary across age groups (Wurtman, Lieberman, Tsay, Nader, & Chew, 1988), the menus and meals offered through nutrition programs will no doubt need to accommodate those differences as well.

Supporting the Future of Senior Nutrition Programs

The delegates at the White House Conference on Aging passed a resolution and strategies that address a number of the challenges previously discussed. The delegates recommended the following to promote the importance of nutrition in health promotion and disease prevention and management:

- Form a public/private nutrition and fitness alliance that would become the authoritative source for seniors and caregiver, and promote through a national media campaign.
- Respond to the special nutritional needs of individual seniors to enhance independent living by reauthorization of the OAA to include the flexibility to utilize non-traditional food sources and strengthening the congregate and home-delivered meal programs to increasing services up to seven days and expanding Seniors Farmers Market Nutrition Program nationwide.
- Through the reauthorization of the OAA (Title III), expand funding to ensure adequate nutrition (eliminate undernutrition) and provide reliable nutrition education/information delivered by registered dieticians and/or technology which can then empower individuals.
- Utilize existing nutrition sciences to concurrently deliver physical activity and exercise information and programs to older adults.

CASE STUDY

Good Nutrition—Making Independence Possible

Manuel, 75, is a shy bachelor who has lived with his mother all his adult life except during two years when he was stationed overseas with the army. After his discharge, he returned home and worked as a cook for the local National Guard for 12 years. Everyone in town talked about the good old-fashioned food that Manuel prepared. When the local National Guard facility closed, Manuel became a self-employed janitor. He continued to work without giving retirement a second thought. His work, his flower garden, and taking care of his mother were his main activities in life. Manuel's income, barely $617 per month, supported his modest lifestyle.

One day, when Manuel was driving to the hardware store to buy garden supplies, a semi-trailer broadsided him. The accident was serious and was Manuel's fault. He was rushed to the hospital with internal injuries and a broken leg and collarbone. During the hospitalization, medical tests revealed that Manuel was diabetic. His diabetes had gone untreated because he had simply ignored symptoms that had plagued him for many years. The untreated diabetes, it now seemed, was the cause of his eyesight deteriorating so rapidly in the year before the accident.

After four weeks, the hospital discharged him to a nursing home, where he spent three months in a skilled care unit. This was a difficult time for Manuel. He was making progress overcoming his injuries, but not the chronic pain in his neck. In addition, his mother died, and he felt terrible that he was unable to be with her before her death. His only remaining family was his estranged sister.

Manuel's greatest desire was to return home. He reminded the nursing home staff and his doctor of that at every opportunity. He desperately missed his garden and the few neighbors with whom he used to chat over the fence. Finally, after weeks of listening to Manuel complain about neck pain and not being able to go home, his doctor ordered more x-rays, which showed that Manuel's neck was broken. He was fitted for a halo cast and told by his doctor that he could return home only if he followed a strict diabetic diet and did not drive.

Case Study Questions

1. Why is nutrition such a central factor in Manuel's plan of care?
2. What community-based food programs would you recommend for Manuel? Which program would you choose as the best option for Manuel? Why?
3. Is Manuel a good candidate for living at home alone if he follows the doctor's instructions? Why or why not?
4. What reasons would you give to defend Manuel's chances for successfully returning home?
5. What reasons would you give to defend Manuel's chances for having to move back to the nursing home?

Learning Activities

1. Have an older adult relative keep a nutrition diary for one week to track what was eaten and when. Keep track of your own nutritional intake for that same week. Examine both diaries. How are they different? Similar? Are there any deficiencies in either diet? What improvements could be made in both diets?
2. Visit or volunteer at the local food bank. How many of the clients are older adults? How often is food distributed? What are the eligibility criteria for participation? How does the food bank obtain food to distribute?

3. Sign up for a congregate meal at a nearby site. How many people attend? How many times during the week are meals served? What is the suggested donation? What was the ethnic makeup of participants? Would the type of meals served attract older adults of different ethnic backgrounds?

For More Information

National Resources

1. National Resource Center on Nutrition, Physical Activity & Aging, Florida International University, University Park, OE200, Miami, FL 33199; phone: 305-348-1517; http://nutritionandaging.fiu.edu; e-mail: nutritionandaging@fiu.edu.

    The National Policy and Resource Center on Nutrition and Aging works with the AoA to improve the nutritional status of older adults by disseminating nutrition information, providing technical assistance and training, and examining nutrition policies.

2. American Dietetic Association, 216 West Jackson Blvd., Chicago, IL 60606; phone: 800-877-1600, ext. 5000 (publications); www.eatright.com.

    The American Dietetic Association is the professional society for dietitians. In addition to other services for its members and a consumer nutrition hotline, the association has numerous publications helpful to consumers, such as *Staying Healthy: A Guide for Elder Americans*, *Older Adults Food Guide Pyramid*, and *Recommendations of Food Choices for Women*.

3. Food and Nutrition Information Center, U.S. Department of Agriculture, National Agriculture Library Building, Room 105, 10301 Baltimore Avenue, Beltsville, MD 20705-2351; phone: 301-504-5719; www.nal.usda.gov/fnic.

    The center provides information to professionals and the general public on nutrition and acquires and lends printed and audiovisual materials dealing with nutrition.

4. Meals on Wheels Association of America (formerly the National Association of Meal Programs), 203 S. Union Street, Alexandria, Virginia 22314; phone: 703-548-5558; www.mowaa.org.

    The Meals on Wheels Association of America provides education and training to those who plan and conduct congregate and home-delivered meals programs.

5. *The Journal of Nutrition for the Elderly*, Haworth Press, www.haworthpress.com/store/product .asp?sku = J052.

    The Journal of Nutrition for the Elderly publishes research on nutritional care for older adults. The journal includes client education suggestions and covers essential aspects of nutrition, from the clinical correlation between the pathophysiology of diseases and the role of nutrition to the psychosocial aspects of eating. In addition to scholarly studies, it also highlights evidence-based interventions for use in community settings.

6. The National Association of Nutrition and Aging Services Programs, 1612 K Street, N.W., Suite 400, Washington, DC 20006; phone: 202-682-6899; www.nanasp.org.

    The National Association of Nutrition and Aging Services Programs (NANASP) is a professional membership organization with members drawn primarily from persons working in or interested in the field of aging, community-based services, and nutrition and the elderly. NANASP is recognized as a primary leadership organization in the field of aging in shaping national policy, training service providers, and advocating on behalf of seniors.

Web Resources

1. Food in Later Life Research Project, University of Surrey, Guildford, Surrey, GU2 7XH, UK; www.foodinlaterlife.org/senior410.html; e-mail: m.raats@surrey.ac.uk.

   The Food in Later Life Research Project is a longitudinal research project funded by the European Union to examine the relationship between food intake, nutritional wellbeing, health, and quality of life among older people and to disseminate and consult with professionals who are in a position to enhance older people's nutritional wellbeing, health, and quality of life through food and service provision. Twelve countries will be involved in the study, including the United Kingdom, Italy, Germany, Sweden, Demark, Portugal, and Spain. The project website contains many resources on the topic of the nutritional wellbeing of older adults.

2. Washington State University Nutrition Education, Farmers Market Nutrition Program, Department of Social and Health Services, Aging and Disability Services Administration, PO Box 45600, Olympia, WA 98504-5600; phone: 800-422-3263; http://nutrition.wsu.edu/markets/sfmnp.html.

   The Senior Farmers Market Nutrition provides fresh fruit and vegetables to lower income seniors and supports local farming by increasing the use of farmers markets, roadside stands, and community-supported agriculture. Eligible participants are issued checks that are used to purchase local produce at authorized farmers' markets or roadside stands, local produce purchased directly from farmers or community-supported agriculture, and delivered to homebound seniors.

NOTE

1. This story is based on true events and provided by the Greater Boston Food Bank and the Food Bank for New York City (2007).

11

Health Care and Wellness

Marge had intended for years to get serious about losing weight. She could not believe it when her physician told her she was diabetic. She had just celebrated her 65th birthday, she felt great, and she was as active as she had ever been. Marge discussed her options for treatment with her doctor and decided to try diet and exercise because her sugar levels were only a little above normal. However, she knew her personality and lifestyle well enough to be aware that she could not do this on her own. Her doctor suggested that she contact the Lifetime Wellness Center through the local hospital. The center encouraged her to enroll in a "Slim for Life" class sponsored by the American Heart Association and attend a class on "Managing Diabetes" sponsored by the hospital. After eight weeks of classes, Marge believes she is on her way to getting control of her weight problem. She also knows the consequences of her actions and that if she needs more help, the Wellness Center is there to support her.

Although changes in physical health are inevitable as individuals age, it is possible to live a healthy life well into the ninth decade. Early detection of conditions such as Marge's diabetes and the assistance of wellness programs will make it possible for her to manage her illness for many years. Indeed, older adults are living longer partly because of the advances in preventive and traditional medical care and improved access to health care services through Medicare. In this chapter, we provide a summary of the health status of older adults, the Medicare and Medicaid programs, and health maintenance organizations (HMOs). We conclude this chapter by describing health promotion and wellness programs available to older adults and looking at future challenges for health care policy and health promotion programs.

HEALTH STATUS OF OLDER ADULTS

Overall, the majority of older adults consider their health to be *good*, *very good*, or *excellent* (National Center for Health Statistics, 2004a). Although self-assessment is certainly one way to measure health status, the presence or absence of chronic or acute disease and the degree of inability in level of functioning are other measures of health status (Kane & Kane, 1981). Population studies of the prevalence of acute conditions reveal that older adults are less likely than younger adults to suffer from acute (i.e., temporary) conditions such as common colds (National Center for Health Statistics, 1990). The consequences of acute illness, however, are more severe for older adults than for younger adults. For example, an equal number of older adults and younger adults get respiratory infections, but death rates are 30% higher for older adults who get these infections (Hooyman & Kiyak, 1996; Hoyert, Heron, Murphy, & Kung, 2006). In contrast, older adults are more likely than younger adults to have chronic illnesses—those that are long term, often permanent, and result in a disability that requires management rather than a cure. Marge's diabetes is a good example of a chronic condition that will require health management for the rest of her life. According to the National Center for Health Statistics (Adams, Hendershot, & Marano, 1999), more than 80% of older adults over 65 have at least one chronic condition. Exhibit 11.1 shows the prevalence of chronic conditions experienced by older persons. The most frequent conditions for Hispanic, Black, and White elders are arthritis and hypertension; however, Black and Hispanic older adults are more likely to suffer from diabetes than White elders. Elderly Blacks are also more likely to suffer from hypertension than are Hispanic and White elders.

The presence of chronic conditions varies across subpopulations of older adults. For example, older women are more likely than older men to suffer from chronic conditions such as arthritis, osteoporosis, hypertension, incontinence, and most types of orthopedic problems (National Center for Health Statistics, 2004b). Similarly, older adults of color suffer from chronic conditions at rates that are often twice those of White older adults.

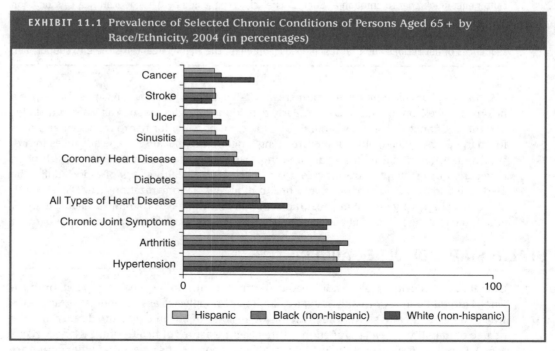

EXHIBIT 11.1 Prevalence of Selected Chronic Conditions of Persons Aged 65 + by Race/Ethnicity, 2004 (in percentages)

Source: National Center for Health Statistics (2004b).

Older Blacks experience hypertension, stroke, diabetes, and kidney failure more frequently than do Whites. Of older Hispanic adults, 85% suffer from at least one chronic condition; by the age of 45, many Hispanics experience chronic health impairments, such as arthritis, heart disease, and diabetes, similar to those of a typical White 65-year-old (Cuellar, 1990). Older Native Americans have even greater rates of chronic conditions. Older Native Americans are more likely to have arthritis, congestive heart failure, stroke, asthma, prostate cancer, high blood pressure, and diabetes than the general population aged 55 and older (Moulton et al, 2005). A more recent health phenomenon among the aging population is the increasing number of overweight and obese individuals. Currently, one in four individuals age 50 and over is considered obese (Rhoades, 2005), and it is estimated that the prevalence of obesity in the 60 + population will increase from 32% in 2000 to more than 37% in 2010 (Arterburn, Crane, & Sullivan, 2004). Exhibits 11.2 and 11.3 show the increasing trends in weight in men and women aged 50–69 from 1985 to 2020. Individuals who are overweight and obese have increased likelihood of being in poorer health, suffering from more chronic health conditions, and being limited in their ability to carry out activities of daily living (ADLs) (Strum, Ringel, & Andreyeva, 2004).

Older adults are also living with and dying from AIDS. According to the National Center for Health Statistics (1993), more people over age 60 died of AIDS than did children. The

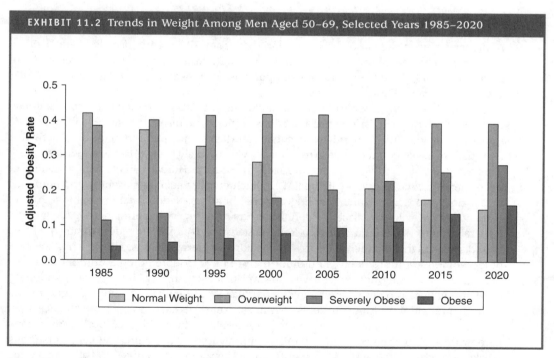

EXHIBIT 11.2 Trends in Weight Among Men Aged 50–69, Selected Years 1985–2020

Source: Strum et al. (2004).

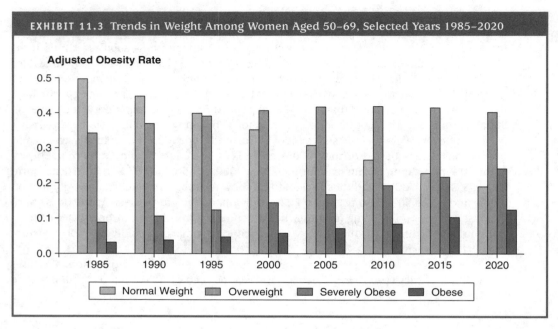

EXHIBIT 11.3 Trends in Weight Among Women Aged 50–69, Selected Years 1985–2020

Source: Strum et al. (2004).

number of persons aged 60 and older who died from AIDS nearly doubled from 1987 to 1992, whereas the number of children who died from AIDS remained stable. As of December 2000, there were some 44,419 persons aged 55 and older diagnosed with AIDS (Centers for Disease Control, 2001).

Persons living with chronic conditions, including HIV-AIDS, experience functional limitations for which they need assistance. Functional limitation, a measure of an individual's health status, is the inability to perform personal care tasks and home-management activities. Personal care tasks, commonly referred to as activities of daily living (ADLs), include tasks such as bathing and grooming, toileting, dressing, and eating. Home-management activities, or instrumental activities of daily living (IADLs), include tasks such as shopping and preparing meals, doing housework, and handling personal finances. National data reveal that 20% of older adults have chronic disability defined as having difficulty in performing ADLs or IADLs (Federal Interagency Forum on Aging-Related Statistics, 2006). More older women are likely to be disabled than older men (43% vs. 40%; Waldrop & Stern, 2003). As shown in Exhibit 11.4, older women are more likely than older men to have trouble doing a number of activities, including walking, light and heavy housework, transferring (e.g., in/out of bed), shopping, and bathing. Just as older women and older adults of different ethnic and racial groups suffer from multiple chronic impairments, they are also likely to have multiple limitations in their everyday activities. In a sample of community-dwelling older adults, 23% of women compared with 13% of men could not do IADLs without assistance (Kramarow, Lentzner, Rooks, Weeks, & Saydah, 1999). A similar disparity existed between older Whites and other racial and ethnic groups in functional abilities. Fifty-three percent of Blacks, 58% of American Indians or Alaska Natives, 49% of Hispanics, and 52% of those reporting two or more races had one or more functional limitations, compared with 40% of non-Hispanic Whites over 65 years of age (Waldrop & Stern, 2003). Furthermore, 40% of older Blacks had functional limitations that were considered to be severe, compared with 27% of older Whites with similar limitations.

A related indicator of functional limitation is the need for assistance in carrying out ADLs and IADLs. Not surprisingly, the need for assistance with daily activities increases with age. As shown in Exhibit 11.5, 6.8% and 14.0% of older adults aged 75 to 84 need assistance with ADLs and IADLs, respectively. The need for assistance increases to nearly 20% and 34% for those over age 85 who need assistance with ADLs and IADLs.

Older women are more likely than older men to need assistance with major activities, such as assistance with bathing, dressing, eating, transferring between bed and chair, and toileting. Although the percentages of women and men aged 70 to 74 who need assistance with everyday activities are similar (47.4% and 45.5%, respectively), by age 80 and older, 68.2% of men and 76.7% of women need assistance with everyday activities (see Exhibit 11.6).

Partly because older adults of different ethnic and racial groups experience a higher number of chronic conditions than do older Whites, they are more likely to need assistance with everyday activities. As shown in Exhibit 11.7, a higher percentage of older Blacks report needing assistance in everyday activities than do older non-Hispanic Whites and Hispanics (McNeil, 2001).

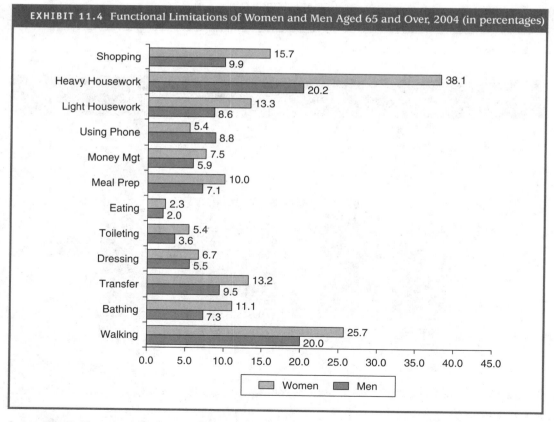

EXHIBIT 11.4 Functional Limitations of Women and Men Aged 65 and Over, 2004 (in percentages)

Source: Compiled from the National Center for Health Statistics (2004c, 2004d).

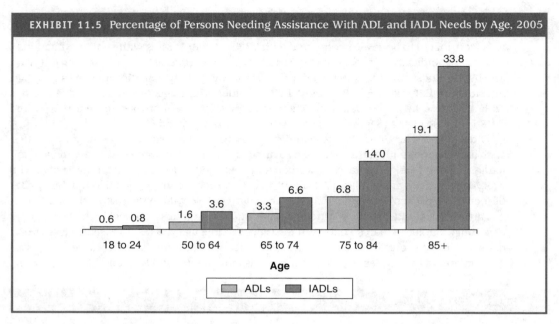

EXHIBIT 11.5 Percentage of Persons Needing Assistance With ADL and IADL Needs by Age, 2005

Source: National Center for Health Statistics (2004f).

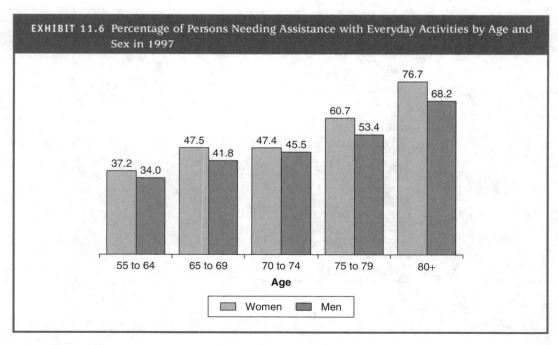

EXHIBIT 11.6 Percentage of Persons Needing Assistance with Everyday Activities by Age and Sex in 1997

Source: McNeil (2001).

In summary, most older adults do enjoy relatively good health well into their seventh decade. As people grow older and move into later life, however, they acquire more chronic conditions and experience fewer acute conditions, although the latter can result in life-threatening illnesses for some. Furthermore, health status varies between older women and men, between Whites and older adults of different racial and ethnic backgrounds, and between persons of different ages. In general, women and racial and ethnic elders have more chronic illnesses and more functional limitations and are more likely to need assistance with major activities.

These health characteristics have significant implications for the delivery of health care and health promotion programs. For example, in later life, adults need health care programs and services that address chronic, rather than acute, conditions. They also need access to and coverage of rehabilitation services, including assistance with assistive technology devices that are designed to maintain functional independence. Furthermore, health promotion programs can assist in preventing illness as well as in maintaining functioning. Later in this chapter, we will discuss the health promotion and wellness programs designed to improve the health status of older adults. In this next section, we provide an overview of the federal health insurance programs—Medicare and Medicaid.

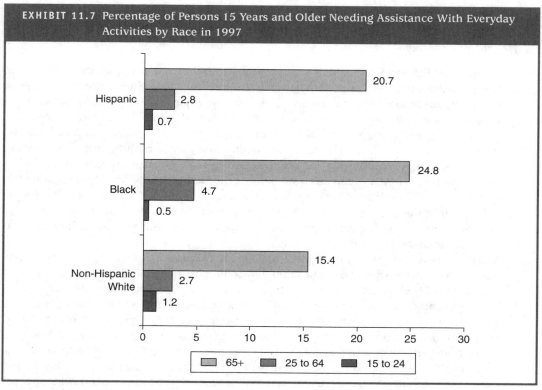

EXHIBIT 11.7 Percentage of Persons 15 Years and Older Needing Assistance With Everyday Activities by Race in 1997

Source: McNeil (2001).

For Your Files: ABLEDATA

Assistive technology devices help people maintain independent living by helping them perform ADLs. Assistive technology devices have been used by persons with disabilities for years; with the growing number of older adults with chronic conditions, however, such devices can effectively assist more older adults with their functional limitations. ABLEDATA, sponsored by the National Institute on Disability and Rehabilitation Research, is a national database of information on assistive technology and rehabilitation equipment from domestic and international sources. ABLEDATA contains information on more than 32,000 assistive technology products that consumers can search on the web or by phone. ABLEDATA also offers fact sheets about devices and topics related to assistive technology, consumer guides to assist with product selection, and other publications for consumers of assistive technology devices. ABLEDATA can refer callers to resources that can help them make their companies accessible. Visit ABLEDATA's fully accessible facilities at 8630 Fenton Street, Suite 930, Silver Spring, MD 20910; phone ABLEDATA for more information at 800-227-0216; or access the website, www.abledata.com.

FEDERAL HEALTH CARE POLICY

Medicare

Medicare is a national health insurance program authorized in 1965 under Title XVII of the Social Security Act as a complement to those receiving Social Security benefits. Originally, Medicare covered older adults over 65, but since its passage, coverage has been extended to persons who are entitled to Social Security disability for 24 months or more, persons with end-stage kidney disease requiring dialysis or transplant, and noncovered persons who elect to buy into Medicare (Health Care Financing Administration [HFCA], 1996b). Beginning in 2001, persons with Lou Gehrig's disease are allowed to waive the 24-month waiting period and can be covered under the Medicare program (Hoffman, Klees, & Curtis, 2006). The Centers for Medicaid and Medicare Services (CMS), formally known as HCFA, administer the program under the direction of the U.S. Department of Health and Human Services. The Social Security Administration is responsible for processing applications and maintaining Medicare records.

There are two original parts to Medicare: *Part A, Hospital Insurance,* which covers costs associated with inpatient hospitalization and some post hospitalization care, and *Part B, Supplemental Medical Insurance,* which covers physician, outpatient care, and other medical services. A new third part of Medicare, sometimes called *Part C*, was established in 1997, and later renamed the *Medicare Advantage Program* in 2003; it expanded beneficiaries' option for participation in private sector health care plans. The 2003 changes in Medicare also introduced *Part D*, which established a new prescription drug program (Hoffman, Klees, & Curtis, 2006; see Exhibit 11.8). Part A is funded by taxes on earnings; employers and employees each pay 1.45% of payroll, and self-employed persons pay 2.9%. Older households pay about 6% of Part A payroll taxes, and Social Security beneficiaries with incomes above a certain amount pay federal income tax, with a portion of these taxes ($4 billion in 1995) being designated for Part A funds. Part B is funded primarily through premiums paid by beneficiaries and general federal revenues. Premiums cover approximately 36% of program costs, and general federal revenues cover the remainder (HCFA, 1996b). Reviewing and paying claims are done by intermediaries, such as utilization review committees (for Part A) and carriers (for Part B), such as Blue Cross and Blue Shield. In 2006, over 43 million people enrolled in one or both of Parts A and B of Medicare, and approximately 6 million have chosen to participate in Part C (Hoffman, Klees, & Curtis, 2006).

Who Is Eligible for Medicare?

All persons who are eligible for Social Security or Railroad Retirement benefits are also eligible for Medicare benefits. In addition, individuals who are entitled to Social Security Disability or Railroad Retirement Disability Benefits for at least 24 months and government employees with Medicare-only coverage who have been disabled for 29 or more months are also entitled to receive Part A benefits. Therefore, individuals qualify for Medicare if they or their spouses worked for 10 years (or 40 quarters) in employment that paid into Social Security. Those who lack a sufficient number of quarters can purchase Part A benefits if they also buy Part B coverage. In 2007, individuals who wished to buy Part A coverage could do so for $410 per month and for $226 if they had 30 to 39 quarters. For individuals who have earned enough quarters, there is no premium cost associated with Part A; older adults choosing to participate in Part B, however, pay a monthly premium. Beginning in January 2007, the amount of the Part B monthly premium is based on the beneficiary's gross income. Individuals with incomes less than $80,000 pay $93.50; those with incomes above $200,000 pay monthly premiums of $161.40. All beneficiaries must meet the $131 per year deductible for physician services (Centers for Medicare and Medicaid Services, 2007).

Coverage

Exhibits 11.9, 11.10, and 11.11 present a detailed explanation of the coverage provided by Part A, Part B, and Part D, respectively. Medicare Part A provides coverage of inpatient hospital services up to 90 days per benefit period[1] plus 60 days of lifetime reserve days, skilled nursing facilities for 100 days following a three-day hospital stay, intermittent home health services if skilled care is needed, and hospice care (HCFA, 2001c). Medicare Part B helps pay for the cost of physician services, outpatient hospital services, medical equipment and supplies, and other health services and supplies. Payments made by Medicare under Part A for inpatient hospital costs are based on the patient's diagnosis (referred to as *diagnostic related group,* or *DRG*). The patient's DRG dictates the payment the hospital will receive as well as the length of stay on which the payment is based. Under the DRG system, payments to the hospital for a given Medicare patient may be more or less than the hospital's cost—thus, the hospital either absorbs the loss or enjoys a profit. Payments for other services under Part A (home health, skilled nursing facility, and hospice) are paid on a "reasonable cost" billed by the provider. Under Part B, Medicare pays physicians on the basis of a "reasonable charge," which is the lowest of either the submitted charges or a fee schedule based on a relative value scale (HCFA, 2001c). If a provider agrees to accept the approved

EXHIBIT 11.8   Overview of Medicare Coverage

Original Medicare Plan	
Part A Hospital	Part B Medical
Medicare provides this coverage. Part B is optional. Beneficiaries have a choice of doctors.	

OR

Medicare Advantage Plans
Sometimes called "Part C," this option combines Part A (Hospital) and Part B (Medical).
Private insurance companies approved by Medicare provide this coverage. Generally, beneficiaries must see doctors in the plan.

+

Part D
Prescription Drug Coverage

Beneficiaries can choose this coverage. Private companies approved by Medicare run these plans. Plans cover different drugs. Medically necessary drugs must be covered.

Part D
Prescription Drug Coverage

Most Part C plans cover prescription drugs; if not, beneficiaries may be able to choose this coverage. Plans cover different drugs. Medically necessary drugs must be covered.

Medigap (Medicare Supplement Insurance) Policy

Beneficiaries can choose to buy this private coverage (or an employer/union may offer similar coverage) to fill in gaps in Part A and Part B coverage. Costs vary by policy and company.

Source: Centers for Medicare and Medicaid Services (2007).

EXHIBIT 11.9 Medicare Coverage, Part A

Services	Benefit[a]	Medicare Pays	Beneficiary Pays
Hospitalization			
Semi-private room, meals, regular nursing services, intensive care, operating and recovering room, drugs, laboratory tests, x-rays, and all other medically necessary supplies;	First 60 days	All approved charges but $992	$992
	Days 61–90	All but $248 per day co-insurance	$248 per day for each benefit period
	Days 91–150	All but $496 per day co-insurance	$496 per day each benefit period
	150+ days– Lifetime reserve days	Nothing	All "Lifetime reserve days" are 60 extra days of coverage that can be used during the lifetime of the beneficiary. Pay $496.00 per day during the 60 days of coverage.
Inpatient mental health care in a psychiatric hospital		Inpatient mental health care in a psychiatric hospital is limited to 190 days in a lifetime	
Skilled Nursing Facility			
Semi-private room and board, skilled nursing and rehabilitative services, and other services and supplies	Days 1–20	100% of covered services	Nothing
	Days 21–100	All but $124 per day	$124 per day
	100 +	Nothing	All costs
Home Health			
Part-time or intermittent skilled care, home-health aide services, durable medical equipment and supplies, physical therapy, occupational therapy, and speech-language pathology	Unlimited as long as Medicare conditions are met	100% of the cost of covered home health care; 80% of approved amount for durable medical equipment	Nothing for services; 20% for durable medical equipment

(Continued)

EXHIBIT 11.9   (Continued)

Services	Benefit[a]	Medicare Pays	Beneficiary Pays
Hospice Pain relief, symptom management, and support services for the terminally ill	For as long as doctor certifies	100% of charges	A co-payment of up to $5 for outpatient prescription drugs and 5% of the Medicare-approved amount for inpatient respite care
Blood When furnished by a hospital or skilled nursing facility during a covered stay	Unlimited if medically necessary	All but first 3 pints per calendar year	For first 3 pints then 20% of the Medicare-approved amount for additional pints of blood

[a]A benefit period begins on the first day a beneficiary receives in-patient hospital benefits and ends after being discharged from the hospital or skilled facility for 60 consecutive days

Source: Centers for Medicare and Medicaid Services (2007).

rate as full payment for services, the provider "accepts assignment." If the provider does not accept assignment for the services provided, the beneficiary is responsible for the remaining balance of the cost of the service and what Medicare will pay. Other services covered under Part B, such as durable medical equipment and clinical laboratory services, are also paid on a fee schedule. Outpatient and home health coverage under Part B is paid on a reasonable cost basis.

According to HCFA (2000a), Part A provided benefits to 33.5 million aged adults and 5.2 million disabled enrollees. Part B provided coverage to approximately 37 million enrollees. Combined benefit payments for Part A and Part B averaged $5,410 per enrollee (HCFA, 2000c).

Medicare beneficiaries can select to receive benefits under the Part C or Medicare Advantage program. To enroll, beneficiaries must live in a locale in which these private sector plans are available. Typically, two types of Part C managed care plans exist: Medicare-managed care plans (PPOs and HMOs) and private fee-for-service plans. Under Medicare-managed care plans, Medicare pays a set amount of money every month to a private insurance company participating in the Medicare Advantage (Part C) program, and beneficiaries must use doctors and hospitals that are members of the plan and must obtain a referral from their primary care provider to see a specialist. Beneficiaries pay the monthly Part B premium, and most plans require a co-payment ($5 to $10) for each doctor visit and possibly an additional monthly premium. Some plans offer additional benefits such as prescription drug coverage.

EXHIBIT 11.10   Medicare Coverage, Part B

Services	Benefit[a]	Medicare Pays	Beneficiary Pays
Medical Expenses Doctors' services, inpatient and outpatient medical and surgical services and supplies, physical and speech therapy, diagnostic tests, durable medical equipment, and other services.	Unlimited if medically necessary	80% of approved amount after $131 deductible	Deductible, plus 20% of approved amount and limited charges above the approved amount
Clinical Laboratory Services Blood tests, urinalysis, and more	Unlimited if medically necessary	Generally 100% of approved amount	Nothing for services
Home Health Care Part-time or intermittent skilled care, home health aide services, durable medical equipment and supplies, and other services	Unlimited as long as Medicare conditions are met	100% of the cost of covered home health care; 80% of approved amount for durable medical equipment	Nothing for services; 20% for durable medical equipment
Outpatient Hospital Services Services for the diagnosis or treatment of illness or injury	Unlimited if medically necessary	Approved amount minus co-pay or co-insurance amount	Co-pay or co-insurance amount
Blood When furnished by a hospital or skilled nursing facility during a covered stay	Unlimited if medically necessary	80% of approved amount after $100 deductible and starting with the fourth pint	For first 3 pints plus 20% of approved amount for additional pints
Mental Health Services	Unlimited if medically necessary	50% of approved amount	50% of approved amount
Ambulance Services	Unlimited if medically necessary	80% of approved amount	20% of approved amount

Source: Centers for Medicare and Medicaid Services (2007).

Private fee-for-service plans are offered by private insurance companies and, as with the managed care plans, Medicare pays a set amount of money every month to the private insurance company. Beneficiaries must go to selected health care providers and hospitals, receive prior authorization for certain medical treatments, and pay Medicare's Part B premium and possibly an additional monthly premium. The insurance company decides how much it will pay and how much the beneficiaries pay for the health services provided.

Cain (1996) has identified a number of advantages that Medicare beneficiaries enjoy when they join HMOs. They usually do not have to pay deductibles or co-insurance payments required under Part A or Part B, and HMOs agree not to charge more than Medicare's approved amount. Therefore, for many older adults, HMOs are an alternative to buying supplemental Medigap policies. In addition, HMOs often provide a wider range of services, including preventive health care, outpatient mental health services, prescription drugs, and eyeglasses. Disadvantages include restrictions on choice of doctor and hospitals who are not associated with the HMO; there is also a fear that older adults will not get the health services they need (Kane et al., 1996). Other problems include misunderstandings among enrollees about the terms associated with HMO enrollment, restrictions, and denial of services (Wilson, cited in National Association of Area Agencies on Aging, 1996).

In 2005, some 4.7 million Medicare beneficiaries chose to be in the Medicare Advantage (Part C) PPO or HMO managed care plans, and 199,000 were enrolled in private fee-for-service plans. Since the creation of Part C, the number of organizations with Medicare Advantage contracts declined from 346 in 1998 to 212 in 2005 (Gold, Hudson, & Davis, 2006; HCFA, 2001b). The decline in the number of private companies offering Medicare Advantage plans to beneficiaries forced over 1.7 million enrollees back to the original Medicare program or another Medicare Advantage provider. In addition, benefits under many of the Medicare + Choice plans have become less generous. In 1998, 78% of enrollees were in Medicare Advantage plans that had no additional premium cost and that included coverage of outpatient prescription drug coverage. By 2001, the percentage of enrollees in such plans dropped to 35% (HCFA, 2001b). In an effort to bolster Medicare Advantage enrollment, Congress increased payment rates to health plans under the Medicare Advantage program, which has been somewhat successful in stabilizing the market and in prompting a modest expansion in the plan and benefits (Gold, Hudson, & Davis, 2006). As of January 2006, enrollment in Medicare Advantage totaled 7.4 million (U.S. Department of Health and Human Services, 2006). Gold, Hudson and Davis (2006) examined the characteristics of benefits and premiums offered by Medicare Advantage plans in 2006 and found that the structure of the benefits and premiums was complex, "presenting beneficiaries with even more Medicare Advantage plan types that vary in how they function and in how benefits and cost sharing are structured" (2006, p. 17). They concluded that, because of the complexities of plans, beneficiaries will need a great deal of support and assistance as they try to choose between the original Medicare Part A & B and Medicare Advantage.

As mentioned earlier, Medicare now provides prescription drug coverage. Drug coverage can be obtained under Part D or included in a Part C plan via a PPO or HMO. Medicare beneficiaries enrolling under Part D are encouraged to join when they are first eligible to do so, or they pay a penalty (1% of national average premium times the number of months eligible and not enrolled) as long as they have Medicare. Individuals who have drug coverage from another source, such as a previous employer, can choose not to enroll in Part D. Beneficiaries may switch prescription drug plans during the enrollment period each year (November 15–December 31) and under other situations as approved by Medicare (e.g., move out of the service area of the plan). Approximately 10 million older adults receive prescription coverage under Part D (U.S. Department of Health and Human Services, 2006).

Each calendar year, those enrolled in Part D pay a monthly premium (the average is expected to be $24 but varies by plan), and a yearly deductible (between $0 and $265 in 2007). No plan may have a deductible higher than an amount set each year. After the deductible has been reached, the plan covers 75% of the next $2,400 of the prescription drug costs and the beneficiaries pay the remaining 25%. After this initial coverage amount has been met, a coverage gap—often referred to as the "donut hole"—is in effect. The "donut hole" is the gap in coverage after the plan and the beneficiary reach a predetermined amount that has been spent on coverage ($2,400 in 2007). Once this amount has been spent, the beneficiary pays 100% of all prescription drug costs and must continue paying the monthly premium. Once beneficiaries spend a predetermined amount on out-of-pocket on prescription drugs ($3,850 in 2007), catastrophic coverage begins. During the catastrophic coverage, the plan covers up to 95% of prescription costs until the end of the calendar year (see Exhibit 11.11). In order for older adults to benefit from Part D, they must be able to sort through a myriad of plans available in their area and identify which plan has better coverage for the prescription drugs they use. Prescription drug coverage in a select plan can also change, thus enrollees may have to reevaluate their plans on a regular basis. Enrollment patterns and benefits will need to be studied in the future. One early study found that over half of respondents reported being confused about the changes and viewed the task of choosing a plan as stressful (Hibbard, Greene, & Tusler, 2006).

EXHIBIT 11.11 Medicare Coverage, Part D

Medicare Part D Coverage—2007		
Prescription Drug Spending	Medicare-Approved Plan Pays	Beneficiary Pays
Up to $265	Nothing	Up to $265 deductible amount
$265 to $2,400	75% of drug costs up to $1,600	25% of drug costs up to $535
$2,400 to $5,451 (donut hole)	Nothing	100% of drug costs up to $3,050
Subtotal		Up to $3,850 out of pocket
Over $5,451	95%	5% or between $2.15 (generic) and $5.35 (brand name)

Source: Adapted from AARP (2007).

Medigap Policies

Many older adults purchase Medicare supplemental insurance policies, commonly referred to as Medigap policies. Medigap policies are designed to assist with the costs of health care services not covered by Medicare. Medigap policies usually pay deductibles, co-payments, and the remaining 20% of the approved charges for physician and hospital services. Limited coverage is sometimes provided for prescription drugs, home care, and preventive care.

Medicaid

In the same year in which Congress enacted Medicare (1965), Medicaid became law as Title XIX of the Social Security Act. Medicaid provides three types of medical assistance for low-income families and individuals: (a) health insurance, (b) long-term care, and (c) supplemental coverage for low-income Medicare beneficiaries for services not covered by Medicare and Medicare premiums, deductibles, and cost sharing. Unlike Medicare, Medicaid is funded through the joint effort of federal and state governments to help states pay for the health care of those who are needy. The federal government provides broad national Medicaid program guidelines and funding to the states. Every state that participates develops its own eligibility standards; determines the type, amount, and scope of benefits and the rate of payment for services; and administers its own program (HCFA, 1996a). In addition, states can apply to the federal government for a Medicaid waiver that allows states to test new benefits or financing or to implement a major restructuring of the Medicaid program. Currently, 30 states and the District of Columbia have been granted a Medicaid waiver by the federal government (Centers for Medicare and Medicaid Services, 2005a). As a result of these variations, Medicaid programs vary by state, and not all low-income individuals are eligible for Medicaid.

Who Is Eligible for Medicaid?

States have some flexibility in setting Medicaid eligibility guidelines. They determine who will be covered and the income guidelines necessary to be eligible. Eligibility falls into two categories—the *categorically needy* and the *medically needy*. Those who are categorically needy must meet certain income and asset guidelines established by the state. Some groups of categorically needy persons, however, are required by federal law to receive Medicaid coverage. For example, persons who receive federal income maintenance assistance, such as current and some former SSI recipients, low-income Medicare beneficiaries, and individuals who were eligible for Aid to Families With Dependent Children (AFDC)[2] as of July 16, 1996 must receive benefits (HCFA, 2001a). States also have the option of covering other categorically needy individuals. These groups include (a) certain aged, blind, or disabled adults who have income above those requiring mandatory coverage but below the federal poverty level; (b) institutionalized individuals with income and resources below specified limits; (c) persons who would be eligible if institutionalized but who are receiving care through home and community-based services; and (d) recipients of state supplementary payments, such as old age pensions (HCFA, 2000c).

Some states opt to include individuals who are considered medically needy but who have too much income to qualify as categorically needy. Under this option, states allow members of selected groups (e.g., aged, blind, and/or disabled persons) to spend down to Medicaid income eligibility guidelines by using their medical expenses to offset their excess income, thus reducing their income level to meet the Medicaid guidelines (HCFA, 2000c). Two groups recently added to the list of medically needy individuals that states may cover are women who have breast or cervical cancer and persons with tuberculosis (TB) who are uninsured (Centers for Medicare and Medicaid Services, 2005a).

Coverage

States participating in Medicaid must provide basic medical services to Medicaid beneficiaries. The following medical services are provided to those who qualify:

- inpatient hospital services;
- outpatient hospital services;
- physician services and medical and surgical services of a dentist;
- nursing facility services;
- rural health clinic services;
- home health care for persons eligible for skilled nursing services;
- laboratory and X-ray services;
- nurse practitioner services.

States also may receive federal assistance if they choose to provide other optional approved medical services. Some optional medical services covered by Medicaid include

- clinic services;
- optometrist services and eyeglasses;
- prescribed drugs;
- prosthetic devices;
- dental services;
- chiropractors;
- psychologists;
- diagnostic, screening, preventive, and rehabilitation services.

Payment for services is made directly to the provider, and the provider must accept the Medicaid payment as payment in full. States may also require beneficiaries to pay co-payments or a deductible for certain services (HCFA, 2001a).

After obtaining permission from the Centers for Medicare and Medicaid Services (formally known as HCFA), states can require beneficiaries to enroll in managed care plans and can offer home and community-based services to those individuals with chronic impairments who are eligible for Medicaid. In 2000, 63% of the Medicaid population was enrolled in a managed care plan, but only 6.3% were age 65 and over (Centers for Medicare and Medicaid Services, 2004). Currently, all states but Alaska and Wyoming have enrolled some percentage of Medicaid beneficiaries in a managed health care plan. Twenty states— Arizona, Arkansas, Colorado, Connecticut, Delaware, Georgia, Hawaii, Idaho, Iowa, Kentucky, Lousiana, Michigan, Nevada, Oklahoma, Oregon, Pennsylvania, South Dakota,

Tennessee, Utah, and Washington—and Puerto Rico, have over 75% of their Medicaid recipients enrolled in Medicaid managed care plans (Centers for Medicare and Medicaid Services, 2005b). States also can request a waiver, called a Program of All-Inclusive Care for the Elderly (PACE), that allows them to offer a package of services to persons who, without community support services, might otherwise be institutionalized. Such services include case management, adult day program services, respite care, and homemaker/home health care.

As mentioned above, Medicaid also provides benefits to persons who qualify for Medicare. For persons who are eligible for both Medicare and Medicaid, called *dual eligibles,* Medicaid pays all the premiums, deductibles, and co-insurance costs associated with Part A and Part B. Medicaid may also pay for services beyond what is covered under Medicare (e.g., hearing aids and skilled nursing after 100 days; HCFA, 2001a). The Medicare program must pay for services before any payments are made by Medicaid.

Other Medicare beneficiaries who can receive assistance from Medicaid are those who have incomes at or below 100% of the poverty line and whose resources are at or below 200% of the SSI guidelines (HCFA, 2001a). Known as *qualified Medicare beneficiaries (QMBs),* these individuals receive assistance from Medicaid in paying the cost-sharing provisions of Medicare. *Specified low-income Medicare beneficiaries* also receive assistance from Medicaid in paying expenses associated with Medicare. Medicaid will pay Medicare Part B premiums for persons who are eligible for Medicare whose incomes are above the QMB levels but below 135% of the poverty level (Centers for Medicare and Medicaid Services, 2005a).

Persons who are over the age of 65 (regardless of their eligibility status) represent 11.2% of persons enrolled in Medicaid and account for 31% of Medicaid spending; however, the percentage of beneficiaries eligible by virtue of being over the age of 65 and meeting income guidelines has declined from 16.7% in 1973 to 9.5% in 2000 (Centers for Medicare and Medicaid Services, 2004). Centers for Medicare and Medicaid Services (2004) data indicate that much of the Medicaid spending for this group is for long-term care—an amount totaling $48 billion, or 34% of total Medicaid spending. Federal medical assistance payments under Medicaid in 2001 were $214.9 billion, with spending on nursing home care totaling $53.1 billion and spending on home health care totaling $20.8 billion. As a result of the growth in the cost of health care for low-income and older adults under Medicaid and Medicare, managed care has emerged as a way to control health care costs. Another way legislators have acted to control Medicaid spending on long-term care costs has been the recent enactment of legislation allowing all states to enact legislation that links the purchase of long-term care insurance with Medicaid. In February 2006 Congress passed legislation that permits Medicaid to cover long-term care needs beyond the terms of the policy, with policy holders not required to "spend down" their assets to meet the Medicaid eligibility guidelines (Capretta, 2007).

Medical Benefits for Retired Veterans

The federal government provides health care coverage for retired members of the uniformed services, as well as their spouses and children, through the TRICARE program. TRICARE provides coverage for civilian hospital services, doctors, and other health care services and supplies. With a few exceptions, retirees who become eligible for Medicare lose their TRICARE coverage, and they become dual enrolled in Medicare and the TRICARE for Life program. Under this program, beneficiaries are required to enroll and pay for Medicare

Part B premiums, and Medicare becomes their primary payer. TRICARE for Life is similar to other Medigap policies that act as a second payer to Medicare, paying for out-of-pocket costs for services provided under Medicare. In addition, TRICARE for Life will pay for some health care services not covered by Medicare, including pharmacy benefits, extended hospital and skilled nursing home care, and mental health counselors (U.S. Department of Defense, 2001).

HEALTH PROMOTION AND WELLNESS

The focus on health promotion and wellness has been driven, in part, by the desire to enjoy a high level of functioning in later life. Growing evidence shows that individuals who engage in healthy lifestyle behaviors have positive health outcomes. For example, 7 of the 10 leading causes of death (e.g., heart disease and stroke) can be reduced by changes in lifestyle, including proper nutrition, exercise, reduced alcohol consumption, and not smoking (Belloc & Breslow, 1972). For older adults in particular, health promotion activities can prevent illness in those who are healthy, prevent those who are ill from becoming disabled, and help older adults who are disabled to preserve function and prevent further disability (Institute of Medicine, 1991). Therefore, numerous health promotion programs targeting older adults have emerged. The Older Americans Act (OAA) has supported the funding of health promotion programs, and the Administration on Aging (AoA) has been instrumental in supporting initiatives designed to enhance the wellbeing of older adults. These efforts will be discussed below.

Policy Background

The 1992 amendment to the OAA authorized the creation of *Part F, Disease Prevention and Health Promotion Services*, under Title III. Under the 2000 amendments, the health promotion programs under Part F were moved to Part D and included funding of the following health promotion programs:

- health risk assessments;
- routine health screenings;
- nutrition counseling and education;
- health promotion programs relating to chronic conditions;
- alcohol and substance abuse, smoking cessation, weight loss, stress management;
- physical fitness programs, group exercise, music therapy, art therapy, and dance movement;
- home injury control services;
- mental health;
- education about the availability of preventive services covered under Medicare;
- medication management;
- information about age-related diseases;
- gerontological counseling;
- counseling regarding social services and follow-up health services.

Funding for preventive health services under Part F for fiscal years 1995 and 1996 was $16,982,000 and $15,623,000, respectively. Although the House proposed eliminating funding for Part F programs in 1997, both the President's and Senate's proposed budgets included funding for preventive health programs. For fiscal year 2001, Congress funded preventive health programs at $21,123,000; in 2006 the funding level was $21,400,000 (Administration on Aging [AoA], 2001e; AoA, 2006d).

During the Past two decades, the AoA has been instrumental in sponsoring a number of nationwide initiatives designed to promote health and wellness of older adults. The National Health Promotion Initiative sponsored by the AoA and the U.S. Public Health Service in 1986 was designed to facilitate collaboration between state and local health departments, state and local area agencies on aging (AAAs), and volunteer organizations in developing and implementing health promotion programs (FallCreek, Allen, & Halls, 1986). The initiative targeted four areas of health promotion—injury control, proper drug use, better nutrition, and improved physical fitness. The initiative was responsible for the development of resource materials, including *Health Promotion and Aging: A National Directory of Selected Programs* (FallCreek et al., 1986), *A Healthy Old Age: A Sourcebook for Health Promotion With Older Adults* (FallCreek & Mettler, 1982), and *Health Promotion and Aging: Strategies for Action* (FallCreek & Franks, 1984).

In 1989, the AoA launched the Historically Black Colleges and Universities Initiatives to address the health promotion needs of older adults of color. Ten schools were awarded grants under this initiative to develop strategies and demonstration projects to promote better self-care habits among minority older persons. Health promotion strategies included church-based health promotion programs, programs for low-income older Blacks living in inner cities and rural areas in Georgia using peer counselors, and the creation of videotapes and instructional guides targeted to older African American audiences through public access television (U.S. Department of Health and Human Services, 1993).

In the 1990s, a major initiative sponsored by the AoA was the Action for Health: Older Women's Project, the National Coalition on Disability and Aging, in 1990. The goal of the Action for Health: Older Women's Project was to demonstrate the feasibility of developing and implementing an innovative community-based, peer educator–facilitated health and wellness promotion program for older minority and low-income women (Herman & Wadsworth, 1992). In 1994, the AoA became a participant in the National Coalition on Disability and Aging to focus attention on the common concerns of aged persons and persons with disabilities. The delivery of care under managed care is just one of the topics coalition members examined. In the present decade, the AoA has collaborated with the Centers for Disease Control to focus on diabetes, cardiovascular disease, and rates of immunization in older ethnic minority groups. The AoA earmarked $1 million to support the initiative called Racial and Ethnic Approaches to Community Health 2010 (REACH 2010) (AoA, 2000). Agencies in four communities were awarded demonstration grants designed to educate older ethnic minorities about diabetes, cardiovascular disease, and immunizations. The four agencies were (a) the Boston Public Health Commission, which targeted its efforts to older African Americans; (b) the Latino Education Project of Corpus Christi, Texas, which targeted older Latinos; (c) the National Indian Council on Aging, which targeted Indian and Alaskan Native populations; and (d) Special Services for Groups of Los Angeles, California, which targeted individuals of Southeast Asian descent. A new effort to fund "evidence-based" health promotion and prevention programs began in 2003. Evidence-based prevention programs use interventions that are based on results from scientific studies published in peer-reviewed journals. During 2003, the AoA funded 12 grants totaling over $2 million per year for three years to implement evidence-based prevention programs in the community. The areas of focus were

- falls prevention;
- physical activity;
- sound nutrition;
- medication management;
- disease self-management; and
- depression (AoA, 2003b).

Examples of programs funded through this initiative included the "Chronic Disease Self-Management for African-American Urban Elders" program in Philadelphia, PA, the "Neighborhood Centers, Inc., Activity Centers for Seniors, in Houston, TX, and the "A Matter of Balance" fall prevention program in Portland, MA. In 2004, the AoA partnered with the President's Council on Physical Fitness and Sports, the National Institute on Aging, the Centers for Disease Control, and other federal agencies to launch the *You Can! Steps to Healthier Aging* campaign, a social marketing campaign designed to increase the number of older adults who are active and healthy by using a partnership approach to mobilize communities. More than 2,700 community organizations have joined the campaign. State and local Area Agencies on Aging, in collaboration with community partners, plan to reach an estimated 4.1 million people through information and 420,000 people through programs (AoA, n.d.). In 2006, the AoA continued to support health promotion and prevention activities in the five areas mentioned above and awarded $13 million to 16 states to implement evidence-based programs in senior centers, nutrition programs, senior housing, and faith-based organizations (AoA, 2006e).

Health Promotion Programs and Users

For many years, older adults were not targets of health promotion programs (McGinnis, 1988). As Walker (1989) pointed out, health promotion programs excluded older adults because it was thought that they could not benefit from activities in which the benefits would emerge in the future. In addition, many believed that health promotion programs would not be successful in changing the lifelong behaviors of older adults. Fortunately, both of these notions have been proven to be incorrect and health promotion programs that target older adults have become more frequent in recent years.

Health promotion programs for older adults have shifted from focusing on the management of specific disease conditions to including prevention of illness and injury and the enhancement of health (Walker, 1989). Thus health promotion programs can address a multitude of concerns and be defined in a variety of ways. For example, Teague (1987) defines health promotion as any combination of health education and related organizational, political, and economic interventions designed to facilitate behavioral and environmental changes which prevent, delay the occurrence, or minimize the impact of disease or disability while promoting the independence and wellbeing of older adults (1987, p. 23).

Health promotion programs can be illness specific, such as programs designed to reduce high blood pressure, or can be broad based and include physical fitness, stress management, nutrition, and environmental awareness. In addition, there are different levels of health program intervention strategies (O'Donnell & Ainsworth, cited in Teague, 1987). *Educational health promotion* programs provide participants with information designed to increase awareness, education, and behavior change. Health education can be delivered through lectures, flyers and posters, health fairs, and resource libraries. *Evaluation screening* programs test past, current, and potential health problems. Fitness assessments are perhaps the most popular evaluation screening programs. *Prescription* programs are used in conjunction with evaluation screening and give participants the information they need to correct or prevent a current health problem. Finally, *behavior change support* programs provide participants with evaluation screening, a prescription for change, and the support system needed for participants to be successful in changing health habits.

Best Practice: Parish Nurse Programs

Parish nurse programs have emerged to reduce health care costs and deliver health promotion education outside the formal health care delivery system. Parish Nurse Programs exist in New Zealand, Australia, Canada, the United Kingdom, and the United States. One example is the Parish Nurse Program of Marquette University College of Nursing, that trains registered nurses and places them to work in churches of all denominations. The role of the parish nurse is to (a) educate members about the relationship between lifestyle, attitudes, faith, and wellbeing; (b) counsel members about health issues, self-care to prevent disease, and coping with chronic illness; (c) refer members to the most cost-effective, appropriate community health services; and (d) facilitate programs within the church to promote healing. Specific health promotion activities include counseling on issues such as cancer, AIDS, and high blood pressure; visiting members in their homes; and offering health screenings and health seminars. Parish nurse programs are being developed across the country.

For more information about Marquette's Parish Nurse Program, contact Parish Nurse Preparation Institute, Marquette University College of Nursing, P.O. Box 1881, Milwaukee, WI 53201-1881; phone: 414-288-3802; www.marquette.edu/nursing/Continuing/Parish.shtml.

Health promotion programs may be sponsored by hospitals, universities, churches, departments of public health, local AAAs or aging network members, insurance companies, and community organizations such as the Red Cross. Programs may be delivered in a variety of settings, including shopping malls, senior centers, hospitals, senior housing, and local schools.

Although information about health promotion activities is widely available, little empirical published research documents who participates in formal health promotion programs. Admittedly, the generalizability of such research is limited because of the wide variation in program content, format, and participant characteristics. A handful of studies, however, can provide a tentative understanding of participation rates and benefits.

Best Practice: Activity Centers for Seniors (ACES)—Neighborhood Centers, Inc. Houston, Texas

The goal of Activity Centers for Seniors (ACES) is to increase the physical activity levels in older adults through a managed physical activity program at senior centers in Houston, Texas. The senior centers are located in impoverished urban settings. Outreach and engagement activities will be implemented, as well as health screenings and assessments. The project targets people age 50 and older who are serviced by the NCI Senior Centers. This population comprises low-income, predominantly African-American, Hispanic, and Asian elderly persons who are at significant risk of chronic diseases. The activity program uses a low-cost, evidence-based exercise program called the EnhanceFitness program (www.projectenhance.org/ind/ fitness.html). There are 320 ACES program participants and their caregivers enrolled in 17 classes at 12 sites. Research conducted at the four-month follow-up testing showed that ACES participants had twice the improvement on average as other EnhanceFitness sites and most participants reported feeling better, having more energy and agility, experiencing fewer aches and pains, and being highly satisfied with the program.

For more information, contact Neighborhood Centers, Inc. (NCI), NCI Activity Centers for Seniors (NCI-ACES), P.O. Box 271389, Houston, Texas 77277-1389; phone: 713-669-5260; www.neighborhood-centers.org//en-us/page.aspx?pageid = 96.

Some evidence suggests that participants in health promotion programs have higher incomes and education, have higher levels of community involvement, and are more often women (Given & Given, 2001; Lefebvre, Harden, Rawkowski, Lasater, & Careton, 1987; Pirie et al., 1986). For example, Buchner and Pearson (1989) examined the characteristics of participants in an HMO senior health promotion program. Demographic factors associated with participation included being older and female, having higher levels of income and education, and being a nonsmoker. Ratings of general health status were not related to participation, and participants were more likely to have lower mental and social health ratings than non-participants. Wagner, Grothaus, Hecht, and LaCroix (1991) evaluated a senior health program involving a sample of people who were 65 years and older and who were enrolled in an HMO. The health promotion program consisted of a nurse educator visit to assess health risks, follow-up classes, written materials, and a review of prescription medications. Researchers interviewed the enrollees who chose not to participate. Non-participants had lower levels of education and family income, were less likely to be members of community organizations, were more likely to smoke, and had more negative self-evaluations of chronic conditions and health status than participants. Other studies comparing participants and non-participants in health promotion programs generally conclude that participants are individuals who already have preventive attitudes toward health care and engage in a variety of preventive health behaviors (Carter, Elward, Malmgren, Martin, & Larson, 1991).

For Your Files: **National Institute on Aging Fitness Guide**

The National Institute of Aging (NIA) has two health and fitness resources that you might find useful when encouraging older adults to engage in fitness activities. One guide is *Exercise: A Guide From the National Institute on Aging.* This illustrated booklet describes ways for older people to exercise safely and stay motivated. Drawings and, in the online version, animations show the correct positions for specific exercises. Also included are tests to help older adults track their progress and a chapter on nutrition. NIA also has developed *Exercise: A Video From the National Institute on Aging.* This 48-minute video demonstrates how to start and stick with a safe, effective exercise program that includes aerobic, stretching, balance, and strength-training routines. It features Margaret Richard, star of *Body Electric*, PBS's most popular exercise show. For more information, visit www.nia.nih.gov/HealthInformation/Publications/ExerciseGuide.

Finally, there is some concern that health promotion programs do not have lasting results (Hickey & Stilwell, 1991; Warshaw, 1988). Lalonde, Hooyman, and Blumhagen (1988) investigated the long-term effectiveness of the Wallingford Wellness Project. This project was a three-year community-based health promotion demonstration project that offered 21 weeks of education and behavior change training to persons 55 and older in physical fitness, stress management, nutrition, and environmental awareness and action. An experimental group ($n = 90$) was recruited from the community and a comparison group ($n = 44$) was recruited through social groups. Follow-up studies revealed that the project was most effective in the short term—up to six months following graduation from the program. Participants reported sustaining behavior changes initiated in physical fitness, stress management, and nutrition; these behavioral changes declined, however, when measured six months later. With regard to retaining health information, participants sustained their increase in health information over pretest levels, except for nutrition information. The project was ineffective in reducing health service use among participants. In contrast, Buchner, Cress, de Lateur, and colleagues (1997) examined the impact of a community-based exercise program where participants engaged in aerobic exercise and strength training. Researchers found that there were positive outcomes in strength, aerobic capacity, and fall reduction at the end of the program. Moreover, 58% of the participants were engaging in unsupervised exercise three or more times per week nine months after they started the program. In a review of 29 physical activity health promotion programs, King, Rejeski, and Buchner (1998) found that the majority of studies reported that the respondents had physical activity levels or fitness levels that were greater than their baseline levels and better than control groups. More recently, researchers have been examining the factors associated with interest in and adherence to health promotion activities. Effective strategies for promoting participation include the use of behavioral or cognitive-behavioral strategies, such as goal setting, along with health education and instruction (Ettinger, Burns, Messier, et al., 1997), locations that are easily accessible (Grove & Spier, 1999), providing individualized assessments and counseling (Fox, Breuer, & Wright, 1997), using a combination of group and home-based program delivery format (King, Haskell, Taylor, Kraemer, & DeBusk, 1991; Rejecki & Brawley, 1997), and taking into account cultural differences (Zhan, Cloutterbuck,

Keshian, & Lombardi, 1998). Clearly, more rigorous studies are needed to evaluate and compare the effectiveness of different types of health promotion and wellness programs offered to older adults.

Best Practice: EnhanceFitness

EnhanceFitness is a health promotion program managed by Senior Services of Seattle/King County in collaboration with Group Health Cooperative and the University of Washington Health Promotion Research Center. The program is a low-cost, evidence-based exercise program that can help active and near-frail older adults become more active, energized, and empowered to sustain independent lives. EnhanceFitness focuses on stretching, flexibility, balance, low-impact aerobics, and strength training exercises. The EnhanceFitness program does not require expensive equipment or a large space and is led by certified fitness instructors who receive training and a detailed manual, which will give them the expertise they need to lead three one-hour classes each week. Empirical research from over 80 sites around the country showed that the program significantly improved overall fitness and health. Results found that 13% of participants reported improvement in social function, 52% reported improvement in depression, and 35% reported improvement in physical functioning. Another study of participants in ethnic community sites with nutrition programs showed that these participants, although less physically fit to start with when compared to majority-White communities, showed greater improvement than those in majority-White sites. EnhanceFitness has won awards from the National Council on Aging, the U.S. Administration on Aging, and the U.S. Department of Health & Human Services. For the results of the research on program effectiveness, see Belza, Shumway-Cook, Phelan, Williams, Snyder, & LoGerfo (2006).

For more information about EnhanceFitness, contact Project Enhance, Senior Services of Seattle/King County, 2208 Second Avenue, Suite 100, Seattle, WA 98121; phone: 206-727-6219; www.projectenhance.org/pro/fitness.html; e-mail ProjectEnhance@seniorservices.org.

CHALLENGES FOR HEALTH CARE AND HEALTH PROMOTION PROGRAMS

Serving Diverse Groups of Older Adults

Extending health promotion and prevention programs to all elderly individuals, especially those hard-to-reach populations, will be critical as the aging population increases in number. Outreach efforts and programs must endeavor to serve elders with lower education and incomes, who are ethnically and racially diverse, as well as those who are physically frail and have multiple chronic conditions. Effective health promotion intervention programs must take into consideration the social and environmental barriers to participation that are unique to those with lower socioeconomic characteristics (Belansky, Belza,

Buchner, Marshall, McTigue, & Prohaska et al., 2006). Health promotion programs must also be sensitive to the cultural characteristics of their participants and be cognizant of differences in language, perceptions, and life experiences (Zhan et al., 1998). For example, Ralston (1993) identified programmatic strategies for health promotion programs targeting older Blacks, including using an educational framework with scheduled classes to deliver information, using Black churches to sponsor programs and using peer leaders to act as liaisons between older adults and the health care delivery system. In addition, health promotion programs must be sensitive to participants' social and environmental context. Something as simple as instructing older inner-city participants to take daily walks may be unsuccessful because they fear walking in their neighborhood or simply lack sidewalks that are safe to walk on (Brawley, Rejeski, & King, 2003; Minkler & Pasick, 1985). Although providing education about preventive health behaviors is an important factor in changing personal behavior, scholars have criticized health promotion programs for focusing too much on individual behaviors while ignoring social factors which negatively impact poor health, including poverty, racism, sexism, ageism, and environmental hazards (Hickey & Stilwell, 1991; Minkler & Pasick, 1985).

Health promotion programs will be meaningless if issues such as access and affordability to health care services continue to be problematic for many low-income older adults. Moreover, older adults should not be overlooked when developing health promotion programs because of an erroneous perception that older adults are unwilling or unable to make healthy lifestyle changes (Chernoff, 2001).

Increasing Research and Program Evaluation

Empirical research must continue to examine the factors associated with participation in and benefits of health promotion programs. Researchers should continue to investigate models that can assist in identifying the motivational forces that are associated with participation in a wide variety of formal health promotion programs (Pascucci, 1992). Professionals designing health promotion programs must also develop evidence-based programs that are based on what research findings show "works," and it is equally important that these programs be evaluated for their effectiveness and sustainability (Bryant, Altpeter, & Whitelaw, 2006). White House Conference on Aging delegates recommended that state health departments and local aging network agencies promote, implement, and evaluate evidence-based health promotion and disease prevention programs at the local level for all citizens.

Supporting Health Programs and Policies in the Future

Traditional health care, with its focus on acute care, does not adequately address the health care needs of older adults who must live with and manage chronic conditions. Older adults need regular primary care to help them prevent illness and maintain their health. Preventive services for the control of high blood pressure, cancer screenings, immunizations, and therapies to help manage chronic conditions are key to extending a healthy life in later life (U.S. Department of Health and Human Services, 1990). Delegates to the White House Conference on Aging (2005) recommended a number of strategies and resolutions designed to enhance the health status of older adults. These included

- expanding Medicare to include oral health services, vision services, and eyeglasses, hearing services, and other emerging preventive services; and
- increasing federal funding to the National Institutes of Health, the Centers for Disease Control, and Title III of the OAA to reduce health disparities and promote health promotion programming for all minority populations, including gays, lesbians, bisexuals, transgender, and seniors with disabilities.

Finally, the delegates adopted four resolutions related to health and health promotion:

- Reduce health care disparities among minorities by developing strategies to prevent disease, promote health, and deliver appropriate care and wellness.
- Improve the health and quality of life of older Americans through disease management and chronic care coordination.
- Prevent disease and promote healthier lifestyles through educating providers and consumers on consumer health care.
- Improve health decision making through the promotion of health education, health literacy, and cultural competency.

Indeed, the challenge facing U.S. society in the next century is creating a health care system that provides all its members, of every age, with accessibility to health care, including regular preventive care, primary care, and health promotion programs.

CASE STUDY

Health Concerns After Retirement

David, 60, retired a year ago from a high-level executive position with a major auto company. His retirement meant the end to 25 years of long hours in fast-paced, high-stress management work. It also meant the end to grueling overseas travel and weeks of separation from his family. During this past year, David has been helping his wife, Evelyn, move into a smaller, but new, home. He has had a lot of time to think about what he would like to do next. David has decided to use his experience by developing a part-time international consulting business that would allow him to work in his home office part time.

Lately, David has been feeling tired and sleeping poorly. He decided that he should have a complete checkup before launching into his new endeavor. He was both anxious and excited about meeting his new doctor, recommended by another retired executive. He told David not to expect to leave this doctor's office with a prescription in hand after a 30-minute visit. The friend was right. The checkup ended up taking two weeks and consisted of a thorough recounting of David's medical history, family medical history, and lifestyle choices. It also included an examination and a series of laboratory tests.

When David returned for the results of his evaluation, he was presented with some startling facts. His doctor told him frankly that he was headed into a lifetime of chronic health problems unless he drastically changed his lifestyle. Specifically, his blood pressure and blood sugar levels were too high, and his insomnia problems were probably due to too much alcohol consumption on a daily basis. The doctor complimented David for quitting smoking 10 years earlier. However, because of the other factors, and because David's father died of heart disease, David was still at risk of heart disease and other complications. The doctor strongly recommended some major lifestyle interventions.

Case Study Questions

1. Would you say that David's doctor is being responsible by strongly recommending lifestyle changes for David? What research supports your answer? Why might David not have encountered such medical recommendations 10 or 15 years ago?

2. In what ways does David fit or not fit the profile of someone who would participate in a health promotion program? Would you say that David has a preventive attitude about his situation?

3. The chapter describes four possible models of health promotion programs. Describe each model and explain how each might apply to David's situation.

4. Without knowing the specific community in which David and his doctor live, where generally might David look for health promotion support for his lifestyle-change work? Find out what health promotion programs are available in your city. Based on what you find, what would you recommend for David?

5. First and foremost, David's doctor is concerned with David's health and wellbeing. In light of current health care trends, how is this case an economic concern for the doctor and for society?

Learning Activities

1. Interview an older adult about his or her physical health. What chronic conditions does the individual have? How do these interfere with activities of daily living? What has the person done to adjust to any impairments? Does the person use any assistive technology devices (low- or high-tech) to help with activities?

2. Ask an older family member or friend to share with you a recent hospital or doctor's bill and the Medicare invoice that corresponds to that health care episode. After gaining the person's permission (and ensuring confidentiality), report to the class the type of health care episode, the amount the health care provider charged, the amount Medicare paid, the amount paid by a Medigap policy (if there is one), and the amount paid by the patient. How easy or difficult was it to gather this information from the invoices sent by each provider?

3. Go to the Medicare.gov site and investigate whether PPOs or HMOs are in your area. If so, check the website and find out what model of PPO or HMO they adhere to and compare the plans with Medicare and a standard Medigap policy. What are the differences in coverage?

4. What health promotion programs are available in your community for older adults? Who sponsors these programs? What services and information are offered in these programs?

For More Information

National Resources

1. American Diabetes Association, 1701 N. Beauregard Street, Alexandria, VA 22314; phone: 703-549-1500 or 800-342-2383; www.diabetes.org.

   The American Diabetes Association works to prevent and cure diabetes and to improve the quality of life of persons affected with diabetes. It provides information about the diagnosis and treatment of diabetes and resources available to assist people with this disease. Local chapters of the association provide support and educational materials. The association publishes *Diabetes Forecast*, a monthly publication about living with diabetes, and numerous pamphlets including *Older Adults: Diabetes and You*.

2. American Heart Association, 7272 Greenville Avenue, Dallas, TX 75231; phone: 214-373-6300; www.americanheart.org.

   The American Heart Association funds research and conducts public education programs on the prevention and control of heart, stroke, and cardiovascular disease. It distributes a number of pamphlets in English and Spanish for older adults, including *Walking for a Healthy Heart* and *An Older Person's Guide to Cardiovascular Health*.

3. The Center for Healthy Aging, c/o National Council on Aging, 1901 L Street, N.W., 4th Floor, Washington, D.C. 20036; phone: 202-479-1200; www.healthyagingprograms.org.

   The Center for Healthy Aging encourages and assists community-based organizations serving older adults to develop and implement evidence-based health promotion/disease prevention programs. Evidence-based programming translates tested program models or interventions into practical, effective community programs that can provide proven health benefits to participants. The website contains information and support for evidence-based health promotion programs in the areas of chronic disease, disabilities, fall prevention, health promotion, medication management, mental health/substance abuse, nutrition and physical activity. Examples of evidence-based programs are also available on the website.

4. Arthritis Foundation, 1330 West Peach Street, Atlanta, GA 30309; phone: 404-872-7100 or 800-283-7800; www.arthritis.org.

   The Arthritis Foundation offers health education programs, brochures, and a bimonthly magazine about resources and programs to help persons with arthritis. Local chapters sponsor exercise programs, support groups, and resource materials.

5. Centers for Disease Control National Prevention Information Network, P.O. Box 6003, Rockville, MD 20849; phone: 800-311-3435; www.cdcnpin.org.

   The National Prevention Network, a referral source for identifying health care resources for persons with AIDS, can help callers locate educational materials. Inquirers can obtain a number of publications, including *AIDS is an Aging Issue: Facts—HIV/AIDS* and *Older Adults and La Edad no le Va a Librar del SIDA [Age Won't Protect You From AIDS]*.

6. The Centers for Medicare and Medicaid (formerly Health Care Financing Administration), P.O. Box 340, Columbia, MD 21045; phone: 410-786-3000 or 800-638-6833; www.cms.hhs.gov.

   The Centers for Medicare and Medicaid coordinate the Medicare program and have publications for consumers, including *The Medicare Handbook* and *Guide to Health Insurance for People on Medicare*.

7. National Caucus and Center on Black Aged, Inc., 1220 L Street N.W., Suite 800, Washington, DC, 20005; phone: 202-637-8400; www.ncba-aged.org.

   The National Caucus and Center on Black Aged has publications on its website including *The Healing Zone Health Update Newsletter* and *Health Status of Older African Americans*.

Web Resources

1. Healthtouch Online: www.healthtouch.com.

   Healthtouch's home page offers health resources and health information. Its website provides a searchable database of prescription and over-the-counter drugs and a health resource directory that provides information about how to contact health organizations for more information about specific health topics. The site also has information about many topics related to health, wellness, diseases, and illnesses.

2. Canadian Fitness and Lifestyle Research Institute: http://www.cflri.ca/eng.

   The mission of the Canadian Fitness and Lifestyle Research Institute is to enhance the wellbeing of Canadians through research and communication of information about physically active lifestyles to the public and private sectors. The site has links to numerous publications on staying active and fit, many directed toward older adults. It's worth the trip to Canada!

3. National Center for Chronic Disease Prevention and Health Promotion: www.cdc.gov/nccdphp.

   The center has a site with links to statistical and educational information about chronic disease, disease prevention and control, and community health promotion.

4. Family Health, College of Osteopathic Medicine at Ohio University: www.fhradio.org.

   The College of Osteopathic Medicine at Ohio University has developed a series of 2½-minute audio programs designed to reach a general audience with practical, easy-to-understand answers to some frequently asked questions about health and health care. Topics currently available include arthritis, frailty and older adults, urinary incontinence, and exercise. Check out this new way of delivering health education via the net!

NOTES

1. Under the Welfare Reform Act called the Personal Responsibility and Work Opportunity Reconciliation Act of 1996, AFDC is replaced by Temporary Assistance to Needy Families (TANF). Under this legislation, states have been given more leeway to determine Medicaid eligibility for families with children.

2. Services to mothers and children under the Medicaid provisions for the categorically needy are not listed.

12

Mental Health Services

Phil, a 78-year-old widower, lived independently until about six months ago. At that time, he realized he no longer could get around without the help of a walker. Just as he was accepting this restriction, his eye doctor told him that nothing more could be done to treat his macular degeneration. Now Phil is legally blind. Because of his independent nature, the eye specialist referred him to a rehabilitation counselor for persons with visual impairments. Although Phil made progress on learning new skills, the counselor became increasingly concerned about his extreme mood swings from anger to despondency and referred him to the mental health center's peer counseling program. After a few weeks of talking one on one with the peer counselor, Phil agreed to participate twice per week in a group of other older adults with similar experiences. Phil likes the idea of talking through his problems with someone his own age. He says, "I am getting the help I need without people thinking I am crazy."

Approximately 7 million people aged 65 and older in the United States have a psychiatric illness, and that number is expected to double to 15 million in the next three decades (Jeste et al., 1999). Some older adults have had serious mental illnesses (e.g., schizophrenia, bipolar disorder) most of their adult lives; others have had periodic episodes of mental illness throughout their lives. For other older adults, like Phil, factors such as a decline in physical health, loss of independence, lower socioeconomic status, multiple stressful life events, and limited social support seriously influence their mental health status for the first time in their lives.

This chapter focuses on mental health services for older adults and their families. We begin by examining federal support for mental health programs and services. Next, we profile older adults with mental health problems and describe the various types of programs designed specifically to address their needs. We conclude this part of the chapter with a discussion of the current and future issues in delivering mental health programs. The second part of the chapter examines mental health services targeted to caregivers of elders with physical and/or cognitive impairments.

POLICY BACKGROUND

The Community Mental Health Act of 1963 created a major change in the provision of mental health services in the United States. It changed the focus of care from long-term, custodial, institutional care in state hospitals to active, outpatient, community-based care. A major goal of outpatient care for all individuals, including older adults, is to encourage maximum independence. This translates into the need for mental health programs and services aimed at keeping older persons within their own homes and communities.

Mental health services for older adults constitute only about 2.5% of Medicare expenditure. Medicare coverage for mental health services was expanded in 1990 (via the Omnibus Budget Reconciliation Act [OBRA] of 1989), but coverage of specialized services is still limited. For example, although there are few limitations on the total number of hospitalization or inpatient days for psychiatric care in general hospitals, coverage for inpatient care in freestanding psychiatric hospitals is limited to 190 days during an individual's lifetime. Outpatient psychotherapy requires a 50% co-payment, while a 20% co-payment is required for medical management, diagnostic services, and professional services for evaluation. A 20% co-payment also is required for partial hospitalization programs that provide structured intensive services for those in acute psychiatric distress who would be hospitalized without these services. OBRA (1989) expanded the coverage for services provided by nonphysician providers. Psychologists and clinical social workers rendering mental health services are now eligible for direct reimbursement; previously, reimbursement was made only when the services provided by these professionals were under the direct supervision of a physician.

In response to the changes put forward by OBRA, the National Association of Insurance Commissioners revised the model Medicare Supplemental (Medigap) insurance regulations. All Medigap policies are now required to cover the 50% co-insurance for outpatient mental health care under Medicare Part B (Finkel, 1993). Unfortunately, this change is prospective, so it does not apply to older adults holding Medigap policies in effect prior to their state's adoption of the new model regulation.

In the 1990s, the number of Medicare participants increased and the cost of maintaining the program rose exponentially. In response to accusations of alleged fraud and abuse of services, the federal government passed the Balanced Budget Act of 1997 to curtail spending and place tighter controls on Medicare providers. As a result, the Health Care Financing Administration (HCFA) (in 2001 renamed the Centers for Medicare and Medicaid Services, or CMS) implemented 16 demonstration sites to test the effectiveness of coordinating care for chronically ill, fee-for-service Medicare beneficiaries. Four of the 11 targeted conditions are mental health conditions: psychoses, Alzheimer's disease, alcohol and drug abuse, and depression. Participating beneficiaries received intervention to improve self-care, identify complications early, avoid hospitalization, and better coordinate treatments and medications for multiple conditions. CMS continues to examine the impact of coordination on clinical outcomes, client satisfaction, quality of life, and the appropriate use of covered services (HCFA, 2001b).

In 1999, the U.S. Supreme Court ruled in *Olmstead v. L.C.* that anyone receiving mental health services was to be served in the least restrictive environment possible. Implications for this ruling required states to develop a system of services to handle the needs of persons with mental illness for whom institutional placement is inappropriate. To meet recipient needs effectively, states were given the latitude to develop programs independently from other states. As a result, Medicaid services vary substantially among states. Coverage includes mandatory and optional services. General hospital inpatient care, physician services, outpatient services in general hospitals, emergency room services, and nursing home care are mandatory. These services focus on the needs of patients with acute illness episodes and persons who need to be in a nursing home. The optional services help persons with chronic mental impairments living in community settings. These services include care by nonphysicians, freestanding outpatient clinics, case management, rehabilitation, and home health care. Many states have not adopted Medicaid's optional elements. In those states that have, providers are often reluctant to participate because of the low rates of reimbursement. In addition, few states have home- and community-based services waivers for individuals with chronic mental illnesses (Lutzky, Alecxih, Duffy, & Neill, 2000).

In response to the Deficit Reduction Act of 2005, which called for further reduction of long-term care spending, CMS announced a new demonstration project to identify how long-term support programs can be rebalanced. *Money Follows the Person* (MFP) is a system of flexible financing for long-term services and supports, which enables available funds to move with the individual to the most appropriate and preferred setting as the individual's needs and preferences change. This approach supports the concept of least restrictive environment and allows the consumer to remain in the community, thus reducing unnecessary institutionalization.

As part of Medicaid reform, Congress passed the Omnibus Budget Reconciliation Act of 1987. This legislation requires that all prospective nursing home applicants who have a primary or secondary diagnosis of a major mental disorder undergo a preadmission screening to determine whether they are appropriate candidates for nursing home admission and if they need active treatment for mental illness. The mental disorders covered by OBRA include schizophrenia, paranoid disorders, major affective disorders, schizo-affective disorders, and atypical psychoses. Nursing homes who admit older adults with designated psychiatric conditions without conducting the prescreening are denied Medicaid payments.

The Social Security Administration administers several programs that provide cash payments or other benefits to persons with mental disabilities. Persons with adequate work histories usually receive monthly cash payments as Social Security benefits, and persons with minimal resources and insufficient work history usually receive a monthly payment under the Supplemental Security Income (SSI) program. Based on the number of SSI recipients aged 65 and older, it is estimated that approximately 20%, or 400,000 people, receive government disability payments because of their mental disorders (Karlin & Norris, 2006; Social Security Administration, 2006b).

Older Americans Act (OAA) funds also may be used to support mental health services for older adults under Title III-B and III-F. Title III-B, which allocates spending for a wide range of supportive services, includes funding for mental health programs. Local Area Agency on Aging (AAA) funds can be used to support mental health programs and services designed to enable older adults to attain and maintain mental wellbeing. Funding also may be authorized under Title III-F, which funds disease prevention and health promotion services. Health promotion services can include screening for the prevention of depression, coordination of community mental health services, provision of educational activities, and referral to psychiatric and psychological services. Thus local AAAs have the opportunity to fund a wide variety of mental health programs and services under the OAA.

USERS AND PROGRAMS

Characteristics of Mental Health Clients

One in four older adults has a significant mental disorder (26%), including 16% with a primary psychiatric illness, 3% with dementia complicated by significant psychiatric symptoms, and 7% with uncomplicated dementia (Jeste et al., 1999). Among the most common mental health problems in older persons are depression, anxiety disorders, and dementia (Narrow, Rae, Robins, & Regier, 2002).

Depression is the most common reason for referring older persons for mental health services (Blazer, 2003). As many as 15% of community-dwelling older adults (Blazer, 1994) and 40% of elders living in long-term care facilities (Parmalee, Katz, & Lawton, 1992) suffer from depressive symptoms. In the majority of cases, their depression is viewed as a reactive depression (i.e., the person is reacting to a major life loss or transition) rather than as stemming from other etiologies. Throughout late life, women report a higher prevalence of depressive symptoms than their male counterparts (Federal Interagency Forum, 2004). Other reasons why older adults are referred for mental health services include Alzheimer's disease and other organic mental disorders, affecting approximately 10% of individuals 65 years of age and older living in the community; suicide behaviors—20% of all suicides are committed by adults 65 years of age and older; and alcoholism, which affects up to 15% of older adults, the same rate as found in the general population (Substance Abuse and Mental Health Services Administration, 2004). Greater percentages of elders from minority groups (i.e., Blacks, Hispanics, American Indians, and Asian-Pacific Islanders) report having mental health problems than do their White counterparts. Within these minority groups, women tend to have higher rates of affective and anxiety disorders, whereas men tend to have higher rates of substance abuse–dependence disorders (Stanford & Bois, 1992).

According to the Surgeon General's report on culture, race, and ethnicity (U.S. Department of Health and Human Services, 2001a), although members of minority groups have a great need for mental health services, they tend not to receive adequate services. In general, minorities have less access to mental health services and those who are treated tend to receive poorer quality of mental health care.

Best Practice: Lifespan's Geriatric Addiction Program

Lifespan, founded in 1971, has provided services to Rochester, New York, area older adults and caregivers for 35 years. In 2001 it began implementing the Geriatric Addiction Program (GAP) after discovering that many older adults did not fit well within traditional treatment programs which are usually geared toward a younger population. GAP provides intervention, assessment, linkage, and counseling within older adult substance abusers' homes. As of 2006, GAP has served approximately 450 older adults and trained more than 850 professionals and 650 nonprofessionals and caregivers in the recognition and dynamics of geriatric addictions. For more information, contact the GAP staff at 1900 S. Clinton Avenue, Rochester, New York 14618; phone: 585-244-8400; www.lifespan-roch.org.

Source: Aging Today (July–August, 2006).

Older adults are less likely than younger persons to self-identify mental health problems and seek specialty mental health services (Corrigan, Swantek, Watson, & Kleinlein, 2003); fewer than 3% report seeing a mental health professional for treatment. This problem of under-identification is further compounded by family members and professional providers who share the misperception that mental disorders are a "normal" part of aging. Several demographic variables are associated with the use of mental health services among older adults (Black, Rabins, German, McGuire, & Roca, 1997; Freiman, Cunningham, & Cornelius, 1993). For example, increasing age is associated with a lower probability of using mental health services, as is minority status. Women and individuals who are recently widowed have a significantly higher probability of health care use for mental problems than do men and married persons. Also, the more acute and chronic the health problems reported by older adults, the more likely those adults are to be using mental health services.

Although rural elders are one of the greatest at-risk groups for experiencing mental health problems (Substance Abuse and Mental Health Services Administration, 2004), only about 5% of rural community mental health centers' patients and 2 to 4% of rural private patients with psychiatric problems are older adults (Karlin & Norris, 2006). Several factors adversely influence the appropriate use of mental health services by rural elders, including sociodemographic, economic, and cultural issues; the lack of mental health professionals to work with aged individuals; and the stigma surrounding mental illness and its treatment (Chumbler, Cody, Booth, & Beck, 2001; Karlin & Norris, 2006).

Estimates of the number of older adults with serious and persistent mental illnesses (e.g., schizophrenia, delusional disorder, mood disorder) range from 2% (Colenda, Bartels, & Gottlieb, 2002) to 4% (Kessler et al., 2002). There is considerable heterogeneity among older adults with serious mental illness with respect to functioning and their need for support. Most older adults with serious mental illnesses live in the community; however, they are three times more likely to be admitted to a nursing home than older individuals without serious mental illnesses (Bartels, Forester, Miles, & Joyce, 2000). For many older individuals with serious mental illness, nursing home placement reflects a lack of community-based alternatives.

Residents of long-term care facilities also benefit from mental health services. The three major nursing home resident groups needing such services are persons who are physically ill but cognitively capable; persons who are mentally ill but cognitively capable; and those with dementia. Although different therapeutic issues arise and different interventions are needed for each group, all long-term care residents face similar situations in which they may require emotional support, including making the transition into the facility, establishing relationships with staff, adapting to the institution's schedule, adjusting to new roles with family caregivers or to a lack of family caregivers, and accommodating to a new activities schedule (Lichtenberg, 1994). Unfortunately, results of a national survey revealed that less than one-fifth of older residents in nursing homes who need mental health services receive them (Smyer, Shea, & Streit, 1994). Those receiving mental health services were more likely to have a specific mental health diagnosis, were exhibiting mood disturbances, and had been transferred from a psychiatric hospital. This suggests that services were more likely to be directed toward individuals with more severe impairments. In addition, age was a factor. Individuals between the ages of 64 and 74 were more likely than older patients to receive care.

Mental Health Programs

Older adults represent 13% of the U.S. population but receive only 6% of community mental health services (U.S. Administration on Aging, 2001d). For most older adults, mental health intervention does not mean going into a counselor's office or receiving help from a specialized mental health care center (see Exhibit 12.1). As few as 2–4% (Karlin & Norris, 2006) of persons seen in private psychiatric offices and only 5% of patients who receive community mental health services are 65 years of age and older (Center for Mental Health Services, 2007). This can be attributed to several factors:

- Most centers are not widely accessible and tend to be isolated from the mainstream of community health and social services for older adults.
- Mental health service programs have not aggressively engaged in outreach and case finding; rather, they tend to rely on referrals and self-identification of potential clients.
- Reimbursement for treatment of mental disorders under Medicare is substantially lower and less comprehensive than for physical disorders (Chumbler, Cody, Booth, & Beck, 2001; Lebowitz & Niederehe, 1992).

The aging service network provides a wide range of mental health services for older adults. The results of a national mail survey of AAAs (Bane, Rathbone-McCuan, & Galliher, 1994) indicated that the most common services available in rural planning and service areas (PSAs) were telephone reassurance, mental health screening, individual counseling, and

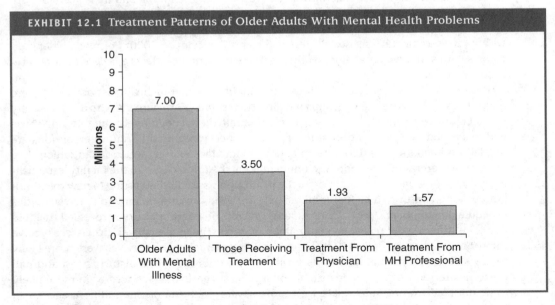

EXHIBIT 12.1 Treatment Patterns of Older Adults With Mental Health Problems

Source: U.S. Department of Health and Human Services/Administration on Aging (2001b).

Alzheimer's support groups. In mixed PSAs (i.e., areas with rural, urban, and suburban counties), the most common mental health services were Alzheimer's support groups, counseling, and mental health referral and materials. Great variability in the community resources that facilitate these services to older adults was found in both the rural and mixed PSAs. For example, more than 80% of respondents in both areas reported the availability of adult protective service intervention for older persons with mental health problems, whereas only 12% of the rural PSAs and 31% of the mixed PSAs reported having a mobile mental health team that traveled to the person's home.

Mental health services and counseling may take place in a health care setting (i.e., physician's office or clinic), the client's residence (i.e., own home or nursing home), a senior center, or an adult day center. For example, in Tallahassee, Florida, a professional counselor is available two days a week at the local senior center to help seniors work through their problems (go to www.talgov.com/dncs/seniors/services.cfm). The Geriatric Service team in Baltimore County, Maryland, provides oversight and consultation for services for older adults with serious and persistent mental illness. Services include the PEERS program, which matches volunteers to elderly people, and the county's Consumer Drop-In Centers (see www.co.ba.md.us/Agencies/health/mental/mhadultsvc.html). The Halton Geriatric Mental Health Outreach Program in Ontario is designed to provide specialized service to older adults with complex mental health needs (e.g., mental health problems accompanied by significant medical illness and/or functional needs; late-onset severe mental illness). Services are brought to where the person resides (e.g., their own home, LTC facility) because the person cannot or will not access the help they need through traditional services (visit http://search.hipinfo.info/details.asp?UseCICVw = 34&RSN = 12647). Mental health specialists in Alabama report that brief, home-delivered psychosocial intervention can be an effective approach for treating rural older adults with emotional complaints such as depression, anxiety, and loneliness (Kaufman, Scogin, MaloneBeach, Baumhover, & McKendree-Smith, 2000).

Relatively few community-based services are available to older adults with serious or chronic mental illness who are at risk, or have a history, of psychiatric hospitalization (Center for Mental Health Services, 2004). A nationwide survey of 73 mental health agencies providing outpatient psychiatric services to this group of older adults provides some descriptive information about the services provided and the problems facing agencies serving older adults with chronic mental illness (Mosher-Ashley & Allard, 1993). The majority of agencies surveyed were community mental health centers (87%). The primary services provided to older adults with chronic mental illness were counseling, crisis intervention, case management, group therapy, case consultation, in-service training, and day treatment. The most common problems agencies faced in providing services to older clients with chronic mental illness were insufficient funds, lack of residential services, lack of transportation, and insufficient staffing.

Although community-based treatment of older adults with mental health problems is preferred by both older adults and mental health professionals, a small proportion of older individuals need more intensive care provided by institutions. In 2005, persons older than age 65 represented 4% of all individuals receiving inpatient psychiatric services (Center for Mental Health Services, 2007). Symptoms of depression, anxiety, dementia, paranoia, delusional ideation, and alcohol and drug abuse are the most likely reasons for admission of older persons to psychiatric hospitals. The need for hospitalization is dependent on the severity of symptoms and the older person's ability to carry out activities of daily living. In addition, patients frequently have concomitant physical illnesses that also must be addressed.

The number of specifically trained individuals to provide mental health services targeted for geriatric patients is small. Four major clusters of professionals treat older adults: psychiatric nurses, clinical social workers, psychologists, and psychiatrists (Halpain, Harris, McClure, & Jeste, 1999). They work in settings such as community mental health centers, inpatient settings, HMOs, public and private agencies, hospitals, nursing homes, and private practice. Mental health services for older adults may also be provided by physicians certified in geriatric medicine, counselors and therapists, and pastoral counselors.

Trained paraprofessionals, known as Qualified Mental Health Professionals (QMHPs), also provide psychological and psychosocial interventions with older adults under the supervision of experienced professionals. Criteria for QMHPs are determined by the states. In some cases they offer formal mental health services, whereas in others they provide informal support. Paraprofessionals work alone, in conjunction with, or under the supervision of trained professionals. One type of paraprofessional program that has grown rapidly during the past two decades is peer counseling programs for older adults. These programs train and supervise older adults to provide counseling and support to other older individuals. Peer counselors typically address a broad range of issues including depression, loneliness, problems that result from physical impairments, and other concerns related to aging, gender, and ethnicity. They receive supervision from a professional counselor employed by the agency sponsoring the program. Programs often begin because they are a cost-effective means of providing mental health services for older adults. The benefits of peer counseling programs for older adults include

- Many older people talk more readily to older people than to professional therapists;
- Peer counselors serve as positive models for their clients;
- Peer counseling enriches the lives of both the client and the counselor; and
- Peer counselors may be more effective than professionals because they are often more aware of the problems of older people (Bratter & Freeman, 1990).

A growing number of mental health and aging coalitions are engaged in efforts to improve the availability and quality of mental health prevention and treatment services to older adults and their families through education, research, and increased public awareness. For example, the National Coalition on Mental Health and Aging (NCMHA) provides guidelines for building state and community mental health and aging coalitions. Older mental health consumers voice their concerns and promote awareness of the need for home and community-based mental health services through participation in the Older Adult Consumers of Mental Health Alliance (OACMHA). The main purpose of OACMHA is to improve the quality of and access to mental health services for older adults (Bazelon Center, 2000). The Substance Abuse and Mental Health Services Administration (SAMHSA) and the National Council on Aging are collaborating to identify ways to engage providers of aging services in substance abuse and mental health education, screening, prevention, treatment referrals, and follow-up activities (Administration on Aging [AoA], 2001d). Working with the Health Resources and Services

Administration and other U.S. Department of Health and Human Services agencies, SAMHSA is evaluating various methods of delivering and financing mental health and substance abuse services for older adults in primary health care settings.

> **Best Practice: Gatekeeper Program**
>
> This program, originally developed in 1978 in Spokane County, Washington, is designed to seek out and offer assistance to at-risk older adults living in isolation. This is accomplished through "gatekeepers," nontraditional referral sources such as postal workers, meter readers, phone operators, and others who come into contact with older adults on a regular basis. Gatekeepers are trained to identify and refer at-risk older adults to appropriate support agencies that can intervene and solve a problem before it becomes a major crisis. For more information about the Gatekeeper Program visit its website at www.smhca.org/gatekeeper.aspx.

CHALLENGES FOR MENTAL HEALTH PROGRAMS

The graying of America and the deinstitutionalization of persons with mental illness have resulted in increased attention to the mental health needs of older adults. Although significant improvements in the delivery of mental health services have been made since the passage of the Community Mental Health Act in 1963 and the funding of mental health programs under the OAA, many challenges remain to improve the delivery of mental health services to older adults (AoA, 2001d).

Connecting the Delivery Systems

The two primary systems involved in providing community services to older adults with mental health concerns are the public mental health system (primarily community mental health centers) and the aging service network. A formal relationship between community mental health centers and the aging network, however, is often the exception rather than the rule. This is unfortunate for older adults because those centers with formal relationships with local AAAs tend to provide a larger range of services to older adults, provide services to older adults in more settings, and provide mental health services to higher proportions of older adults than do those without formal affiliations (Kuiken, 2004). Thus, joining forces appears to be the most effective and efficient means of reaching and serving older adults with mental health concerns.

Reaching Diverse Groups

Older adults from minority groups use mental health services to a lesser extent than their White counterparts, yet they appear to have the same, if not greater, need for such services. Use is affected by language barriers, limited access to information regarding available services, transportation, cultural dissimilarity, and reduced social and economic resources (Abramson, Trejo, & Lai, 2002). Because individuals from ethnic minority groups represent a rapidly increasing segment of the total older adult population, mental health services must recognize the importance of cultural sensitivity and cross-cultural training of mental health professionals as one means of eliminating the barriers to, and promoting the use of, mental health services by ethnic minority elders.

The rural older adult population also is vastly underserved by the mental health system (Karlin & Norris, 2006; Neese, Abraham, & Buckwalter, 1999). As in most other service sectors, rural providers are faced with the issues of availability, accessibility, and acceptability of mental health services. In addition, the closure of rural physician practices and hospitals has forced rural citizens either to use local emergency services, regardless of whether they are capable of responding to mental health problems, or to seek health care in distant urban areas (U.S. Congress, Office of Technology Assessment, 1990).

Training Providers

The demand for mental health services is likely to increase as baby boomers tend to utilize mental health services more frequently than the current cohort of older adults and are less stigmatized by seeking mental health care. The number of health care professionals available to treat the growing number of older adults with mental health problems is inadequate. At least 5,000 additional board-certified geriatric psychiatrists and geropsychologists are needed to meet the needs of this growing population (Jeste et al., 1999). Similar needs are projected for the other specialists constituting the core disciplines of geriatric mental health—including counselors, social workers, and psychiatric nurses. Continuing education programs also are needed for current mental health practitioners, many of whom lack the knowledge and skills necessary to effectively work with older adults needing mental health services.

Providing Mental Health Programs in the Future

During the 2005 White House Conference on Aging, delegates passed a resolution to improve recognition, assessment, and treatment of mental illness and depression among older Americans. Strategies for implementing this resolution include

- parity coverage for mental health and substance abuse as compared to physical health in Medicare and all other health programs;
- assuring access to affordable, comprehensive, quality mental health and substance abuse services in a variety of settings including senior centers, housing, nursing facilities, assisted living centers, adult day care, and independent living;
- promoting training and education for early intervention;
- integrating culturally competent older adult mental health and substance abuse services into primary care and other wrap-around service systems; and
- promoting older adult mental health research and coordinating and financing evidence-based and emerging best practices and collaboration between research institutions and community-based service delivery.

Because the vast majority of older adults exist in and interact with a family network, the mental health needs of those within the family network must also be addressed. We now turn our attention to the mental health needs of family caregivers.

MENTAL HEALTH SERVICES FOR FAMILY CAREGIVERS

Almost one in four caregivers provides assistance to a family member with dementia, Alzheimer's disease, mental confusion, or forgetfulness (National Alliance for Caregiving/AARP, 2004). One potential consequence of providing care for older adults with physical and cognitive impairments is an increased risk of mental health problems among family caregivers. Caregivers are highly vulnerable to stress-related physical and emotional complaints. Approximately 20% of family caregivers suffer from depression, twice the rate of the general population (Family Caregiver Alliance, 2002).

Although caring for one's spouse or parent is fairly common practice, particularly for midlife and older women, a family care situation receiving greater attention is that of grandparents assuming full-time parenting responsibilities for their grandchildren. Approximately 2.4 million grandparents have primary responsibility for their grandchildren, of whom 840,000 have been caring for their grandchildren for five or more years (U.S. Bureau of the Census, 2003, October). The majority of grandparents rearing grandchildren are between the ages of 30 and 59 (60%), married (73%), and female (62%). More than half of them are in the labor force and about one-fifth have incomes below the poverty threshold. Although older adults representing all race and ethnic groups are raising grandchildren, minority grandparents are two to three times as likely as their White counterparts to assume the parenting role (Fuller-Thompson, Minkler, & Driver, 1997). Some grandparents report increased physical and mental health problems as a result of assuming parenting responsibilities for their grandchildren (Grinstead, Leder, Jensen, & Bond, 2003).

Community services for caregivers include educational programs, support groups, respite care, and assistance with handling their emotional reactions to the changes in their loved ones. These services may be partially funded or supported by various state, local, and nonprofit voluntary agencies. In this section, we describe the characteristics of caregivers who use mental health services and the types of services available to them. We end with a discussion of the challenges facing programs trying to reach and serve these caregivers.

USERS AND PROGRAMS

Characteristics of Caregivers Using Mental Health Programs

Family caregivers who seek support from mental health professionals present a wide array of problems and concerns. A study of 51 family caregivers who participated in weekly individual counseling sessions revealed nine pressing issues and problems: improving coping skills (time management, dealing with stress, and other coping mechanisms); family issues regarding spouse, siblings, and children; responding to the older person's emotional and behavior needs; physical wellbeing and safety; legal and financial affairs; quality of relationship with the care receiver; eliciting formal and informal support; feelings of guilt and inadequacy; and long-term planning (Smith, Smith, & Toseland, 1991). These problems and issues are consistent with reviews of more recent studies of caregiving demands (c.f., Dilworth-Anderson, Williams, & Gibson, 2002; Schulz & Martire, 2004; Torti, Gwyther, Reed, Friedman, & Schulman, 2004; Yee & Schulz, 2000) and suggest areas in which practitioners need to be prepared to help caregivers with a broad range of problems and concerns.

Mental Health Programs for Family Caregivers

Programs designed to meet the mental health needs of family caregivers include individual counseling, support groups, and educational programs (Bourgeois, Schulz, & Burgio, 1996; Cooke, McNally, Mulligan, Harrison, & Newman, 2001; Zarit, 1996; Zarit & Zarit, 1998). Evaluations of these intervention strategies suggest positive outcomes for the caregivers who participate (Schulz, 2000; Yin, Zhou, & Bashford, 2002).

With respect to individual counseling, spouses of persons with Alzheimer's disease reported less depression after their participation in brief psychodynamic psychotherapy. This approach offered caregivers the opportunity to understand how past conflicts influenced their reactions and responses to their current situation (Trotman & Brody, 2002) After completion of brief cognitive-behavioral therapy (CBT), whereby participants were taught to identify and modify the negative thoughts that contributed to the development and maintenance of depression, caregivers reported a significant reduction in symptoms associated with depression (Walker & Clarke, 2001). Similarly, caregivers enrolled in a CBT intervention demonstrated a significant reduction in anxiety over time (Akkerman & Ostwald, 2004). Reductions in anxiety were maintained over a six-week follow-up period, suggesting that CBT may offer caregivers skills that will help in modulating anxiety throughout their caregiving career. A review of studies conducted with primary care partners for physically frail elders also revealed positive outcomes for those who received treatment, compared with a no-treatment group (Cooke, McNally, Mulligan, Harrison, & Newman, 2001). Caregivers participating in counseling demonstrated more effective coping skills, improved psychological wellbeing, and improved relationships with care receivers as compared to caregivers who did not receive counseling.

Support groups—a popular form of caregiver intervention—are widely available. Most groups are limited to six to eight sessions. Almost all include both education and support, focusing on seven major themes: information about the care receiver's situation; the group and its members as a mutual support system; the emotional impact of caregiving; self-care; problematic interpersonal relationships; the development and use of support systems outside the group; and home care skills. The typical support group is comprised of predominantly middle-class women, mostly the wives and daughters of individuals with some form of cognitive impairment (Bourgeois et al., 1996). Support groups are generally not well attended by minority individuals caring for older relatives. In some minority families, lack of participation may be due in part to the caregivers' reliance on other family members or informal helpers for caregiving assistance and strong cultural norms of family responsibility (Qualls & Roberto, 2006).

Numerous educational programs have been developed to meet the needs of individuals faced with the challenges of providing care for frail, aging relatives. Most of these programs are for spouses and adult children who have assumed the primary responsibility for a family member experiencing physical or cognitive decline. Programs cover a variety of topics, including community resources, sensory changes, communication skills, normal aging, behavioral changes, living arrangements, coping with stress, and chronic illness. Among the few program descriptions and evaluations published in family and gerontology journals, several commonalities exist. First, the presentation formats are similar. A two-hour session offered during several weeks is the most popular model. Second, almost all programs use a multiple-topic approach. Third, although the majority provide similar content, most programs are designed for a specific target population (Brubaker & Roberto, 1993). Because psychoeducational programs typically do not carry the stigma often associated with counseling or other invention programs, they often have greater appeal to ethnic and racially diverse caregivers. For example, Hispanic and Latino caregivers who participated in an eight-week class designed to teach specific cognitive and behavioral skills for coping with the frustrations of caregiving assessed the program favorably and reported increased knowledge, hope, and self-confidence along with decreased guilt and despair (Gallagher-Thompson, Arean, Rivera, & Thompson, 2001).

A large multi-site research project funded by the National Institute on Aging and National Institute for Nursing Research in the late 1990s investigated the efficacy of several interventions for reducing the burden on diverse groups of family caregivers to older adults while improving the quality of care (Schulz, Belle, Czaja, Gitlin, Wisniewski, & Ory, 2003). Each site in the Resources for Enhancing Alzheimer's Caregiver Health (REACH) study tested distinctive interventions targeted at particular caregiving populations with individually designed interventions including home visits, psychoeducational support classes, family interventions, and telephone-linked computer tools to foster communication among professionals and family caregivers. Overall, the findings suggest that active interventions were superior to control conditions in reducing (a) caregiver burden, (b) caregiver depression, (c) burden for women and those with high school or lower education, and (d) depression for Hispanic caregivers, non-spouses, and those with less than a high school education. Further description of the study sites, conditions, and multi-site outcomes are published in a special section of *Psychology and Aging* (2003, no. 3), and site-specific methodologies and findings are published in a special section of *The Gerontologist* (2003, no. 4).

Many Cooperative Extension programs provide support in meeting the mental health needs of caregivers of frail elders. Through the facilitation of formal educational programs and support groups, family members learn how to more effectively carry out their roles and responsibilities as primary caregivers while reducing feelings of stress and burnout. For example, North Carolina Cooperative Extension agents and specialists are part of a statewide network using the *Powerful Tools* curriculum to educate caregivers about taking care of their family members as well as themselves (Hampton, 2006). The program focuses on coping with stress, communicating with family members and care receivers, decision making, and arranging for caregiver down time. *Replenishing the Working Caregiver*, a program developed by the Kansas State University Cooperative Extension Service, educates family caregivers on the process of caregiving for older people and the importance of partaking in a support group to prevent or decrease potential caregiver burnout. Upon completion of the three-month support group, caregivers leave with a care buddy who continues to provide support through one-on-one telephone calls or chat room exchanges (Cooperative Extension System, 2006).

For Your Files: Caregiver Support Groups in America

The Self-Help Support Group On-Line is a searchable database that includes information on over 800 national, international, and demonstrational model self-help support groups, ideas for starting groups, and opportunities to link with others to develop new national or international groups. This database uses information provided by the American Self-Help Clearinghouse, a department of the Behavioral Health Center of Saint Clare's Health Services in Denville, New Jersey, which publishes *The Self-Help Sourcebook*. For more information, call the American Clearinghouse at 973-625-3037; www.mentalhelp.net/selfhelp.

Over one-half (59%) of family caregivers are employed at least part time (Pandya, 2005). Since the pioneering efforts of the Travelers Companies in the mid-1980s, workplace support for caregivers has increased (Wagner, 2003). Employers provide support for their employees with elder care needs through their policies (e.g., job-sharing options, flextime, and medical, personal, or family leave time), benefits (e.g., insurance, tax credits, dependent care reimbursement plans, and subsidized care), and services (education, information and referral, counseling, and case management).

CHALLENGES FOR FAMILY CAREGIVER MENTAL HEALTH PROGRAMS

As the number of frail older persons increases and more family members occupy the role of caregiver, the emotional support provided by mental health services will be in greater demand. A number of challenges need to be addressed to meet the mental health needs of family caregivers.

Increasing Participation in Programs

A limited number of caregivers attend mental health–related programs or use services that may enhance their ability to provide care. This may be because many do not identify themselves as caregivers or because they may lack a caregiving alternative that would allow them to attend therapy or other types of programs. When caregivers do access these services, it usually is because they have reached a crisis stage. Health care and other service providers need to inform caregivers of the availability of supportive services and encourage their use before caregivers experience distress. Caregivers need to be continually reminded to "take care of themselves." They also need reassurance that using services does not mean that they are failing to meet their caregiving responsibilities but rather that through the use of such services, they are maintaining and enhancing their coping abilities. Employers also need to recognize the benefits of mental health programs for their employees who are family caregivers and to make those services available through employee assistance programs.

Reaching Diverse Groups

Despite research demonstrating that minority caregivers experience burden and depression, they are less likely to participate in caregiver support programs. Because cultural norms may make it difficult for caregivers to turn to the formal network for support, services must be sensitive to the differing personal and cultural expectations held by caregivers of various ethnic and racial groups (AARP, 2001). The American Psychological Association's (2002) guidelines for providing service to culturally diverse populations provide a foundation from which to design effective interventions for families providing care. Specific principles include awareness and acknowledgment that culture is a primary aspect of human existence, and that culture and ethnicity inevitably shape behavior. Sensitivity, knowledge, and understanding of the cultural backgrounds of both the intervener and the family member are required in persons and programs seeking to assist individuals. Of particular importance is sensitivity to the individual's cultural background and preferences, including language, family values, community, and religious systems.

Providing Mental Health Programs in the Future

The delegates of the 2005 White House Conference on Aging passed two resolutions specifically addressing the needs of family caregivers:

- to develop a national strategy for supporting informal caregivers of seniors to enable adequate quality and supply of services; and
- to support older adult caregivers raising their relatives' children.

With respect to caregivers of older adults, proposed strategies included

- Refine definition of kinship care to include designated non-related caregivers in the Older Americans Act, Family and Medical Leave Act, and other federal and state laws that pertain to family caregiving.
- Amend Medicaid regulations at the federal level to allow family caregiving as a paid service.
- Support working caregivers by encouraging and providing incentives for employers to provide information and referral, geriatric care management, caregiver leave, flextime and other work–life programs, and to help working caregivers prepare for their own retirement by providing retirement education, advice, and availability of long-term care insurance and other benefits
- Conduct extensive outreach to (boomer and younger) caregivers to ensure they know what supports, education, and training are available and when and how to access these services.

Strategies to support grandparents raising grandchildren included

- Provide for adequate funding for grandfamilies.
- Provide outreach and education that are culturally and socioeconomically sensitive, directed at caregivers, schools, and the public at large.
- Educate caregivers of children to establish legal guardianships and establish programs to assist caregivers to negotiate the legal system.
- Make state laws more malleable and less restrictive for grandparents to take care of individual children's needs (a "loosening up" of government control of health care issues, school issues, and leisure activities).

CASE STUDY

Schizophrenia Complicates Care Needs

Katherine is a 77-year-old divorced woman who has a diagnosis of schizophrenia. Although Katherine has most likely been a schizophrenic since her early 20s, she was not formally diagnosed until her mid-50s. Since her diagnosis and subsequent treatment, Katherine has enjoyed long periods when she has felt good. Like many mental health patients, however, when Katherine is feeling good she stops taking her medicine. Gradually, mood changes occur that escalate to hostile and paranoid behavior. On many occasions, she has had to be hospitalized in the psychiatric care unit of the local hospital. The length of time under such care varies, depending on how long it takes to regulate her medication.

Despite her illness, Katherine raised four sons. Two of her sons are dead, one lives out of state and takes no interest in his mother, and the fourth and youngest son, Tom, lives nearby. Tom tries to help his mother, but it isn't easy. She keeps to herself and does not let people—even her son—get close to her. In her community, she is known as a character who doesn't mince words. Although she is fiercely independent, she is dedicated to her church. One of her favorite rituals is communion, which she always takes twice a year.

Now age has compounded her problems. Katherine is overweight, is unsteady on her feet, and has arthritis and poor vision. It is increasingly difficult for her to get around. At this stage, her isolated, simple life is also becoming problematic. She requires more services such as transportation, shopping assistance, and daily monitoring to make sure she is taking her medication. Although her disease has leveled out some, she continues to have relapses when she is noncompliant with her medicine. These events are more frequent than necessary. Both her son Tom and her mental health worker of three years are concerned about her future.

Case Study Questions

1. Which mental health research data discussed in this chapter best describe Katherine?

2. Do you think Katherine's mental health diagnosis, coupled with her physical problems, makes her more at risk of institutionalization? Why or why not?

3. Katherine probably would not qualify for nursing home care as a Medicaid recipient solely because of her physical health. Under what circumstances described in the chapter could Katherine receive nursing home care paid for by Medicaid?

4. Fortunately, Katherine has the services of a professional mental health worker. From which of the mental health programs described in the chapter has Katherine most likely been receiving services?

5. What types of support may be available for Tom to help him understand and care for his mother?

Learning Activities

1. Interview a mental health professional who works with older adults. What are some of the primary issues with which many older adults seek or need assistance? What are some of the difficulties in getting older adults to participate in mental health services? Why has this professional decided or been chosen to work with older adults? How might the skills needed be similar to or different from those needed to work with other populations?

2. Ask a mental health service provider to share with you copies of the assessment tools that are used for younger and older adults. Are they similar or different? Would you have difficulty in answering some of the questions?

3. Sit in on a peer counseling or other type of mental health training. What was the topic? How did it relate to older adults, family caregivers, or those providing services to them? What did you learn?

4. What do you believe are the benefits and issues related to mental health services for older adults and their family caregivers? What did you learn were some of the barriers, and what might the agency and the community do to break down the barriers? What might keep you from accessing mental health services currently and in the future?

For More Information

National Resources

1. National Institute of Mental Health, Public Information & Communications Branch, 6001 Executive Blvd, Room 8184, Bethesda, MD 20892-9663; phone: 1-866-615-6464; www.nimh.nih.gov.
    The National Institute of Mental Health conducts and supports research to learn more about causes and treatment of mental and emotional disorders. Available are free publications including *Facts About Anxiety Disorders,* and *Older Adults: Depression and Suicide Facts.*

2. National Mental Health Association, 2000 N. Beauregard St., 6th Floor, Alexandria, VA 22311; phone: 703-684-5968 or 800-969-6642; www.nmha.org.

   The National Mental Health Information Center, established by the National Mental Health Association, provides inquirers with information about mental health topics and has a wide variety of written information about mental health topics.

3. The Geriatric Mental Health Foundation, 7910 Woodmont Ave, Suite 1050, Bethesda, MD 20814; phone: 301-654-7850; www.gmhfonline.org/gmhf.

   The Geriatric Mental Health Foundation was established by the American Association for Geriatric Psychiatry to raise awareness of psychiatric and mental health disorders affecting older adults, eliminate the stigma of mental illness and treatment, promote healthy aging strategies, and increase access to quality mental health care. Review the Foundation's website for mental health information for older adults and their families, to find a geriatric psychiatrist, and for information about programs and events.

4. Alzheimer's Association, 225 North Michigan Avenue, Floor 17, Chicago, IL 60601; phone: 800-272-3900; www.alz.org.

   The Alzheimer's Association sponsors education programs and support services to patients and families who are coping with Alzheimer's disease. The Association offers a 24-hour hotline with information about Alzheimer's disease and local chapters and resources. Educational materials are also available.

5. *Clinical Gerontologist.* The Haworth Press Inc., 10 Alice St., Binghamton, NY 13904; phone: 800-429-6784; www.haworthpress.com/store/product.asp?sku = J018.

   This journal presents timely material relevant to the needs of mental health professionals and all practitioners who deal with older clients and their families. All articles in this practitioners' journal feature timely, practical material relevant and applicable to the assessment and management of mental disorders in later life.

6. *Aging & Mental Health,* 325 Chestnut Street, Suite 800, Philadelphia, PA 19106; phone: 800-354 1420; www.tandf.co.uk/journals/titles/13607863.asp.

   This journal provides a leading forum for this rapidly expanding field, which investigates the relationship between the aging process and mental health. It encourages an integrated approach between the various biopsychosocial processes and etiological factors associated with psychological changes in the elderly and emphasizes the various strategies, therapies, and services which may be directed at improving the mental health of older adults.

Web Resources

1. Mental HealthNet: www.cmhc.com.

   This is quite a site! It offers more than 4,200 individual resources on mental health issues. Links to a reading room, professional resources, self-help resources, and other mental health web resources are listed. Definitely worth the visit when you have some time to spend between classes!

2. Psych Central, Dr. John Grohol's Mental Health Page: www.psychcentral.com/web.htm.

   This psychWeb pointer helps visitors locate information on the web and is organized by topic or alphabetically. There is an incredibly lengthy list of general support resource links to other sites on the web with a brief description. It's the most comprehensive mental health listing we have found.

3. National Mental Health Association: www.nmha.org.

   The National Mental Health Association's website contains information on depression, coping with loss, and other topics of interest.

4. National Clearinghouse for Alcohol and Drug Information: Prevline (Prevention Online): www.health.org/about/sitemap.aspx.

    This site provides general statistics, referrals, resources, research, publications, and a list of other sites that deal with alcohol and drug abuse. Publications may be ordered online free of charge by visiting http://ncadistore.samhsa.gov/catalog/results.aspx?h = drugs&topic = 24.

5. National Family Caregiver Support Program Resource Room: www.aoa.gov/prof/aoaprog/caregiver/caregiver.asp.

    Sponsored by the U.S. Administration on Aging, the Caregiver Resource Room provides information for families, caregivers, and professionals providing support for older adults and grandparents, and relative caregivers of children not more than 18 years of age. Resources include caregiving tips, fact sheets, findings from national studies of caregiving, and contact information for state Family Caregiver Support Programs.

6. The U.S. Center for Mental Health Services: http://mentalhealth.samhsa.gov/cmhs.

    This center provides annual statistical and demographic information about consumers of mental health services. Go to the Center's website at http://mentalhealth.samhsa.gov/cmhs/MentalHealthStatistics to get the latest report. Select your state within the report and review how it compares with the national average.

13

Legal Services

Fernando telephones the local area agency on aging requesting emergency food. The agency staff member arranges for food to be delivered and then asks Fernando why he has none. It seems that he has not received his Social Security check for two months. He did get a couple of letters from Social Security a few months ago, but he does not read well, so he set them aside and forgot about them. He did not pay his rent this month or last and ran out of medicine two days ago. The agency staff member arranges for Fernando to receive daily meals and medication. She also calls the local senior legal assistance program and makes an appointment for Fernando. With the assistance of a senior legal aid attorney, his Social Security checks are reinstated, and his landlord has agreed not to evict him.

$\mathbf{F}$ernando's situation illustrates how one problem—in this case, a lack of food—can in turn reveal a cascade of other additional problems, many of which are or become legal issues. Older adults may experience legal problems brought about by changes in work, family, and physical health. These problems can have devastating consequences on their quality of life. For example, a retired person may be unable to collect an expected pension. After the divorce of a child, the ex-son- or daughter-in-law might refuse to let grandparents visit grandchildren—or, because of other circumstances, grandparents may effectively find themselves parents once again, caring for grandchildren. Upon the death or divorce of a spouse, tangible property must be divided, and when physical or mental capacity wanes, substitute decision makers may need to be appointed to make decisions on behalf of an older adult. Legal problems may also occur because older adults do not have access to legal advice before signing legal documents (Moore, 1992).

In this chapter, we review the federal policies that facilitated the development of legal programs serving older adults. We then briefly discuss the legal problems that older adults often encounter and with which they consequently need assistance and take a look at the different types of legal programs designed to serve older adults. We conclude the chapter by discussing the challenges that legal programs face in meeting the legal needs of older adults.

POLICY BACKGROUND

In 1974, Congress passed legislation that created the Legal Services Corporation (LSC). Its purpose is to provide low-income individuals with minimum access to legal assistance. The LSC is a private, nonprofit organization directed by an 11-member board appointed by Congress and the President. Currently, the LSC funds 138 local legal services programs in all 50 states.

Individuals can receive legal assistance through a local legal services office, provided that their income does not exceed 125% of the poverty line and their legal problem is civil rather than criminal. The majority of cases handled by legal services staff on behalf of older adults include housing issues, such as landlord–tenant disputes and subsidized housing complaints; family issues, such as divorce; and public benefits issues, such as Social Security and SSI. Of the 906,338 cases closed by legal services advocates in 2005, 11.3% involved legal assistance to clients older than age 60 (Legal Services Corporation, 2006).

Since its inception, the LSC has not been without its critics. Every year during the Reagan and Bush Administrations (1980 to 1992), the budget submitted by the White House proposed to eliminate the LSC and its programs. Severe cuts in LSC funding through the years have resulted in fewer attorneys and paralegals available to handle cases. Staff reduction has caused many offices to limit the type of cases accepted and the number of people served. For example, the LSC Act of 1974 defined minimum access to legal assistance as having two legal services attorneys for every 10,000 poor persons. Funding levels to meet minimum access standards were obtained in 1980 and 1981 ($300 million and $320 million, respectively); currently, however, there is only one attorney for every 10,000 poor persons. This compares with approximately 28 attorneys for every 10,000 persons with incomes above the poverty line (U.S. Senate Special Committee on Aging, 1993). Funding levels steadily improved in the latter 1990s. For the fiscal year 1995, Congress appropriated $415 million to fund the LSC programs. Appropriation was $278 million for the fiscal year 1996 and by 2005, funding was at the same level it was in 1981—approximately $330 million (Legal Services Corporation, 2006). As a result, the number of local legal services offices has dropped from 269 in 1999 to 138 in 2005. In addition, a number of national and state support centers that provided technical legal assistance and expertise on a variety of poverty law issues were eliminated.

Older Americans Act Support of Legal Assistance

Legal programs became eligible for funding under the Older Americans Act (OAA) in 1973. Amendments to the OAA in 1981 required that Area Agencies on Aging (AAAs) spend an "adequate proportion" of Title III-B dollars on legal services. A subsequent amendment in 1987 required State Units on Aging (SUAs) to set minimum percentages that AAAs must spend on providing legal assistance. The amendments in 2000 simply require that AAAs provide an adequate proportion of their funds for legal assistance. AAAs are also required to give priority to older adults with income, health care, long-term care, nutrition, housing, utilities, protective services, defense of guardianship, abuse, neglect, and age discrimination assistance legal problems (§ 305[11][E]). AAAs must contract with legal providers who have experience in delivering legal assistance, and must involve the private Bar in efforts to improve older adults' access to legal assistance. In 2004, $23 million in Title III funds was spent on legal assistance, providing more than 1 million legal assistance hours to older adults (Administration on Aging [AoA], n.d.).

In addition to Title III-B dollars allocated to fund legal assistance programs, the Vulnerable Elder Rights Protection Activities program (Title VII), authorized in 1992 and again in the 2006 amendments to the OAA, directs funding for legal assistance support. Title VII monies are also used for states to establish focal point programs at the state level for elder rights policy review and advocacy. These state programs, called Legal Services Developers, must create statewide standards for legal service delivery, provide technical assistance to AAAs and legal service providers, promote training to representative payees and guardians, and promote pro bono programs in cooperation with the private Bar. Title VII monies are also used for programs that are designed to prevent elder abuse, neglect, and exploitation. The 2006 amendments introduced a new term—"elder justice." When used in a collective sense, elder justice means efforts to prevent, detect, treat, intervene in, and respond to elder abuse, neglect, and exploitation and to protect individuals with diminished capacity while maximizing their autonomy. Elder justice also means the recognition of the individual's rights, including the right to be free of abuse, neglect, and exploitation. Funding is made available for programs that

- conduct public education about elder abuse and outreach to help identify possible cases of abuse and exploitation;
- promote the development of information and data systems for elder abuse reporting systems and conduct analyses of state information concerning elder abuse;
- conduct training on the identification, prevention, and treatment of elder abuse and exploitation as well as conduct training that assists the victims of elder abuse;
- promote the development of an elder abuse, neglect, and exploitation system to identify, investigate, and resolve cases;
- examine various types of shelters serving older adults, called "safe havens" and testing various "safe haven" models that recognize the rights of older adults; and
- address underserved elders in rural locations, in minority populations, and low-income elders.

In addition, the 2006 amendments to Title VII added grants to promote statewide development and implementation of comprehensive multidisciplinary elder justice systems. These systems are characterized by an integrated, multidisciplinary, and collaborative system for preventing, detecting, and addressing elder abuse, neglect, and exploitation. Funds are designed to specifically support programs that provide widespread, convenient public access to the range of available elder justice information, programs and services; that reduce duplication and gaps in the elder justice system; and that provide a uniform method for the standardization, collection, analysis, and reporting of data.

Finally, the AoA supports the delivery of legal assistance under Title IV that provides discretionary funds to support research and demonstration projects. Since 1998, Title IV dollars have supported the creation of legal hotlines for older adults. As mentioned in Chapter 2, OAA funds are used to provide national support and consultation to those who deliver legal assistance to older adults. For example, the Center for Social Gerontology and its National Support Center in Law and Aging, the National Senior Citizens Law Center, the American Association of Retired Persons' National Training Project, the Pension Rights

Center, and the National Bar Association's Black Elderly Legal Assistance Support Project are some programs that have been supported by OAA dollars.

USERS: LEGAL PROBLEMS OF OLDER ADULTS

Obtaining a profile of who uses legal assistance programs is a difficult task because many programs do not compile detailed information about client characteristics (e.g., marital status, age, income, and education) or are hesitant to publicly reveal client characteristics to protect client confidentiality, or such data are provided only to local AAAs or SUAs and not published in academic journals. Thus, statistical information on Title III-B legal assistance clients is inadequate. Some inferences about client characteristics can be made, however, by examining the type of legal problems for which clients seek assistance. In addition, the type of cases that legal programs accept will affect the type of clients served by those programs. Moreover, legal assistance programs funded under the OAA target socially and financially needy older adults. An older adult with a sizable estate will no doubt be served by the family attorney or be referred to an estate lawyer rather than to a Title III legal aid program. In the next sections, we will review the civil and criminal legal problems of older adults and, when available, the extent to which older adults report having those problems.

Legal problems emerge in various ways. Older adults who lack an understanding about what constitutes a legal problem or how laws originate may not be able to identify that a legal remedy exists when problems occur. Persons who work with older adults also must be aware of potential legal problems so that referrals can be made to appropriate legal services.

Legal problems can be categorized as either civil or criminal. Civil legal problems are disputes between individuals or organizations, whereas criminal legal problems are those acts that threaten the well-being of the state and include crimes against the person such as assault, homicide, rape, and robbery. Civil legal problems commonly experienced by older adults are presented next, followed by criminal problems.

Family Issues

Divorce

In the year 2005, only 7.9% of individuals 65 and older were divorced, but more older women were divorced than older men (8.5% vs. 7%, respectively; U.S. Bureau of the Census, 2006b). Although divorce is uncommon in later life and less frequent than in other age groups, its consequences can be financially devastating to older women who divorce. Many women in the current cohort of older adults have been lifelong homemakers who often have no financial support apart from those benefits associated with being a spouse. When husbands file for divorce, lifelong homemakers may discover that the house, utilities, bank accounts, credit cards, and automobiles do not have both names on titles and accounts. Divorce might even exclude the wife's access to her husband's pension. Such arrangements leave them financially vulnerable and in need of legal assistance to protect their rights to marital property.

Grandparent Visitation and Grandparents Raising Grandchildren

Of older adults, 80% have children, and of those, 94% are grandparents (Hooyman & Kiyak, 1996). Researchers have documented that grandparents occupy important roles within the family network. For example, grandparents provide emotional and instrumental support, offer stability in times of crisis, assume parental responsibilities for grandchildren when parents are unavailable, and serve as the keepers of family history (Matthews & Sprey, 1984; Minkler & Roe, 1996). Strong emotional bonds are not uncommon between grandparents and grandchildren (Hodgson, 1995; Roberto & Stroes, 1992).

Various disruptions in the nuclear family can fracture the relationship between grandparents and grandchildren. For example, divorce, death of a parent, adoption of a grandchild by a friend or relative, or termination of parental rights may sever intergenerational bonds. Until recently, grandparents had no legal recourse to aid them in re-establishing contact with their grandchildren. Now, however, all 50 states have enacted laws that allow grandparents to petition the court for visitation rights. State statutes vary with regard to who can petition, the circumstances that must be present in the nuclear family before visitation rights are considered, and how the court determines whether grandparent visitation would be in the best interests of the grandchildren.

Other grandparents have a different set of problems concerning their grandchildren. Growing numbers of grandparents have found themselves parenting their grandchildren (Minkler & Roe, 1996). According to the U.S. Bureau of the Census (2003, October), 2.5 million grandparents are responsible for the basic needs (e.g., food, shelter, clothing) of the grandchildren they live with; these grandparents represent 43% of all grandparents who live with their grandchildren. Grandparents take on the parental role when, for a variety of reasons, parents are unable to care for their children. Grandparents who become parents often need assistance in filing for additional health or income benefits or in filing for adoption or custody.

Estate Planning

A will provides a means to specifically identify and distribute tangible property after death. Dying without a will (intestate) results in the distribution of property among family members in accordance with state law. Thus the distribution of the assets of a person who has died intestate can be complicated, time consuming, and subject to conflicts among family members regarding the value and ownership of the property. Therefore, many older adults—even those with small estates—can benefit from drafting a will. In a statewide survey of the legal needs of older adults in Georgia, problems with wills and estates were one of the top three legal issues with which older adults wanted help (Thomas, 2006).

Income

Many older adults live on fixed incomes and rely wholly or in part on public income programs such as Social Security, SSI, Railroad Retirement, or veterans' benefits. Some 20% of older adults rely on Social Security for their sole source of income; 2 million receive SSI benefits (Social Security Administration, 2004). Given the complex and complicated regulations that govern the administration of these programs, it is not surprising that many legal problems can arise.

Legal problems occur when program intake workers refuse to process applications because older adults do not have the documents needed to prove their age, work history, marital status, or financial status. In addition, eligibility criteria are often excessively complicated, confusing, or easily misinterpreted. State and federal programs such as old age assistance programs and SSI base eligibility on financial need, and applicants must prove that their income and asset levels are below eligibility amounts. Definitions of income and assets can create confusion because in-kind assistance, such as gifts of food, can count as income. An otherwise qualified individual may be denied access to critical financial assistance. Finally, legal problems can surface even after individuals are receiving benefits. For example, because eligibility for Social Security is based on work history, an error in an earnings record can result in a smaller benefit amount. Mistakes occur in an estimated 2–3% of earnings records (Matthews & Berman, 1990).

A second type of legal problem related to income assistance programs occurs when participants receive a notice of overpayment or notice of termination of benefits. Overpayments occur when income amounts exceed eligibility criteria or when the benefit amount paid to the recipient is miscalculated. For example, the father of one of the authors of this book sought legal assistance after he received a $13,000 overpayment notice from Social Security (the notice suggested that he send Social Security a check for the entire amount within 30 days!). Further investigation revealed that an error made by a Social Security technician in recording his working income into his monthly Social Security benefit amount for a three-year period had caused the overpayment. A legal services paralegal was able to negotiate with Social Security a repayment plan that took a small amount of money from his monthly check until the overpayment was paid.

Overpayments also can result when older adults receive income benefits from more than one program. Consider the case of Mary Espinosa, who received a small Social Security check, based on her husband's earnings, together with an SSI check, for a total monthly income of $425. Following Mr. Espinosa's death, Mary went to the Social Security office to report his death so that her technician could adjust her benefit amount. Mary continued to receive both checks until one day she received a notice of overpayment demanding that she repay $3,000 in SSI benefits. Mary did not realize that, although her SSI intake worker sat next to her Social Security intake worker in the same office, she needed to notify both workers of her change in circumstances. A legal advocate can determine whether the overpayment actually occurred and, if the situation warrants, can appeal the overpayment decision or, if necessary, can negotiate a repayment schedule.

Although older adults can appeal these adverse decisions, they may not understand why they have been denied benefits or have had their benefits reduced and may assume that nothing can be done. A reduction or termination of benefits could place the older adult in a position of being unable to pay for rent, food, or necessary medical assistance. Therefore, it is critical that older adults consult legal advocates when there are changes in benefit eligibility or amount. In the Georgia study mentioned earlier (Thomas, 2006), problems with government benefits was the top legal need of older adults.

Employment

Age Discrimination

In 2005, persons aged 65 and older represented 14.5% of the nation's workforce. Some 5.3 million workers over 55 were employed part time as well (U.S. Bureau of the Census, 2001b; U.S. Bureau of Labor Statistics, 2006b, U.S. Bureau of Labor Statistics, 2006c; U.S. Department of Labor, 2000a). Older adults who wish to remain working or to obtain work may encounter age-based discriminatory employment practices. Although the number of older adults who have experienced workplace discrimination is unknown, researchers report that many managers have negative stereotypes about older workers. These include the perception that older workers will not perform as well as younger workers, that older workers are not cost-effective, and that older workers are not suitable for training (Rix, 1994; Sterns & McDaniel, 1994). Such attitudes and beliefs, although not supported by empirical research (see Commonwealth Fund, 1993), can lead to discrimination against older workers.

To counter age discrimination against older workers, Congress enacted the Age Discrimination in Employment Act (ADEA) in 1967. Although some exceptions exist, the ADEA prohibits employment discrimination against persons aged 40 or older. Under the Act, employers must not refuse to hire individuals on the basis of their age; discriminate with respect to compensation, terms, conditions, or privileges; limit, segregate, or classify employees in a way that adversely affects their employment status or opportunities because of age; or retaliate against employees who exercise their rights under ADEA (Strauss, Wolf, & Schilling, 1990). The ADEA also prohibits employment agencies from engaging in discriminatory employment practices. Older workers who feel they have been discriminated against can file a claim with the Equal Employment Opportunity Commission and may also have claims under state law. In 2005, the commission received 16,585 age discrimination complaints (U.S. Equal Employment Opportunity Commission, 2006). The number of age discrimination complaints is likely to increase with the aging of the baby boomer cohort.

Pensions

For some older adults, private pension plans provide additional income in retirement. According to the Employee Benefit Research Institute, the number of private pensions has increased from 340,000 in 1975 and 870,000 in 1987 to 730,031 in 1998 (cited in Strauss et al., 1990; Employee Benefit Research Institute, 2003). In 2004, 41.9% of all workers participated in an employment-based retirement plan (Employee Benefit Research Institute, 2005). As of 1998, 71% of private sector workers over age 55, 84% of state and local public sector workers, and almost all federal workers were covered by a pension plan (Lichtenstein & Verma, 2003). Unlike Social Security, whose regulations apply uniformly to all older adults, pension plans vary from employer to employer. We reviewed the types of pension plans in more detail in Chapter 9.

The Employee Retirement Income Security Act (ERISA) of 1974 regulates the administration of pensions. Retirees can file a federal suit if pension benefits have been unfairly denied, if future benefits are affected by changes in the pension plan, if the plan or funds have been improperly managed, if other rights outlined in the plan are breached, or if the plan does not disclose information required by ERISA (Matthews & Berman, 1990). Although retirees have various legal safeguards to their pension funds, it is probable that the majority of retirees are unaware of their rights under ERISA.

Health Care

Medical Insurance

As with income assistance programs, older adults can encounter legal problems with Medicare and Medicaid. (We discussed these in greater detail in Chapter 11.) Most legal difficulties with Medicare Part A can occur when coverage is denied for services rendered. A denial most often occurs when the Medicare insurance carrier determines that services were not medically necessary, that services could have been provided on an outpatient basis, or that services were custodial rather than medical (Matthews & Berman, 1996). Disputes of payments under Part B usually concern the scope of coverage or the amount approved for payment by Part B carriers. Appeals against adverse decisions are made to the Social Security Administration.

Because Medicare does not cover all medical expenses and older adults must pay for deductibles and uncovered services out of pocket, many purchase supplemental insurance (Medigap) policies to help pay medical expenses. Unfortunately, older adults are often victims of Medigap insurance fraud—pressured to switch companies or to purchase duplicate policies, denied coverage because of pre-existing clauses, or refused for renewal of a policy for reasons other than nonpayment. In recent years, the selling of Medigap policies has come under scrutiny and regulation. Federal law requires each state to adopt standardized Medigap benefit policies. When violations in these regulations occur, advocates can pursue legal remedies with the state insurance commissioner or through a civil court.

Medicaid eligibility is based on income and asset levels and on being age 65 or older, blind, or disabled or having dependent children. Because Medicaid is a state and federal program, income and asset levels for eligibility vary among states. Under the Medicaid program, adverse decisions with regard to eligibility and coverage can be appealed. Legal difficulties with health care insurance were mentioned as a legal problem experienced by 24% of elders in Georgia (Thomas, 2006).

Advance Directives for Health Care

Readers may remember hearing about the case of Terri Schiavo. Terri, age 26, collapsed in her home in 1990 and never regained consciousness. After she had been in a vegetative state for eight years, Terri's husband petitioned the court to have her feeding tube removed, but her parents opposed this decision. In part because Terri had only made oral declarations of what her end-of-life decisions would be, and because her parents did not believe she was in a vegetative state, legal appeals—including involvement by the Florida Legislature and the U.S. Congress—continued until February 2005. A final legal decision to remove the feeding tube from Terri was made on March 18, 2005, and Terri died on March 31, 2005 at the age of 41 (University of Miami Ethics Program, 2007). Due to this and two other similar end-of-life cases that have gained national attention—the Karen Ann Quinlan case in 1975 and the Nancy Cruzan (*Cruzan v. Harmon*) case in 1990—and the increase in the number of persons who wish to remain in control of health care decisions after they are unable to articulate their desires, states have enacted laws that allow for the creation of *advance directives*. Advance directives are legal documents that convey the wishes of an individual regarding personal health care decisions and that must be executed while the individual is still competent. Two types of advance directives are the durable power of attorney for health care and the living will.

Older adults who want to articulate their health care wishes can do so in many states by executing a durable power of attorney for health care decisions. A durable power of attorney appoints an agent to make health care decisions outlined in the document. A living will also provides a legal mechanism that enables individuals to express their wishes regarding life-sustaining treatment. Living wills are more narrow in scope because they authorize the withdrawal of certain life-sustaining procedures only in situations in which the individual has a terminal illness or is comatose (Alexander, 1991). Only a small percentage of older adults report that they have executed a living will. In a national study of community-dwelling older adults, Hopp (2000) found that 29% had executed either a living will and/or a durable power of attorney. She also found that there was a greater likelihood of having a living will or a durable power of attorney among Whites and those with higher levels of income and education. Providing preventive legal assistance to older adults by drafting these documents before they are needed can reduce the occurrence of problems in the future.

Consumer Fraud

Older persons are prime targets of consumer fraud and deceptions. According to the FBI, the amount of money being scammed primarily from older adults is approximately $500 million a year from telemarketers and $25 billion a year on bogus health products (U.S. Senate Special Committee on Aging, 2000; Federal Bureau of Investigation, 2005). Older adults tend to be more vulnerable to certain types of telemarketing fraud. In 2003, 66% of reports of sweepstake fraud, 59% of lottery club scams, and 52% of magazine sales scams were made by older adults (National Fraud Information Center, 2004). For a variety of reasons, older adults may be more likely than others to be victims of consumer fraud. First, physical frailty or mental impairments may leave older adults at a disadvantage in understanding and negotiating with persistent salespersons. Second, older homebound persons may welcome opportunities to shop at home and may enjoy the company of friendly visiting salespersons and be more likely to be at home when the telemarketer calls. Third, older adults with low incomes may be especially susceptible to apparent opportunities to increase their incomes, take advantage of promised low prices, or send away for prize money. Federal and state consumer protection laws provide legal remedies for consumer fraud cases. Older victims of consumer fraud need to consult legal advocates to help them recover the costs of their fraudulent purchases.

Nursing Homes and Long-Term Care

Of older adults, 5%, or approximately 1.5 million persons, reside in long-term care facilities at any one time; of adults aged 65 and older, however, 43% can expect to stay in a long-term care facility (Murtaugh, Kemper, & Spillman, 1990). A variety of legal concerns may unfold during a resident's stay in a long-term care facility. One source of legal problems can be the admission agreement. Studies evaluating the legality of nursing home admission agreements found that many contained illegal or questionable provisions (Amborgi & Leonard, 1988; Wacker, 1985). Unfortunately, when problems do occur with the provisions set forth in the admissions agreement, older adults or their family members may not realize that they have a valid legal challenge to those contracts.

A second concern is the enforcement of residents' rights. Federal and state governments have enacted numerous laws to protect the rights of nursing home residents and to promote a high standard of care. Nursing homes must provide care and services to residents in a way that promotes and maintains the residents' physical, social, and mental wellbeing (Eldeman, 1990). Federal law protects residents' rights, including the right to privacy, the right to speak freely, the right to refuse treatment, and the right to freedom of association (see Chapter 19). Although nursing home residents and their family members can call on an ombudsman to advocate on behalf of the resident, there may be instances when a breach of residents' rights calls for a legal remedy.

Substitute Decision Making

Imagine for a moment that you have failed to open your mail for a couple of months. What would be the consequences of such a seemingly innocent mistake? No doubt your utilities would be on the verge of being turned off. Your car payment and insurance bills would be overdue, and letters threatening repossession would be in the stack of unopened letters. Checks would go undeposited. Bank accounts would be left unattended and important notices left unanswered. Such a scenario is not hard to imagine happening to older adults who are cognitively impaired and unable to manage their personal affairs.

Older adults who need assistance managing their personal affairs have legal ways to appoint a substitute decision maker. Legal documents such as a power of attorney or durable power of attorney are used to appoint someone to manage financial affairs. Individuals must be mentally competent before they can execute these documents. A durable power of attorney, unlike the power of attorney, continues to remain in effect upon the incapacity of the executor.

Another type of substitute decision maker is a guardian or conservator. Courts can appoint guardians or conservators who have the authority to make personal or financial decisions on behalf of an incompetent adult. Before a guardian or conservator can be appointed, the individual must file a petition with the court and prove that the older adult, called a ward, is mentally incompetent. Once appointed, guardians have the power to make decisions about every aspect of the ward's life, including living arrangements, financial affairs, health care, and social relationships. Because of the extensive nature of the guardian powers, guardianships should be sought only when other less restrictive options are unavailable (Keith & Wacker, 1994).

Criminal Legal Problems

Criminal legal problems include assault, robbery, rape, burglary, larceny, and motor vehicle theft. Many researchers report that older adults are more fearful of crime than are younger adults, and a higher percentage of older Blacks express a fear of crime than do older Whites (62% vs. 28%, respectively; Lee, 1983; Lindquist & Duke, 1982; Michigan Offices of

Services to the Aging, cited in Kart, 1997). Nevertheless, older adults are far less likely to be victims of crimes (Catalano, 2006). As shown in Exhibit 13.1, the crime rate for selected crimes against older adults is markedly less than the rate for adults under age 65. Although older adults are less likely to be victims of crime, the outcome is often more physically, emotionally, and financially devastating than for younger victims of crime (Covey & Menard, 1988; Crandall, 1991). One of the more significant crimes affecting older adults is elder abuse.

EXHIBIT 13.1 Victimization by Type of Crime and Age (rate per 1,000 persons)

Age	All Crime	Sexual Assault	Robbery	Assault	Purse Snatching/Pocket Picking
12 to 15	45.3	1.2*	3.5	39.3	1.3
16 to 19	45.8	3.2	7.0	33.9	1.6
20 to 24	48.4	1.1*	5.5	40.3	1.5
25 to 34	24.6	0.7*	3.1	19.9	1.0
35 to 49	18.4	0.6*	1.9	15.0	1.0
50 to 64	12.0	0.6*	1.4	9.3	0.6
65+	2.8	0.0*	0.6	1.9	0.4

Source: Catalano (2006).

*Based on 10 or fewer sample cases.

Best Practice: National Association of Triads, Inc.

Representatives from the American Association of Retired Persons, the International Association of Chiefs of Police, and the National Sheriff's Association developed the concept of triads in 1988 to promote older adults' safety, reduce their criminal victimization, and enhance the delivery of law enforcement services to them. In 1989, the first triad partnership was created in St. Martin Parish, Louisiana. Local triads are guided by SALT (Seniors and Law Enforcement Together) Councils, which plan activities and programs that are designed to benefit both law enforcement and older adults. There are triads in 32 states, England, and Canada. The National Association of Triads, Inc. is the organization that provides advice, support, technical assistance, and training to local triads.

For more information, contact the National Association of Triads, Inc. (NATI), 1450 Duke Street, Alexandria, VA 22314; phone: 703-836-7827; www.nationaltriad.org.

Elder Abuse

Elder abuse most often occurs within the family context, and perpetrators are usually the elders' primary caregivers (Pillemer & Finkelhor, 1989). Elder abuse includes physical, psychological, and financial abuse as well as neglect. Victims of physical and psychological abuse are often in poor emotional health; the victims of neglect are usually older women, with multiple frailties, who are cognitively impaired and socially isolated (Wolf, 1996). The prevalence of older adults who have been injured, exploited, or mistreated by someone on whom they rely on for care is estimated to be between 2% and 10% (Lachs & Pillemer, 2004). The first national study of elder abuse conducted by the National Center on Elder Abuse at the American Public Human Services Association (formerly the American Public Welfare Association) found that some 551,000 older adults living in domestic settings were abused or neglected, or experienced self-neglect (AoA, 1998). All 50 states have legislation that allows for intervention and protection of vulnerable, disabled, or incapacitated adults. The responsibility for investigating such cases rests with either the state Social Services Department or the SUA (Wolf, 1996). Because a family member is most often the abuser, and because the older adult is often frail and dependent on the caregiver for assistance, intervention can be difficult. It is estimated that for every one case of abuse, neglect, exploitation, or self-neglect reported to authorities, five cases go unreported (American Public Human Services Association, 1998). For competent older adults, legal assistance can help evict or restrain the abuser; for incompetent victims, protective services can be implemented. The designated state agency, usually the Department of Social Services, offers protective services to help the victim resolve the abuse or, as a last resort, may seek a guardianship to protect the victim from exploitation. Protective services are also called to intervene in cases of self-neglect.

For Your Files: **The Clearinghouse on Abuse and Neglect of the Elderly (CANE)**

The Clearinghouse on Abuse and Neglect of the Elderly (CANE) at the University of Delaware is the nation's largest digital library of published research, training resources, government documents, and other resources on elder abuse. You can obtain citations and brief summaries of peer-reviewed journal articles, books, agency reports, transcripts of hearings, news articles, videos, memoranda of understanding (MOU), and online resources addressing the abuse and neglect, self-neglect, and financial exploitation of elders. CANE is a partner of the National Center on Elder Abuse (NCEA). NCEA is funded by the U.S. Administration on Aging, Department of Health and Human Services. You can access the database at http://db.rdms.udel.edu:8080/CANE/index.jsp.

LEGAL ASSISTANCE PROGRAMS

Despite the creation of legal programs through the OAA and the LSC, many older adults—particularly low-income and minority elders—do not receive legal assistance with civil problems. This is particularly true for those older adults who have incomes just above the

LSC guidelines yet cannot afford the costs of a private attorney. Furthermore, the limited numbers of attorneys and paralegals staffing legal assistance programs are serving fewer clients and accepting fewer numbers and types of cases. To address the lack of available legal assistance for older adults, SUAs and local AAAs have developed unique methods of delivering legal assistance and have formed partnerships with state and local private bar associations to broaden their involvement in the delivery of legal services for older adults. These different methods of delivering legal assistance are discussed below.

Legal Hotlines

According to Moore (1992), improving access to legal assistance must begin with improving the entry point to legal assistance and increasing the provision of preventive legal assistance. Legal hotlines have emerged as one way to address both problems. There are currently legal hotlines operating in 28 states, the District of Columbia, and Puerto Rico, which are supported by funding from the AoA. Residents of the state who are aged 60 and older can call a toll-free number and speak directly to an attorney. Attorneys offer legal information or advice, refer those who need representation and can afford to pay for it to attorneys who charge a fixed rate per hour, or refer those who cannot afford legal assistance to a local legal services program. Users of hotline services, who frequently have low income, report high levels of satisfaction, and the majority would recommend the services to a friend. In 2005, a nationwide study of 23 legal hotlines reported a total of 96,005 calls with each hotline program handling an average of 4,572 calls (AARP Foundation, 2006). Advantages of a telephone hotline service include being accessible to persons who are homebound or without transportation, being able to give prompt information and thereby reduce the anxiety level of older adults, and being able to resolve simple problems quickly.

For Your Files: The Samuel Sadin Institute on Law

The Samuel Sadin Institute on Law at the Brookdale Center on Aging at Hunter College acts as a legal support program for social workers, paralegals, attorneys, and other professionals engaged in advocacy assistance to older persons who are poor. An interdisciplinary staff of attorneys and social workers has expertise in Medicare, Medicaid, SSI, Social Security disability, home care, health care decision making, adult protective services, Medigap, and long-term care insurance. The staff is available to provide technical assistance on public benefit laws and regulations to elected public officials and staff of other not-for-profit agencies. More than 2,500 professionals are trained annually, and telephone case consultations average 1,000 calls per month. The institute publishes many publications, including the *Benefits Checklist for Older Adults* and training manuals. For more information, contact the Samuel Sadin Institute on Law, Brookdale Center on Aging, Hunter College, 425 East 25th Street, 13th Floor North, New York, NY 10010; phone: 212-481-3780; www.brookdale.org.

One example of a legal hotline program is the Northern California Senior Hotline. Older adults over 60 living in northern California can call or e-mail about a legal problem and receive legal advice. In 2000, they handled approximately 500 cases per month (Legal Services of Northern California, 2001). Moore (1992) described a hotline program tested by the Legal Counsel for the Elderly that targets older adults of color. Minority volunteers are trained to act as mediators between the older adult and the hotline attorney. A volunteer conducts the preliminary interview of the older adult and gathers an understanding of the problem. The volunteer then contacts the hotline attorney, obtains information about the proper course of action, and has the responsibility of helping the client follow the advice given.

Bar Association Services

Edelstein (1996) outlined Bar association services that may be useful to older adults. These include lawyer referral services, referral and information services, reduced-fee panels, volunteer lawyer panels, and outreach programs.

Lawyer Referral Services

A lawyer referral service is typically composed of a panel of attorneys who will give advice or represent individuals with legal problems. Callers are referred to an attorney who has some expertise with the type of legal problem encountered and who is located nearby. The initial consultation is provided free of charge or for a small fee, with no obligation to continue with that particular attorney. No prescreening is done on the legal merits of the case.

Lawyer Referral and Information Services

A lawyer referral and information service is similar to the lawyer referral service except that calls are screened more carefully for legal merit, and simple problems are often resolved before the referral is made. The service is provided at no cost or for a nominal fee, and there is no further obligation by the client to continue with the attorney.

Reduced-Fee Panels

Reduced-fee panels are coordinated by local or state Bar associations and are composed of attorneys who will provide legal assistance in specialized areas of law. For example, the Maryland State Bar Association sponsors a Sixty-Plus Legal Program through which participating attorneys offer low-cost assistance with wills, living wills, powers of attorney, and small estate administration for older adults with moderate or low incomes.

Volunteer Lawyer Panels

Some communities have created pro bono legal programs staffed with volunteer attorneys who provide free legal assistance to older adults. These pro bono programs usually require clients to meet some financial guidelines and often limit the type of legal problems they accept. One pro bono program enlists volunteer paralegals who deliver free legal services at "Saturday clinics" at a different site each month in minority communities (Moore, 1992).

State and local Bar associations also are involved in educating older adults about potential legal problems. Bar associations may sponsor continuing education sessions about legal problems germane to older adults, produce legal handbooks for senior citizens, and sponsor "law days" for older adults (Coleman, Wood, Sabatino, Nelson, & Baker, 1986).

Outreach Programs

The American Bar Association's Commission on Law and Aging funds a number of legal outreach programs through its Partnerships in Law and Aging Program. Outreach programs are designed to deliver legal services to isolated older adults. One example of such a program is the Legal Services of Eastern Missouri's Homebound Elderly Outreach Project, which recruits and trains volunteer attorneys and law students to provide legal services (primarily wills, powers of attorney, and advance directives) to the socially and economically needy, homebound, elderly population in St. Louis. And in San Luis Obispo County, California, the Latino Elders Outreach Program targets Spanish-speaking elders in rural areas to explain legal aspects of problems and to provide legal assistance if needed.

Dispute Resolution Programs

Mediation services offer individuals an alternative to the costs associated with traditional court litigation. Mediation is done through a neutral third party who guides the parties to a mutual resolution. Mediation is usually less expensive, less time consuming, and less stressful than traditional legal methods, and mediation settlements tend to be more lasting than settlements imposed by the courts (Edelstein, 1996).

Dispute resolution programs are emerging across the country as a viable alternative to going to court. Many dispute resolutions programs are sponsored by local or state Bar associations and university law school programs. For many older adults who have legal problems, a dispute resolution program may be a better option than the traditional court system, although the extent to which older adults use dispute resolution services is unknown.

Money Management Programs

For some older adults, paying bills and managing finances becomes an overwhelming task because of health limitations or inexperience. Although family members frequently assist with money management tasks (Stone et al., 1987), many older adults who do not have an informal support network to turn to are not able to easily secure this type of assistance. Money management programs have been created to assist older adults with their financial activities.

These programs help clients with bill paying and check depositing, sorting through medical bills and filing claims to insurance companies, budgeting, and preparing durable powers of attorney or burial trusts (Tokarek, 1996).

Best Practice: Dispute Resolution Center

The Dispute Resolution Center in Saint Paul, Minnesota, is a private nonprofit organization founded to provide mediation, facilitation, training, and referral services in the Twin Cities. As a community resource, the center assists individuals, families, community groups, government agencies, and businesses in resolving conflicts. A majority of the individuals served by the center are people in lower income ranges. Through constructive means such as mediation and facilitation, the center has helped in thousands of matters to prevent the need for costly litigation.

The Dispute Resolution Center is a Certified Community Dispute Resolution Program under the guidelines administered by the Supreme Court. The center works with social service and government agencies, and handles between 400 and 500 cases on average each year. Community problems handled include matters of public safety concerning traffic and parking; rental arrangements; consumer-merchant disputes; neighborhood conflicts about noise, pets, and property lines; and small claims concerning money, property damage, or breach of contract.

To accomplish its goals of fostering open communication and encouraging positive responses to conflict, the Dispute Resolution Center recruits and trains a diverse group of volunteer mediators. The center benefits from more than 50 volunteers who represent a broad cross-section of the community. In 1998, the volunteers contributed approximately 2,000 volunteer hours as mediators, office workers, and board members.

The Dispute Resolution Center also provides workshops and presentations on conflict resolution and communication for community groups and organizations such as schools, colleges, landlord or tenant unions, community councils, block clubs, youth centers, and other audiences.

For more information, contact Dispute Resolution Center, 974 West Seventh Street, Saint Paul, MN 55102; phone: 612-292-7791; www.disputeresolutioncenter.org.

CHALLENGES FOR LEGAL PROGRAMS AND SERVICES

Removing Barriers to Legal Services

One important challenge for legal assistance programs is to identify and remove the barriers that impede older adults in obtaining legal relief. Although no empirical research has documented the reasons why older adults might hesitate to seek legal assistance, anecdotal information from individuals providing legal assistance suggests that numerous barriers act to keep older adults from seeking legal services. Among them are personal factors, such as a lack of knowledge about legal rights, fear of the legal system, embarrassment, and structural factors, such as geographic distance, that act to limit access to services.

Best Practice: Jewish Family and Children's Services

The Jewish Family and Children's Services offer a personal affairs management program for frail older adults who live in San Francisco and San Mateo counties. The fee-for-service program provides different levels of assistance to clients. In "no authority" cases, staff members assist clients in paying bills, budgeting, and processing medical claims. When a client's physical health makes it difficult to write checks or sign documents, a durable power of attorney is executed by a staff member. This enables the staff member to sign documents on behalf of the client. If the client becomes or is unable to make decisions on his or her own behalf, a staff member can seek a conservatorship. A court-ordered conservatorship awards a staff member legal authority to manage a client's assets. The program has approximately 95 clients and is staffed by two full-time employees.

One case involved an older man who had been isolated in his apartment because of his difficulties with emphysema. When program staff members met with him, they discovered $60,000 worth of undeposited Social Security, pension, and disability checks, as well as a year's worth of unprocessed medical claims. In addition to taking care of the client's financial needs, staff arranged to have meals delivered to his home.

For more information about the Personal Affairs Management program, contact the Jewish Family and Children's Services, 2150 Post Street, San Francisco, CA 94115; phone: 415-449-3700; www.jfcs.org/Services/Seniors.

Source: Tokarek (1996).

As mentioned earlier, if older adults are not aware that a problem they are experiencing has legal remedies, they will not be inclined to seek out legal advice or assistance. Even when it is apparent that the problem encountered needs a legal professional, for many older adults the legal system seems complicated, foreign, and intimidating. It is often difficult to find an appropriate attorney, and frail older adults might not have the physical or mental stamina to fight what they imagine will be lengthy litigation, with its complications and confusing legalese. Furthermore, having a legal problem can elicit feelings of embarrassment, especially when the legal problem has occurred because of poor judgment or lack of foresight.

Making Legal Programs More Accessible

Another challenge is to make legal programs easily accessible. Programs that do provide legal assistance are often not readily accessible to those without transportation or people who live in rural areas. Although legal services may be available in a given community, if they are located away from low-income neighborhoods or segregated neighborhoods, such programs will be less available to these at-risk populations. Language barriers and a lack of cultural sensitivity can keep many older adults from various ethnic backgrounds from seeking legal assistance. This is especially significant because racial and ethic minority elders have greater unmet legal needs than do their White counterparts (American Association of Retired Persons, cited in Moore, 1989).

Supporting Legal Programs in the Future

Finally, in recent years, legal assistance programs have been underfunded and understaffed. If the legal needs of low-income and middle-class older adults are to be addressed, funds for legal programs that serve older adults should be increased. The 2005 White House Conference on Aging delegates recommended resolutions that supported a number of new policies that ensured authorization of and adequate access to legal assistance programs. In addition, delegates recommended the implementation of programs and policies that affect older adults in a number of legal concerns. Some of the strategies included the following:

Access to Legal Services

- Ensuring access of seniors to legal services through funding of legal service providers.
- Providing access to legal counsel for elderly in fraud and abuse situations.
- Providing more adequate federal funding for civil legal aid nationwide for low- and moderate-income older Americans of diverse cultural backgrounds.

Advance Directives

- Educating the public and legal and health care providers on end of life, and the legal and ethical obligation to follow advance care directives.
- Developing health care and community collaborations with faith-based communities, aging service, and other community providers to promote advance care planning and completion of advance directives for all individuals.
- Providing, through public education, mandatory courses on aging and end-of-life issues targeting elementary, junior high, and high school students.

Preventing Elder Abuse and Fraud

- Enacting and fully funding comprehensive justice legislation to address elder abuse, guaranteeing protection for older Americans and building the capacity of APS programs in every state.
- Developing innovative prevention and intervention programs for elder mistreatment. Such programs should be culturally sensitive.
- Enacting laws which specifically protect Native American Elders from financial exploitation and abuse.
- Establishing public–private partnerships for detection of abuse, neglect, and exploitation—for example, banks, utility companies, post office, press, and aging network.
- Strengthening laws for prosecuting mail fraud from other countries using P.O. box clearinghouses.
- Increasing training about elder abuse to all relevant professionals, including law enforcement and prosecutors to ensure maximum prosecution of offenders.

Guardianships

- Expanding guardianship and protective services to include a complete and integrated set of services such as financial management, legal assistance, and cognitive evaluation.
- Developing adequate systems to regulate and oversee guardians/conservators of incapacitated adults.

As the number of older adults increases in the coming decade, there will no doubt be a greater demand for legal assistance programs and services. This increase in demand for services will likely occur without an increase in funding levels, and legal service providers and AAAs will be challenged to develop creative methods of legal education and service delivery.

CASE STUDY

A Widow in Legal Trouble

Jean is a 66-year-old woman who was widowed at age 65. She and her husband, Fred, had been married for 42 years when he died suddenly of a heart attack. For most of their working years, they managed apartments. Jean assumed the office duties, and her husband maintained the physical building and grounds. This employment gave them an apartment, utilities, and an income of approximately $20,000 per year. It was a dependable existence, and they were well liked and respected by their renters.

Like many husbands of that generation, Fred paid the bills and balanced the checkbook. Jean always depended on Fred to handle the couple's finances. After Fred's death, Jean, of necessity, had to take over the finances. Within two months, Jean realized that she was in deep trouble. Unbeknown to her, Fred had been taking cash advances from eight credit cards to support a gambling habit. The credit card receipts were arriving, it seemed to Jean, almost daily. To her horror and distress, the cash advances totaled $40,000. Now unemployed and frail from her advancing emphysema, Jean was barely getting by on $812 Social Security per month. Quickly, Jean realized that, after rent, utilities, groceries, prescription drugs, and other necessities, she could not pay off this incredible debt.

Jean's daughter, Susan, was sympathetic and supportive but unable to provide financial assistance. A few years earlier, Jean and Fred had invested the little savings they had in a grocery business for their daughter. This was an unsuccessful venture that eventually went bankrupt. The first credit collection calls have begun, and Jean is completely distraught. She finally mustered up the courage to tell her best friend what had happened, but then it took her another two weeks to pick up the telephone and call the senior paralegal program at the local area AAA.

Case Study Questions

1. Jean, like Fernando in the introduction to this chapter, has multiple problems. List all possible problems that could be brought on by Jean's husband's actions.

2. Which of Jean's problems are legal issues? Which fall into other service categories?

3. Of all Jean's problems and worries, what is the single thing that could be addressed that would bring her the most peace of mind? Defend your choice.

4. Considering the chapter's discussion of why older adults might hesitate to seek legal assistance, what factors in Jean's case substantiate her reluctance to call an attorney?

5. Jean's health situation suggests that possible end-of-life legal issues could be addressed. Referencing the chapter, suggest one or two other legal areas that could be approached with Jean.

Learning Activities

1. Make an inventory of the legal aid programs that serve older adults in your community. What type of cases do they accept? Where do these programs refer people when they cannot take their cases? What is the breakdown of the cases they accept in a given year?

2. Contact your local District Attorney's Office and arrange an interview to find out about cases of elder abuse and fraud involving older adults that the office prosecutes each year. Does the office sponsor any public education for older adults about consumer fraud or elder abuse?

3. Make a list of the legal problems discussed in this chapter. Obtain permission from 10 older adults to ascertain whether they have had any of these legal problems in the last year. If so, ask them if they sought legal advice for the problem and the outcome of the situation. Be sure to keep your interviewees' names confidential when reporting your findings.

For More Information

National Resources

1. American Bar Association, Commission on Law and Aging, American Bar Association, 740 15th Street, N.W., Washington, DC 20005-1019; phone: 202-662-1000; www.abanet.org.
   The commission focuses on the legal concerns of older adults and provides technical assistance, models of legal assistance projects, telephone and written assistance, publications, and speakers.
2. American Association of Retired Persons Foundation Legal Advocacy, 601 E Street N.W., Washington, DC 20049; phone: 888-687-2277; www.aarp.org/research/legal-advocacy.
   AARP Foundation Legal Advocacy is one of the few national organizations that defends and supports the legal rights of older Americans across the United States—assuring that they have a voice in our judicial system. Their legal work encompasses areas of federal and state laws that affect older Americans' day-to-day lives, including, age and disability discrimination in employment, pensions and financial fraud including predatory lending, health and long-term care, disability, and government and public benefits

3. National Senior Citizens Law Center, 1101 14th Street, N.W., Suite 400, Washington, DC 20005; phone: 202-289-6976; www.nsclc.org.

    The center offers advice, litigation assistance, and training and program development assistance to legal services providers and state and local area agencies on aging.

Web Resources

1. AoA's National Aging Information Notes on Legal Services for Older Adults: www.aoa.gov/prof/notes/notes_legal_services.asp.

    This is a great place to start when looking for legal resources for older adults. AoA has compiled links to legal resources and resources about elder abuse. Updates to the page are made regularly.

2. SeniorLAWCenter Home Page: www.seniorlawcenter.org.

    SeniorLAW Center, in Philadelphia, provides free legal representation and legal education to older adults. The site provides information about a variety of legal issues of concern to older adults and also describes a number of special projects the centre has, including the Legal Services for Hispanic Elders, Community-Based Neighborhood Legal Services and Community Clinics, KinCAN—Kinship Caregiver Assistance Network, and The Homebound Elderly Legal Project.

3. National Senior Citizens Law Center: www.nsclc.org.

    The center has information about its services, manuals, and publications, as well as information about Social Security and SSI, Medicare, Medicaid, nursing home residents' rights, home care, pension rights, age discrimination and mandatory retirement, and OAA services.

4. National Committee for the Prevention of Elder Abuse Page: www.preventelderabuse.org.

    The National Committee for the Prevention of Elder Abuse (NCPEA) is an association of researchers, educators, and practitioners who conduct research and provide professionals with information about intervention strategies. The website contains links to critical issues, what communities can do to prevent elder abuse, help for victims and vulnerable persons, and a bibliography.

5. ABA Commission on Law and Aging: www.abanet.org.

    The Commission examines a wide range of law-related issues, including legal services to older persons, health and long-term care, housing needs, Social Security, Medicare, Medicaid, and other public benefit programs, and offers a number of online legal resources.

6. *Senior Citizens Handbook*: Prairie State Legal Services: www.pslegal.org/Publications/Senior_Handbook/Index.htm.

    Prairie State Legal Services is a not-for-profit corporation that provides free legal help to senior citizens and low-income persons in 36 counties in northern and central Illinois. The *Senior Citizens Handbook* offers information about a variety of legal issues such as health care, family issues, consumer issues, and long-term care. It's one good example of the many consumer senior legal handbooks available to elders and their advocates in many states.

7. National Center on Elder Abuse: www.elderabusecenter.org.

    The National Center on Elder Abuse is funded by the AoA and is operated through a partnership with a number of national organizations. The center's comprehensive website provides information about elder abuse and resources. Visitors can also access the quarterly newsletter, *NCEA Exchange*.

14

Transportation

An older man in a wheelchair was picked up by a paratransit system in El Paso, Texas, to go from the nursing home where he resided to K-Mart. The trip did not take more than 15 minutes. During the trip, the man expressed how pleased he was to be getting out. He said that he had been a resident of the nursing home for seven years and that this was his first outing during that time that was not medically related (Peterson, 1995, p. 12).

It is difficult to understand how most of us would feel if we could not do something as common as take a trip to K-Mart. We jump in our cars at a moment's notice to run this or that errand. For most Americans, taking several trips per day to a variety of locations is a common occurrence. This gentleman, however, was grateful that accessible transportation was available and thrilled to be enjoying a nonmedical outing. The actual purpose of his trip may have been less important to him than the opportunity for an outing.

Mobility attained through the private automobile is the American way of life. We all remember the anticipation of getting our first driver's license. Most teenagers are excited to obtain a driver's license, and having a car is a rite of passage. Aside from deriving enjoyment from car travel, without transportation we could not meet our basic needs. Going to work, buying groceries, seeing the doctor, going to the park, visiting with friends—all become difficult and often impossible without transportation. Thus we enter later life being accustomed to having the ability to come and go as we please.

Transportation plays a critical role in the physical, social, and psychological well-being of older persons. Physical health depends on access to medical facilities and other social services. The ability to maintain an active social life in old age depends on accessibility to family and friends as well as recreational and cultural activities. Key ingredients of psychological health that are enhanced by mobility are the ability to choose one's range of activities and promoting the feeling of belonging to the community (Wachs, 1979).

In this chapter, we review the legislative history of transportation services, the transportation patterns of older adults, and the different models of transportation services available. We conclude by identifying some of the challenges in meeting the transportation needs of an aging society.

POLICY BACKGROUND

Twentieth-century growth patterns, coupled with America's emphasis on travel by personal automobile, have contributed greatly to decline in travel options. Private transportation has come to dominate travel in this country to such an extent that the United States is less connected via public transportation in the 1990s than it was in the late 1920s. Previously, through a series of easy transfers, passengers could travel from Burlington, Iowa, in the southeast corner of the state, along the Mississippi River, to Waverly in central Iowa—a distance of more than 150 miles—and back in the same day. The same journey today would be impossible ("Community Service is Key," 1994). In an attempt to reverse this trend, federal and state transportation legislation has been enacted during the past 25 years to increase transportation options for persons who are transit dependent.

Responsiveness to mobility needs began in the 1970s when the United States made significant gains in providing transportation options for elders and persons with disabilities. Beginning in 1970, an amendment to the Urban Mass Transportation Act of 1964 advanced the cause of transportation for older adults and persons with disabilities by mandating that these individuals have the same right as other persons to use mass transportation facilities and services. Spurred on by demands made by older adults, persons with disabilities, and their advocates, approximately 4,000 or more special-purpose transportation systems were in operation by the end of the decade (Ashford, Bell, & Rich, 1982). These programs varied from a single vehicle to a fleet of buses serving urban and rural areas, resulting in a mosaic of transportation programs across the country. During this same period, transportation was the "sleeper" issue at the 1971 White House Conference on Aging, ranking third in importance, preceded by income and health.

Another important statute of the 1970s, the Rehabilitation Act of 1973 (§ 504), directed federally assisted transit providers to offer half-fare service to older persons in off-peak periods. These regulations also required that local transit planning processes make special efforts to plan public mass transportation facilities and services that could effectively be used by older and disabled persons. Transportation planners and operators responded to Section 504 mandates by implementing special transportation systems for the older adults and persons with disabilities. These systems used smaller buses and vans, and could provide door-to-door service. Such systems became known as *paratransit* operations.

During the 1980s, the United States entered a second generation of specialized transportation developments. Although the 1970s were a decade of growth and development of specialized transportation systems, the 1980s were a decade of retrenchment in response to a general tightening of the availability of financial resources at all levels of government (Ashford et al., 1982). The 1980s were also a time when transportation systems emphasized cost-effectiveness and efficiency in providing public transportation. Federal legislation required that programs applying for federal transit funds develop a transit development plan. These plans identified present and future needs and how transportation would be coordinated with other providers. Only with an approved plan could local or regional transit groups compete for federal transit funding. Today, transit development plans are still a requirement to receive federal transit funding.

In the 1990s, two laws were passed that greatly influenced public transit. The first was the Americans with Disabilities Act (ADA), signed into law in July 1990. This far-reaching law prohibits discrimination against people with disabilities in almost all aspects of American life and extends comprehensive civil rights to people with disabilities similar to those conferred on racial minorities by the Civil Rights Act of 1964. ADA requirements cover transportation services, facilities, and equipment of all entities, public and private. A key requirement of the ADA is that all new transit vehicles must be accessible to persons with wheelchairs. Fixed-route systems must offer a paratransit or specialized service for persons with disabilities who cannot access the fixed-route system. Furthermore, this paratransit service must be comparable to the fixed-route service in fares, hours and days of operation, response times, and geographic areas covered. The ADA also provides specific eligibility criteria for the comparable paratransit service for what constitutes disability.

Prior to the ADA, many paratransit systems transported elders because of age or disability. Ironically, because age alone is not a factor in determining ADA eligibility, the passage of the ADA may have proved to be a barrier for older adults who rely on public transportation services. Could older passengers who do not meet the stricter disability guidelines lose their mobility so that the program has the resources to meet the ADA obligations? The Act, it was feared, would motivate transit operators to reduce service because they would lack the resources to respond effectively to all mobility needs (Rosenbloom, 1993a). A 1992 study commissioned by the American Association of Retired Persons (AARP) looked at 300 ADA implementation plans and interviewed 18 communities for an in-depth analysis of how they would approach ADA implementation. The study found that most of the 18 case study cities admitted that many older persons would be found ineligible by new screening and certification procedures (Rosenbloom, 1993b). How many older Americans meet the stricter ADA requirements, how many will actually be displaced by the ADA from paratransit service, and how local communities will ultimately respond to this situation all remain unanswered questions at this time. Further research is needed to understand how the ADA has affected older Americans.

The Intermodal Surface Transportation Efficiency Act (ISTEA) of 1991 made several significant changes to the federal transit program. One obvious change was renaming the federal agency that oversees the transit industry.

The agency that had been called the Urban Mass Transportation Administration since its birth in 1964 was renamed the Federal Transit Administration (FTA). This name change reflected an awareness by Congress and the federal government that public transportation is vital to all citizens, urban and rural (Rucker, 1995a). ISTEA specifically addressed the mobility needs of older persons, persons with disabilities, and those who are economically disadvantaged. The legislation also placed great emphasis on local, regional, and state planning and coordination; it made funding of capital and operating costs dependent on assurances that local transit systems were coordinated with regional and state transit plans. The most current transportation legislation was signed into law in 2005: the Safe, Accountable, Flexible, Efficient Transportation Act—A Legacy for Users (SAFETEA-LU). The Act provides $286.4 billion for transit programs through the year 2009 (American Public Transportation Association, 2005).

USERS AND PROGRAMS

Transportation Patterns of Older Adults

Older Americans largely rely on private vehicles for their transportation needs. In 1997, 92% of all men and 67% of all women age 65 and over had a driver's license (Rosenbloom & Waldorf, 1999). Up to age 75, the majority of older adults have good driving records and appear to perform as well as middle-aged drivers. However, older adults age 85 and older have a fatality rate that is nine times higher than drivers between the ages of 25 and 69 for each mile driven (National Highway Transportation Safety Administration, 2001). Exhibit 14.1 shows the percentages of older urban, suburban, and rural adults who rely on various forms of mobility. The majority of older adults, regardless of location, rely on private vehicles rather than public transit for transportation needs. Almost 90% of trips taken by older adults over age 65 are in a personal vehicle (National Cooperative Highway Research Program, 2006).

However, compared with younger drivers, a higher percentage of older adults do not drive. Twenty percent of older adults over age 65 do not drive compared with 6.9% of people between the ages of 19 and 64. Isolation is greater among older non-drivers than older drivers, as over half of non-drivers, compared with 17% of older drivers over age 65, or 3.6 million people, stay home on any given day and make fewer trips for social, family, religious, and medical reasons (Bailey, 2004; National Highway Transportation Survey, 2001). Moreover, isolation of older non-drivers is greater among racial and ethnic minority elders and those living in the southern and Midwestern states (Bailey, 2004).

Not surprisingly, a small percentage of older adults report using public transportation. When examining the use of public transportation among older adults, only 11.5% of older adults reported using transit, 34% indicated that there was no transit available to use, and 53.8% indicated that transit was available, but they did not use it (National Cooperative Highway Research Program, 2006). Those most likely to use transit were non-White and

EXHIBIT 14.1 Travel Modes by Gender and Residence for Persons Aged 65 Years and Older (in percentages)

Mode	Urban	Suburban	Rural
Private vehicle	77.3	93.7	94.8
As driver	54.9	71.7	68.1
As passenger	22.4	22.0	26.7
Public transit	8.5	0.9	0.3
Walking	13.3	4.6	4.6
All other modes	0.9	0.8	0.3

Source: Rosenbloom and Waldorf (1999, p. 107).

those living in city centers, and those least likely to use public transit were the oldest old, rural persons, and those with two or more ADL limitations.

Gender

Among the current cohort of older adults over the age of 65, women are less likely to hold a driver's license, less likely to drive than men, and take fewer and shorter trips than do men (National Cooperative Highway Research Program, 2006). Twenty-seven percent of women over age 65 indicate that they do not drive (National Cooperative Highway Research Program, 2006). Overall, both urban and rural older women are less likely to rely on a private vehicle, and more likely to use public transportation, than are older men. Higher percentages of older men and women, regardless of residence, rely on walking more than they do on public transit systems (Murakami, 1994).

Health

Many factors influence the mobility of older persons, and consequently the use or nonuse of public transportation. The most obvious is health. Of the more than 30 million Americans aged 65 or older, 16% (almost 5 million) report some sort of mobility limitation because of a health condition that has lasted for six or more months and has resulted in difficulty going outside the home alone. The incidence of health-related mobility problems is substantially higher for women and is higher among rural residents (21%) than among urban residents (12%; National Eldercare Institute on Transportation, 1994). Fifteen percent of those who do not ride public transportation, even though it is available, said it was because of a health limitation (National Cooperative Highway Research Program, 2006). Thus older adults with mobility limitations are among those who are transit dependent.

Geographic Location

Geographic location also affects mobility options. Rural residents who are aged, disabled, or poor are particularly transit dependent. Nationally, 76 million people are considered transit dependent, and rural areas account for 29 million, or 38% of the total. Specifically, 32% of all rural residents are classified as transit dependent (U.S. Bureau of the Census, 1996b). By contrast, only 30% of urban residents are so classified. Another factor resulting in rural transportation deficiency is the loss of long-haul bus services to 15% of rural communities. More than 50% of the nation's rural residents live in areas with no federally assisted public transit service (National Eldercare Institute on Transportation, 1994).

One way to analyze transit ridership by older adults is to break ridership patterns into urban, small urban, and rural components. This is useful because there are differences among these areas. A study prepared for the Administration on Aging (AoA) showed that in the 33 largest cities (those with populations of more than 1 million), transit resources were substantial, yet many of the mobility needs of older adults were still unmet (National Eldercare Institute on Transportation, 1994). In those areas, only 6% of the total ridership and 13% of the noncommuter ridership were composed of older persons. In small urban areas (areas of 50,000 to 200,000 persons), the total served was substantially less than in the large urban areas. Furthermore, the total amount of service per senior was substantially less: 12.5 trips annually in small urban areas, 20 trips annually in areas with a population between 200,000 and 1 million, and 37 trips annually for the largest urban areas. Transit ridership by older adults in rural areas was even more limited. Of the 7.9 million persons aged 65 and older living in nonmetropolitan areas, 36% (2.8 million) lived in places without public transportation. Another 48% (3. million) lived in areas in which use of public transit services was less than two rides per year.

Income and Race

Economic problems also magnify transportation problems. In 2000, 10.2% of older adults, or 3.4 million, in the United States were living in poverty. Elders living in rural areas were poorer than their urban counterparts (13.2% of older adults living in rural areas were poor, compared with 12.4% living in urban areas). Racial and ethic minority elders are more at risk of being poor than are their white peers. For example, in 2000, approximately 8.9% of white elders were living in poverty, whereas nearly a quarter of all African Americans aged 65 or older were poor. For Native American elders, the poverty rate was 29%; for Hispanic elders, it was 23% (Administration on Aging [AoA], 2001f). Thus, the expense of maintaining a private vehicle is beyond the means of many low-income older persons and low-income non-White elders. Twenty-eight percent of older African-Americans, 19% of older Latinos, and 9% of Asian Americans live in households without a car (Bailey, 2004).

As shown in Exhibit 14.2, non-driving among older adults is greatest among those over age 85, women, non-Whites, poor, those living alone and in center cities, and those with a greater number of ADL limitations (National Cooperative Highway Research Program, 2006).

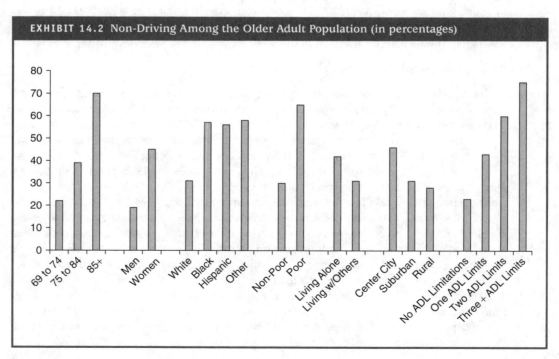

EXHIBIT 14.2 Non-Driving Among the Older Adult Population (in percentages)

Source: National Cooperative Highway Research Program (2006, p. 19).

Availability and Use of Public Transit

Non-drivers who have transportation needs must rely on either friends or family or use public transportation. Unfortunately, 51% of all Americans report that they do not have access to public transportation services (Bailey, 2004). Interestingly, less than half of the baby boomer population is located within three-quarters of a mile of a fixed-route transportation system (National Cooperative Highway Research Program, 2006). Access to all forms of public transportation is markedly less in sprawling suburbs, small towns, and rural areas compared to urban areas.

Barriers to Public Transit Use

Why is the rate of public transit use by older adults so low in areas in which public transportation is available? A variety of barriers exist to keep older adults from using public transportation when it is available. If you have some free time one afternoon, try getting from your house or apartment to the senior center, grocery store, or medical clinic *via public transportation*, and try to envision yourself as an older adult. While on your trip, think about the following:

- How difficult was it to figure out the route you needed to take to get to your destination? What times did the bus service not run?
- How long did it take you to get to the bus stop? What would it be like waiting there in bad weather?
- How high was the first step into the bus? Were the seats comfortable?
- Could you get in and out of them easily?
- How many transfers did you have to make during your trip?
- How close did the bus drop you to your final destination?
- How long did it take you to complete your trip?

If you are a veteran of using public transportation, you probably do not think twice about making your way across town and completing your journey without much trouble, but how would an older adult fare? Those of you who use your car to get around probably experienced some uncertainty—we hope you did not get lost! But from an older adult's perspective, using public transportation can be challenging.

Health and Physical Barriers

Health problems or other physical impairments can keep older adults from using fixed-route transit systems. Fifteen percent of older adults reported that they did not ride transit systems because of a health problem (National Cooperative Highway Research Program, 2006). Older adults report that they have to walk long distances to the nearest bus stop and that bus stops have inadequate shelters, no benches, and poor lighting. The buses themselves may pose problems because steps into the bus are often high and narrow, the seats are difficult to get into and out of, bus windows are so dirty that they are difficult to see out of, and buses are often overcrowded (Patterson, 1985; U.S. Department of Transportation, 1980).

Fear of Crime

Fear of crime is also a concern for many older adults (Lowy, 1980; Patterson, 1985). In his study of older transit riders, Patterson found that older adults' fear of crime was significant in all aspects of the trip. For example, 77.3% reported fear while waiting at the bus stop, 69.5% were afraid while walking to and from the bus stop, and 64.8% were afraid while riding the bus. Other research has shown that most perceived crime-related experiences are classified as "quality-of-life" offenses, such as obscene language, verbal abuse, public drunkenness, vandalism, and disorderly conduct (Hardin, Tucker, & Callejas, 2001).

Bus Schedules

Another barrier to riding transit systems relates to bus schedules. Most transit systems are designed for commuters going to work, rather than to hospitals, clinics, and senior centers (Huttman, 1985). In Patterson's (1985) study, many older transit riders reported a lack of frequency of bus service during the daytime (66.9%) and evenings (78.0%). Insufficient destinations was the most frequently cited reason why older adults over age 65 in southern California did not use the transit system (Ong & Haselhoff, 2005).

Best Practice: Lane Transit District, Eugene, Oregon

Lane Transit District (LTD) operates a one-on-one training initiative called the Bus Buddy Program. The program teaches seniors how to ride the bus in a relaxed way by breaking down barriers and building confidence. LTD recruits regular bus riders to serve as volunteers, known as Bus Buddies, and partners with local senior centers to match individual seniors with these volunteers. Bus Buddies teach seniors about the LTD transit system, as well as how to plan trips and navigate routes. Each Bus Buddy and senior then ride the bus together. Afterward, the pair discusses the trip and the Bus Buddy answers any remaining questions about using public transportation in Eugene. In addition, seniors aged 62 and older can ride LTD buses free every Tuesday, courtesy of community sponsors. Seniors schedule doctors' appointments, visits with friends, and shopping trips on Tuesdays to take advantage of this offer. This has become an extremely popular program. For individuals aged 70 or older, LTD offers a "Pass for Life" card.

For more information, contact LTD, P.O. Box 7070, Eugene, OR, 97401-0470; phone: LTD Guest Services at 687-5555; www.apta.com/easyrider/workfiles/documents/gettingstarted.doc.

Source: American Public Transportation Association (2005).

The National Eldercare Institute on Transportation (1992) conducted focus groups of older adults around the country to ascertain anecdotal information about transportation barriers. Older adults reported that the ideal transportation system would have drivers who were courteous and patient, travel shorter distances to destinations located within their neighborhoods, have smaller buses that were for seniors and persons with disabilities only, not require transferring, have bilingual staff, and have more flexible bus schedules to meet the needs of community people, not just workers.

Social Barriers

Minority and ethnic elders may face additional barriers that result from cultural perceptions and a lack of sensitivity by the transportation service system. For example, many minority elders shy away from all services, including transportation, because they have experienced hurtful discriminatory practices in the past. Other barriers include language and literacy barriers, discomfort if the rider is the only minority person using the transportation system, fixed route services that do not adequately serve minority neighborhoods, and service providers who assume that minority elders rely on their families for transportation (Heath, 1993). In addition, transit providers must be able to convey to a wide demographic of individuals the knowledge and information that the service exists, where the service travels, where and how to catch the bus or light rail, the arrival and departure times, and where to disembark (Hardin, Tucker, & Callejas, 2001).

Transportation Programs

Community transportation programs vary greatly in funding and design. Transit resources available to older persons have been described as a mosaic rather than as an integrated network. This mosaic is made up of public systems supplemented by transportation programs provided by nonprofit organizations, human service agencies, caregivers, and communities of faith (National Eldercare Institute on Transportation, 1994). A transportation program could be as basic as a group of volunteers working on their own or under the auspices of an umbrella human service agency to transport older adults to medical appointments and other important destination points in their community. At the other end of the spectrum, the transportation program could be a sophisticated, multifaceted system including a fixed-route service with a complementary paratransit service that is scheduled through a fully computerized central dispatch component. In each community, it is the challenge of the human service professional to find out what programs exist, and who is eligible for service and under what circumstances.

To best understand any discussion about transportation programs, one must have a basic knowledge of a few transportation terms that describe general types of transportation delivery systems (see Exhibit 14.3). Public transportation and specialized transit have been referenced several times in this chapter. *Public transportation* is defined as service that is available for any trip purpose to any person of any age and is operated by public agencies or supported by public funds to some extent. *Specialized transit,* on the other hand, is service that is provided for a variety of trip purposes and is open to older, disabled, and/or low-income persons but usually not to the general public. Specialized operators range from urbanized operators with large fleets of more than 30 vehicles to rural systems with only one van and volunteer drivers. Another term, *incidental transit* or *human service agency transportation,* describes those programs in which transit is "incidental" to the agency's main program purpose. For example, mental health centers, senior centers, hospitals, and nursing homes often provide some transportation for their clients. The transportation, however, most likely is an optional service that the organization is providing to enhance its main program. *Commercial service* is defined as service provided by for-profit entities on a for-hire basis. Taxi services, shuttles, limousines, and charter services fall into this category.

EXHIBIT 14.3   Selected Transportation Terms

ADA: The Americans With Disabilities Act, a federal law requiring that facilities and services be made accessible to persons with disabilities

APTA: The American Public Transit Association, representing the interests of public transit agencies, particularly those in large urbanized areas

Complementary paratransit: A service that must be offered by fixed-route public transportation operators to persons with disabilities who cannot access or use regular fixed-route service

CTAA: The Community Transportation Association of America, representing the interests of specialized transit operators and those who operate in rural and small urbanized areas

Curb-to-curb service: A demand-responsive service system in which the passenger must come out to the vehicle

Deadhead: The time and/or distance that a transit vehicle does not spend in revenue service or moving passengers (e.g., the travel from a garage to the beginning of a route)

Demand-responsive service: A personalized, direct transit service usually provided for persons who are older or disabled on either an immediate demand basis or an advanced reservation basis; often used interchangeably with *paratransit, dial-a-ride,* or *specialized service*

Deviated fixed route service: A fixed-route service that will deviate from its regular route to pick up special riders such as older or disabled persons and then return to its regular route without significantly detracting from its schedule

Door-through-door service: A demand-responsive system in which the driver goes into the home and/or final destination to provide more assistance, especially for frail or disoriented individuals

Door-to-door service: A demand-responsive service system in which the driver goes to the door of the passenger's residence and provides assistance if needed

E&D: Elderly and disabled; in the past, the more common term was E&H ("elderly and handicapped")

Fixed-route service: A regularly scheduled transit service operated over a set route

FTA: Federal Transit Administration; a federal agency in the U.S. Department of Transportation that provides funding for various transit services; formerly known as the Urban Mass Transportation Administration

Human services transportation: Transportation provided to persons served by human service programs such as Medicaid and Title III of the Older Americans Act; most transportation is provided to older, disabled, or low-income persons on a demand-responsive basis

Incidental provider: An organization that provides transit only to its own clients, mainly as a service incidental to its primary service

Paratransit: Transportation that is more flexible and personalized than conventional fixed-route, fixed-schedule mass transportation service but does not include exclusionary services such as charter or sightseeing trips (see also *demand-responsive service*)

SAFETEA-LU: Safe, Accountable, Flexible, Efficient, Transportation Equity Act—A Legacy for Users, signed into law in 2005 is the federal legislation for transit and highway programs. The Act provides funds for capital investment and programs that address special transit needs as well as research on transit issues.

Source: Mauser (1994); APTA (2005).

Best Practice: Partners in Care and the Ride Partners Program

Partners in Care is a service credit exchange program located in Severna Park, Maryland, designed to create community by linking frail elderly and disabled adults with neighbors who volunteer their time to help with occasional tasks and errands. The goal of these services is to help seniors and disabled adults remain independent in their own homes. Participants may provide services, receive services, or both. For each hour of service donated by a volunteer, an hour of service credit is earned. The credit may be used by the individual at a later time or donated back to the program for others in need. Groups of volunteers are encouraged to combine their efforts for larger projects. The majority of tasks members provide involve transportation for a variety of needs. In 2006, members of Partners in Care drove over 90,000 miles to complete a variety of tasks for individuals, including transportation to medical appointments, laboratory testing, mammograms, and pharmacy pickup. Partners in Care provides niche transportation support for those seniors who need extra help getting from their homes into a car, for trips at the edge of the normal work day, and for trips that may not be accommodated by family members or the Department of Aging van system.

The Ride Partners Program is a result of a collaboration among the Annapolis Department of Transportation, Americorps, and Partners in Care and provides out-of-county transportation. Members are encouraged to participate in these much-needed trips through a mileage reimbursement incentive and a sliding fee scale for participants. In 2005, Partners in Care provided 123 trips under the Ride Partners Program.

For more information, contact Partners in Care, Inc., 348 Ritchie Highway, Severna Park, MD 21146; phone: 410-544-4800, 301-682-5588, or 800-227-5500.

Within these general categories of transportation programs are several types of service in terms of organization. A *fixed-route* service is a regularly scheduled service operated on a set route. A *deviated fixed-route* service is a fixed-route service that will deviate from its regular route to pick up special riders such as persons who are older or disabled, depending on its passengers' requests. Let's suppose a county transportation program runs several routes a week on scheduled days and at particular times to the county's rural senior centers to transport groups of seniors to a major shopping center. Depending on the needs of the seniors, the driver will pick up or drop off seniors in neighboring towns that are off the route. The driver is also able to change the destinations according to the needs of the group being transported. This system can modify the usual route to meet the needs of the riders. Opposite to fixed-route and deviated, or modified, fixed-route services is the *demand-responsive* system, a personalized service usually provided for older and disabled persons. It is provided on an immediate-demand basis or on an advance-reservation basis. This term is often used interchangeably with *paratransit, dial-a-ride,* or *specialized service.* This service can be curb to curb (the passenger must come out to the vehicle), door to door (the driver goes to the door of the passenger's residence and provides assistance if needed), and/or door through door (the driver goes into the home and/or final destination to provide more assistance, especially to frail or disoriented individuals). An important feature of demand-responsive service is that transportation services are tailored to the needs of individual riders. Most demand-responsive systems operate minivans, vans, or minibuses to provide this service. Passengers call, usually a minimum of 24 hours in advance, to schedule a van for an appointment. The transit scheduler will match the request with the appropriate vehicle and routes. Whether a transportation system is fixed route, modified fixed route, demand responsive, or a combination of service modes depends on the needs of the community and the resources available to meet those needs (Mauser, 1994).

Federal Transit Administration

Of the types of transportation described above, most visible are the programs funded with federal funds, which provide over half of all public money for transportation for older persons. Most of that money comes from two sources: the FTA and the U.S. Department of Health and Human Services (Lee, 1993; USDHHS). This network provides an estimated 95 million trips per year in rural areas and 7.7 billion trips per year in urban areas (Rucker, 1995b).

Four principal funding sources through the FTA are critical to meeting the mobility needs of older and disabled persons. One FTA program, called Formula Grants for Other Than Urbanized Areas or Section 5311, apportions funds to states for public transportation in rural and small urban public transportation areas. In most Section 5311 programs, however, the majority of riders are older persons or persons with disabilities. Section 5311 transit systems provides an estimated 154.2 million trips per year and elderly riders account for 31%, while 23% of riders are persons with disabilities. Section 5311 programs are made up of a network of approximately 1,200 public, private for-profit, and private nonprofit agencies that cover a service area of 3.5 million square miles and 91 million people (Community Transportation Association of America, 2001). Demand-responsive service is the most common mode of service among Section 5311 providers (85%). Fixed-route service is provided by 51% of providers and route and point deviation services are offered by 50% of providers (Community Transportation Association of America, 2001). The remaining service is fixed route or modified fixed route. Funding for Section 5311 in 2006 was $388 million (U.S. Department of Transportation, 2005a).

Section 5310, Formula Grants for Special Needs of Elderly and Disabled Individuals, is another FTA program that offers funds to assist with the purchase of capital equipment to agencies serving older persons and persons with disabilities. Each state determines specific program eligibility criteria since the legislation does not define "elderly" or "disabled" (Koffman, Raphael, & Weiner, 2004). Funds can be awarded to private nonprofit organizations and to public organizations as well. The SAFETEA-LU legislation increases coordination requirements and projects must coordinate with human service transportation plans (U.S. Department of Transportation, 2005b). Seven states—Wisconsin, Alaska, Minnesota, Oregon, and three other states yet to be identified—will participate in a pilot program that will increase the amount of funds that can be used for operating assistance in hopes that this will improve services to elderly adults and individuals with disabilities. Nearly 3,700 transportation providers in the United States receive Section 5310 funds and over a 10-year period (1992–2001) 18,000 vehicles were purchased with Section 5310 funds (Koffman, Raphael, & Weiner, 2004). Funding for Section 5310 in 2006 was $112 million (U.S. Department of Transportation, 2005b).

Section 5307 makes federal monies available for public transportation in urbanized areas. Formula grants are available to communities of 50,000 or larger for transportation planning, equipment costs, and operation costs. Recipients of these funds may not serve nonurbanized areas and are not required to serve the entire urbanized area they represent. For example, unincorporated areas surrounding a large city may not be served by the city's Section 5307 program (Mauser, 1994).

A new program enacted under the new SAFETEA-LU legislation is Section 5317, "New Freedom Program." The purpose of this program is to provide funds to encourage service and facility improvements to address the transportation needs of persons with disabilities that go beyond what is required by the Americans with Disability Act. Projects must coordinate with locally developed human service transportation programs. Funding for 2006 was established at $78 million (U.S. Department of Transportation, 2005c).

Department of Health and Human Services

Under the USDHHS, transportation programs are funded primarily through the Older Americans Act (OAA), the Community Services Block Grant, and Title XIX of the Social Security Act (Exhibit 14.4). Title III, Part B of the OAA authorizes transportation services to facilitate access to supportive services, nutrition services, or both. How these monies flow to the states and local area agencies on aging (AAAs) is explained in Chapter 2.

The network of Title III–funded older adult transportation providers includes more than 2,400 agencies using an estimated 15,800 vehicles. Some 30% of these Title III agencies also receive FTA Section 5310 funding, and another 10% to 12% receive other FTA funding, including Section 5307 described above. Program data for the fiscal year 2004 show that Title III programs provided 2,007,470 one-way assisted trips (AoA, 2006f). Expenditures under Title III of the OAA in 2004 for transportation for older adults totaled $201,446,586, representing 8.5% of Title III expenditures. Because the AoA discourages the use of Title III funds for the purchase of vans, the major portions of these monies were allocated for operational rather than capital expenses (National Eldercare Institute on Transportation, 1994). Transportation services are also funded under Title VI which provides funds to Native American Indian Tribes. Often, OAA funds are part of a public–private partnership to increase transportation services. A private or corporate entity will work with a government entity—in this case, the local AAA—to deliver a service to needy older adults. In 2000, $107 million in state and local funds were used to match OAA funds used for transportation services (AoA, 2002b). This is a growing trend to maximize resources.

An example of such a public–private venture is in Springdale, Arkansas, where the AAA issues coupons to elderly adults with low incomes and persons with disabilities to offset a portion of the cost of a taxi trip with the local taxi company. The city gains a valuable service for its older adults and residents with disabilities. Meanwhile, the taxi company increases its ridership (Area Agency on Aging of Northwest Arkansas, 2006).

Two other important sources of support for public transportation are the Community Service Block Grant and Title XIX Medicaid, both USDHHS programs. Under the block grant program, states and Indian tribes receive funding to provide a broad range of social services for low-income persons. These funds are awarded on a formula basis to states, which pass the majority of these funds on to local nonprofit community action programs. Transportation services commonly are provided by many of these local programs.

EXHIBIT 14.4 Important Sources of Transportation Support Through the Federal Department of Health and Human Services

Funding Source	Eligible Recipients	Program Description
Title III	State Agencies on Aging and local Area Agencies on Aging who subcontract with local providers	Funds are available through Title III, Part B of the Older Americans Act to provide community-based systems of transportation, legal, and in-home services for elders, as well as for multipurpose senior centers.
Title VI	Tribal organizations and public or private nonprofit organizations which service Native American elders	Funds are available through Title VI of the Older Americans Act to provide nutrition, information and referral, transportation, and other services to Indian elders.
Community Services Block Grant	Funds are available to local agencies, often county based, to serve low-income persons.	Funds may be utilized for employment, education, housing, nutrition, energy, emergency assistance, and related needs such as transportation for elders, low-income persons, and the disabled.
Title XX Social Services Block Grant	State and local social service agencies	Enables states to address goals of reduced dependency on social programs. Services can include transportation.
Medicaid	State and local medical assistance agencies	Funds available through Title XIX of the Social Security Act to enable states to provide health care services to medically needy low-income persons. States are to assure transportation to medical services for Medicaid beneficiaries.
Developmental Disabilities Basic Support Grants	State and local developmental disabilities agencies, often called Community Center Boards	Funds provide medical services, support services—programs that enable persons with developmental disabilities to become independent and productive; transportation is a key service for independence.

Title XIX of the Social Security Act, the Medicaid Program, establishes and supports essential health care for low-income people—primarily older persons, persons with disabilities, and single-parent households with dependent children. Nonemergency medical transportation (NEMT) has been part of the Medicaid program since 1969, when federal regulations mandated that states ensure access to medical services for all Medicaid recipients who have no other means of transportation available to them. However, the ways in which transportation services are delivered vary widely from state to state. Some states offer a comprehensive array of transportation services that include taxis, vans, and public transportation passes, whereas other states simply provide gasoline vouchers or mileage reimbursement (Koffman, Raphael, & Weiner, 2004). A Community Transportation Association of America study in 2000 (Raphael, 2001) reported that state and federal funding for NEMT services totaled $1.75 billion. States spend about 1% of Medicaid expenditures on transportation services and provide more than 100 million trips. Rural transit agencies are particularly reliant on Medicaid NEMT which provides between 8% and 70% of their transportation budgets.

Successful transportation programs can tap many other sources of funding to meet the needs of mobility-dependent persons. Examples include other federal sources, foundations, advertising, rider fees, and special fundraising events (see Exhibit 14.5).

EXHIBIT 14.5   Some Other Federal Sources of Transportation Funding

Funding Source	Eligible Recipients	Program Description
Congregate Housing Services Program	Public bodies and private nonprofit corporations managing housing for elders and persons with disabilities	Funds are available to provide meals and non-medical support services, including transportation services, to allow frail elders or disabled persons to maintain maximum independence in a home environment.
Foster Grandparent Program	Sate and local government agencies, private nonprofit organizations	Funds may be used to provide stipends, transportation, and other support services for low-income elders working as volunteers in programs serving infants, children, or youth with special needs.
Retired Senior Volunteer Program	State and local government agencies, private nonprofit corporations	Funds may be used to provide transportation and other support services for elders to work as volunteers in community-service activities.
Senior Companion Programs	State and local government agencies, private nonprofit corporations	Funds may be used to provide transportation and other support services for low-income elders to work in community service activities serving elders with physical, mental, or emotional impairments.
Other Sources	Other sources of funding may include United Ways, fares, local tax initiatives, service clubs, foundations, contracts with programs to provide services to a specific group of recipients, and in-kind donations, to name a few.	

Source: Adapted from the *Community Transportation Reporter* (January 1994); and Diebert (1996), used with permission.

> **Best Practice: Partnering With Taxi Services**
>
> Many local communities that have taxi service have been partnering with these companies to provide transportation services to elderly and disabled adults. However, many vary in terms of their eligibility and cost.
>
> Ozaukee County in Wisconsin offers a shared taxi service. Trips can be arranged in advance or for travel the same day services are needed. The county is divided into five zones and the cost is based on how many zones you travel. Riders share a taxi with others and the cost of round-trip travel for older adults and persons with disabilities within one zone costs $4.50 and between four zones costs $10.50, which is slightly less than the full fare. You can find out more by visiting www.co.ozaukee.wi.us/Aging/OutOfCountyTransportation.htm.
>
> Fairfax County Virginia Department of Transportation offers the "Seniors-On-the-Go" taxi program. The taxi cab service is available countywide, and older adults can call one of three taxi cab services to arrange a ride. The program is limited to individuals over age 65 who are considered to have low incomes. Eligible seniors purchase taxicab coupons booklets worth $30 at a cost of $10 per booklet. The difference is subsidized by the Fairfax County government. You can find out more by visiting www.fairfaxcounty.gov/fcdot/seniors.htm.

CHALLENGES FOR TRANSPORTATION PROGRAMS

Currently close to 7 million older adults do not drive and more than half do not drive because of health reasons (Houser, 2005). Furthermore, much of rural America remains without transportation services. Of the nation's rural residents, 38% live in areas without any public transit service, and another 28% live in areas in which the level of transit service is negligible. The per capita rural transit service levels lag substantially behind service levels available to urban residents (Rucker, 1995b). In urban areas with populations of more than 1 million, public transit resources are substantial compared with rural areas; the mobility needs of many urban older adults, however, are still unmet.

Elderly Drivers

Before we discuss the challenges in providing public transportation in our communities for older adults, we should first consider the challenges that will face a society in which there will be an increase in the number of elderly drivers. Realistically, travel by car will continue to be the primary mode of transportation for many older adults in the foreseeable future. Older persons in 2020 will have grown up during a period when use of the automobile became an integral part of everyday life. They will be more likely to retain their driver's licenses compared with the current cohort of older adults and to have high expectations about driving (Eberhard, cited in Committee for the Study on Improving Mobility and Safety for Older Persons, 1988). Jette and Branch (1992) conclude that future generations of older drivers are likely to be even older and drive more miles than the older drivers of today by virtue of their increasing numbers and their continued reliance on the car in old age. Because America has supported a national policy during the past 60 years that places high priority on private automobile transportation, some argue that roadway design, automobile engineering, and licensing and retraining of drivers are all critical considerations in enabling older adults to use their automobiles as long and as safely as possible.

Many planners and policy makers are investigating how communities can maximize the ability of older adults to meet their mobility needs safely. One way to improve the safety of older adult drivers is to improve roadway characteristics. This would include such things as improving roadway markings, making highway signs more legible, improving vehicle safety, and establishing, among other things, better standards for left-hand turn lanes (older drivers in particular have difficulty with left-hand turns). A specific example is the current standard highway signage. The standard assumes that an inch-high letter is legible at 50 feet. This standard corresponds to a visual acuity of 20/25, which exceeds the visual acuity of about 40% of drivers aged 65 to 74. This is just one example of how a better designed road-way system that takes the needs of older adults into consideration would go a long way in maintaining the mobility of older adults. At some point, however, when seniors can no longer drive, programs that assist in helping older drivers make the emotional transition from driving to being dependent on other means of transportation will be critical in reducing the isolation that comes with the inability to drive (Stephens et al., 2005). The success of this type of program depends, of course, on the availability of other community transportation alternatives.

Barriers to Public Transportation Use

In communities where public transportation is available, barriers to service use discussed earlier in the chapter must be addressed to increase ridership of young and old alike. As noted earlier, one barrier to using existing public transit includes a perception that using public transportation isn't a safe means of travel. Improving lighting and increasing monitoring of transit stops could help address these fears. Adding transit stops in neighborhoods and providing more comfortable stops (with covers and benches) and adding transit stops at locations frequented by older adults could help improve access and use of public transportation. Often overlooked is the need for personal assistance getting on and off buses or vans. Many transit services require riders to use services independently, and this simple detail can keep some older adults with minor mobility issues from using public transportation.

Meeting Transit Needs

The key to providing effective community transportation systems will mean that communities must seek to offer a variety of transportation options—from walking to providing fixed-route, demand-response service, deviated fixed route, and specialized services—that are responsive to the varying levels of independence and social and medical needs of older adults. Although walking is often overlooked as a means of transportation, many older adults could access basic services if walking or low-speed transit options (golf carts or scooters) were better accommodated. Fixing and widening walking paths (with places to rest), and improving the safety of crosswalks, including providing more time to cross streets, would help many older adults achieve mobility independence.

Utilizing volunteers and promoting ride-sharing services can be a viable alternative in meeting community transportation needs, particularly in underserved rural and suburban areas. Delegates from the 2005 White House Conference on Aging, recommended strategies that would help promote volunteer transportation services, including

- tax incentives for community-based volunteer transportation programs; and
- removal of legal barriers for volunteers including protection of unreasonable increases in automobile insurance rates when volunteers use their own cars to drive older adults.

Although many transit vehicles can accommodate persons with disabilities, there are specific changes to transit vehicles that could promote the use of public transportation among older adults. Transit vehicles with lifts to ease boarding, buses that "kneel" at curbside, and buses or light rail with cars that have low floors and low platform boarding will be needed to attract and serve an increasing number of elderly riders (American Public Transportation Association, 2003).

Transportation services in the suburbs will become critical in the coming years as baby boomers age in place in suburbs that have little or no access to public transportation. More older people now reside in suburbs where reliance on the automobile is greater, and as people age they are less likely to change residential location, so researchers expect that the graying of the suburbs will continue (U.S. Senate Special Committee on Aging, 1991a).

Of course, increasing public transit options will require an increase in local, state, and federal funding. Transportation advocates across the country have called for an increase in the amount of federal and state funding, including an increase in the amount of money earmarked in the OAA, for public transportation (White House Conference on Aging, 2005).

Improving Coordination of Resources

One of the biggest challenges that face public transit systems in our communities is the lack of transportation coordination. Transportation coordination includes activities such as the formation of partnerships, sharing of planning resources, joint identification of consumer needs, identifying and sharing available services, costs, and revenues and reporting (Burkhardt, 2005). Any one or a combination of these efforts can lead to an increased level of service that provides improved mobility and access to a range of activities and services. The U.S. General Accounting Office (1991a) conducted a study of special transportation services for older adults. The authors reported that, of the 19 special transportation programs studied, 18 showed that fragmentation of special transportation is a pervasive, long-standing problem and that in many communities agencies operate in isolation from one another. This fragmentation occurs despite federal legislative mandates to encourage coordination. Multiple funding sources for special transportation services result in differing program guidelines for operational practices. For example, the Federal Transit Act encourages the charging of fares, whereas the OAA explicitly prohibits charging for services but allows voluntary donations. Another problem affecting coordination and efficiency is that many social service community agencies such as adult day programs, nursing homes, and senior centers purchase vans to respond to the needs of their clients. Often, these vans sit idle for long periods or are not at full capacity when in use. Not only does lack of coordination result in a community not being served adequately within its own boundaries, but there is an incredible imbalance in service levels from community to community and in traveling from one community to another when public transportation is required. One community can be served adequately by a transit program while a neighboring community has no transit service at all. Even large metropolitan areas, which overall have better coverage from public transportation, have unserved population pockets, including suburban areas surrounding central cities. Less likely to be found is public transit service between communities, particularly small to midsized communities. Currently, the federal government, through the SAFETEA-LU legislation, places a heavy emphasis on local transportation coordination and a balanced, flexible funding approach to transportation.

Coordination will continue to be critical as funding for transit programs declines or stays flat. Without adequate transportation to and from social and health care services, most social delivery programs lose much of their impact, and any reforms made in health care will be pointless without health care access. Another future funding challenge is the uncertainty of Medicaid and the transportation services it provides, as the federal and state governments debate how to make this program more cost-effective. The future of Medicaid transportation funds is uncertain at best. In addition, there is speculation that many other federal programs will be "block granted" to the states in the future, leaving the states with considerably more flexibility than they currently have to determine how federal monies are expended. Will transportation for older and disabled persons be a priority against a myriad of other pressing human needs and limited budgets that states are facing?

In light of the social and demographic changes that loom ahead, the U.S. Department of Transportation (1997) released a report that identified the long-range proactive strategies needed to accommodate the transportation needs of older adults in the twenty-first century. Recommended new alternatives included (a) added emphasis on mobility alternatives for older adults, (b) development of medical practice parameters and guidelines when conducting evaluations for licensure, (c) improvement of highway travel, (d) improvement of the identification and evaluation of problem drivers, and (e) introduction of technologies that will enhance the safety and ease of vehicle operation. Ideally, future planning for the mobility needs of all populations will not center on transit versus cars but will focus on how to build communities that give older adults a range of mobility options that they can select on the basis of their particular capabilities and situation.

CASE STUDY

A Need for Transportation Planning and Coordination

Daylight, Inc., is a small, social-model adult day program. Daylight's mission is to help older adults remain independent in the community and to give caregivers time apart from the daily stresses of caregiving. At first, the Daylight staff and board of directors thought that they would have to close due to lack of interest. But 15 years later, with consistent marketing, great personal effort by the executive director, and excellent support from an active board of directors, Daylight has increased its average attendance from 6 to 17 persons per day. Family calls and agency referrals to the program are coming in weekly. Two years ago, Daylight opened a satellite program 35 miles away to serve seven rural communities in the southern half of the county. Now there is a need for a modern facility and expansion of services to include weekend and overnight respite. Daylight has embarked on a major capital development project in partnership with a home health care agency. The proposed facility will house both agencies and permit program expansion and flexibility that are not currently possible.

At a recent annual planning retreat, the staff receptionist commented about the many callers who ask about the program but who ultimately do not enroll their family members in Daylight. After much discussion, the board directed the executive director to conduct a follow-up survey with those callers to learn why they chose not to use Daylight. A telephone survey was prepared, and volunteers called 37 families.

The survey results showed that 42% of the families contacted did not choose Daylight as a respite option because of the lack of transportation. Nearly 55% of those surveyed in the southern part of the county listed transportation as the principal barrier to enrollment. Transportation barriers were due to age, disability, and conflicting work schedules. When the executive director brought this information to the next board meeting, the board decided to form a task force to develop a plan of action for board consideration that would address the transportation problem.

Case Study Questions

1. Assume that you are a member of the task force. What additional information would you want to know before you proceed with the development of a plan of action to address these transportation barriers?

2. Daylight is planning to build a new facility. What relationship does this transportation issue have with the success or failure of the new facility, if any?

3. On the basis of what you have learned from reading the chapter, what types of transportation programs might you need to contact? What questions would you need to explore with these entities to write your report and proposal for the Daylight board of directors?

4. What transportation options should the task force explore? Describe at least three transportation options for Daylight and list the advantages and disadvantages of each option.

5. How is this situation relevant to the chapter's discussion of the relationship between mobility needs of frail elders and home and community-based services?

6. List the transportation terminology that best describes the typical Daylight passenger and the type of service most suited to this passenger.

Learning Activities

1. Contact your state transportation association. To find the name and phone number of the transit association in your state, go to the Community Transportation Association of America's website, www.ctaa.org. Find out the association's stance on transit issues, gaps in service for older adult riders, and future public transit plans.

2. Select a destination to which an older adult might travel, such as the bank, Social Security office, senior center, grocery store, or doctor's office. Use the local public transportation system to get there. Try to select a location that is not close to your home. If you are familiar with riding public transportation, select a location you have not been to before. Record your observations and make note of the following:
   a. How long did it take for you to get to the bus stop?
   b. How long did you have to wait?
   c. How long did it take to get to your final destination?
   d. How many older adult riders were there?
   e. How many barriers to riding public transportation could you identify that you think would make it difficult for older adults to ride the bus? Look for things such as these:
      - bus stop location and condition;
      - height of steps into the bus;
      - seating; and
      - ability to see upcoming stops.

   Make a note of your general feelings. Did you feel any apprehension? How hard was it to figure out your route and bus stop location? On the basis of your observations, what suggestions do you have for making public transportation older adult friendly?

3. Interview an older adult who is currently driving and one who uses public transportation. Ask the current driver how his or her driving has changed through the years, who he or she would rely on if he or she were no longer able to drive, and whether he or she would consider using public transportation, and if not, why not. Ask the public transportation user what he or she likes and dislikes about public transportation and what suggestions he or she has for improving transportation services.

For More Information

National Resources

1. Community Transportation Association of America, 715 15th Street N.W., Suite 900, Washington, DC 20005; phone: 202-628-1480; www.ctaa.org.
   The association's website has links to state and local transportation systems, federal transportation news and budget information, and transportation funding sources that describe more than 90 transportation grants available, along with links to other related transportation sites.

Web Resources

1. *Metro Magazine*: www.metro-magazine.com.

   Metro Magazine's home page is geared primarily to transportation professionals but does have a good resources page that offers links to ADA paratransit coalitions, news groups, and transit-related sites.

2. Wandsworth Community Transport: www.wandsworthcommunitytransport.org.uk.

   Take a trip to the United Kingdom and check out the transportation services offered by the Wandsworth Community Transport System.

3. Federal Transit Administration (FTA): www.fta.dot.gov.

   The FTA's home page is a great place to start to access a tremendous amount of information about transportation. Visitors can search the National Transit Library by using key words; read reports about transit accessibility, the history of transit, public participation, and outreach; and access directories and references.

4. National Aging Information Center, Aging Internet Information Notes—Transportation and Mobility: www.aoa.dhhs.gov/NAIC/Notes/transportation.html.

   Check out this site for information about community transportation, driving and mobility issues, and reports and articles about transportation and older adults.

15

Housing

It has been a year since Lois sold her home and moved into a federally subsidized senior housing complex. The move was a difficult decision, and the two years she waited for an opening were challenging and frustrating. But once settled into her new apartment, she had no regrets. Her modest income of $623 per month had been totally inadequate to meet the expenses of keeping up her home and paying for her heart medication, groceries, and utilities. She rarely had as much as a dime left over at the end of the month. She couldn't even begin to consider a major roof repair that was sorely needed. She misses her old neighborhood, but she doesn't miss the worries of taking care of a house and yard. Now that her money goes a little further, she can enjoy some outings with her new friends.

The majority of older individuals perceive their home as one of their most prized possessions. A home is much more than physical shelter. It gives those who dwell in it a sense of security, privacy, comfort, and independence. It also plays a major role in facilitating social interaction with family and friends (Kochera, Straight, & Guterbock, 2005). A home holds for its residents a multitude of memories and a sense of continuity in life. Findings from a recent AARP study suggest that the vast majority of older adults want to stay in their homes for as long as possible (Kochera et al., 2005). The quality and type of dwellings in which older adults live depend on many things, such as their income, age, marital status, gender, and race, as well as their health and functional status.

We begin this chapter by describing the theoretical concept of *person–environment fit* as a framework for understanding the relationship between older individuals' place of residence and their physical, psychological, and social needs. We then discuss the various independent and supportive housing arrangements in which older adults reside and policies that support these arrangements. The chapter concludes with a discussion of several emerging issues that are likely to influence the housing options and needs of older adults in the future.

THE PERSON–ENVIRONMENT FIT MODEL

For older individuals to be satisfied with their environment, an appropriate "fit" needs to exist between their level of competence and the demands of their environment (Lawton, 1980;

Lawton & Nahemow, 1973). *Competence* refers to the upper limits of an individual's abilities and extends across several areas of functioning, including health, sensory-cognitive abilities, capacity for self-care, ability to perform instrumental activities, mastery, and social skills (Lawton, 1982). If the environment is too demanding for an older adult's competence, or if the environment puts too few demands on the older adult's competence, there is a poor fit.

Elders enjoy a range of comfort and display adaptive behavior when their physical and social living environments are compatible with their personal abilities and resources. A moderately challenging environment is beneficial because it encourages growth, and therefore stretches the person's abilities. Too wide a discrepancy between personal competence and the demands of the environment results in maladaptive behavior and personal stress, and can impede the person's abilities to carry out activities of daily living (ADLs). For example, we know that living in their own homes is the preferred housing choice of most older adults. If, however, the home becomes too costly to manage or the older person is physically unable to maintain it, the demands of the environment may be too stressful. Relocation decisions often occur when older adults, or others in their support network, decide that they are no longer competent to remain living in their current housing environment.

When selecting a new housing option, older persons should avoid moving to a residence that requires too little from them or lacks the stimulation necessary to challenge their existence. When older adults find that their skills and abilities are limited by their environment, they often become bored and give up doing many things for themselves. Overstimulation by the environment can cause distress, but understimulation can be just as stressful for the individual, and can result in greater dependence and feelings of helplessness (Lawton, 1982).

In summary, when one is considering outcomes related to the person–environment fit model, the preferences of the individual and the nature of the environment must be taken into account. The older adult's decision to move often is prompted by a need for greater physical, psychological, and/or social security (Parmelee & Lawton, 1990). An older person's security needs, however, may be in direct conflict with that person's need for autonomy and independence. To successfully adapt to a new, more structured living environment, older adults need to actively pursue a level of autonomy appropriate to their personal resources and competencies. We now turn to a discussion of the different types of housing environments that older adults occupy.

USERS AND PROGRAMS: INDEPENDENT LIVING ENVIRONMENTS

Independent living environments are designed for older adults who are able to manage daily activities, such as housekeeping, cooking, and personal care, with little assistance from others. Widely varying living environments exist that allow older adults to live independently. Each of these will be discussed below along with the programs and services that help older adults remain in their independent living environment.

Single-Family Dwellings[1]

The majority of noninstitutionalized, community-dwelling older adults own or rent their dwellings. The majority live in detached, single-family dwellings (68%), whereas the remainder live in multi-unit buildings (20%), mobile homes (7%), and semidetached houses (5%) (see Exhibit 15.1).

EXHIBIT 15.1 Types of Dwellings of Older Adults

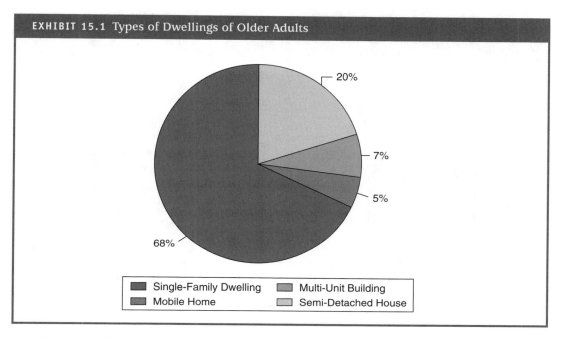

20%

7%

5%

68%

Single-Family Dwelling   Multi-Unit Building
Mobile Home   Semi-Detached House

Source: U.S. Bureau of the Census (2006c).

More than two-thirds (70%) of older adults who own their homes have no mortgage debt, while 30% are making mortgage payments. Approximately 20% of elders are renters.

Personal variables such as age, race, gender, marital status, and income influence home ownership in later life (Kochera et al., 2005). Approximately 41% of individuals aged 65 to 74 and 39% of individuals aged 75 and older are homeowners. Ownership levels are higher for married-couple families (39%) than for men (8%) or women (23%) who live alone in later life. Older persons with incomes greater than $25,000 and White elders are more likely to be homeowners than their less financially well-off and minority counterparts (see Exhibit 15.2). Approximately 85% of non-Hispanic White elders are homeowners compared with 68% of Black older adults and 63% of Hispanic elders.

About two-thirds (63%) of elderly people reside in the suburbs; 37% live in central cities and 26% live in non-metropolitan areas. Forty-nine percent of persons 65 or older moved into their current place of residence before 1980. Five percent of these residents have moderate or severe physical problems.

Although many older homeowners do not have a mortgage and consequently spend less on housing than do younger and middle-aged adults, a greater percentage of aged homeowners spend 30% or more of their income on housing than younger homeowners spend (see Exhibit 15.3). Of minority elders who own their homes, 75% of Black elders and 83% of Hispanic elders spend 30% or more of their income on housing. Low-income

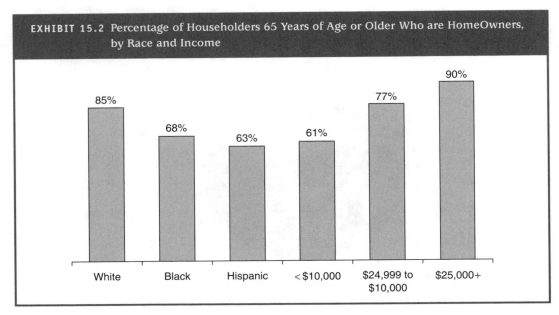

EXHIBIT 15.2 Percentage of Householders 65 Years of Age or Older Who are HomeOwners, by Race and Income

Source: U.S. Bureau of the Census (2006c).

elders are especially hard hit when it comes to the percentage of their income spent on housing costs. Among older persons living below the poverty line, 77% spent 30% or more of their income on housing. This pattern—in which low-income elders spend a higher percentage of their income on housing costs than higher income elders—holds true regardless of ownership status. For example, older householders with an annual income of less than $10,000 are likely to spend $250 or more per month on housing costs, leaving them with $583 or less for living expenses. These older adults clearly represent the predicament of being "house rich" but "cash poor."

Housing Programs

As we mentioned at the beginning of the chapter, the majority of older adults, such as Lois, want to remain living in their own homes for as long as possible. This may be more difficult for older adults with low and middle incomes and those with houses in need of repair. Most communities offer programs that can provide economic and tangible assistance to make housing costs and repairs more affordable.

Home Equity Conversion Mortgage Programs

Older adults who own their homes can convert part of their home equity into cash while still living in their home through home equity conversion mortgage programs (HECM). To be eligible for a HECM, a homeowner must be 62 years of age or older, have

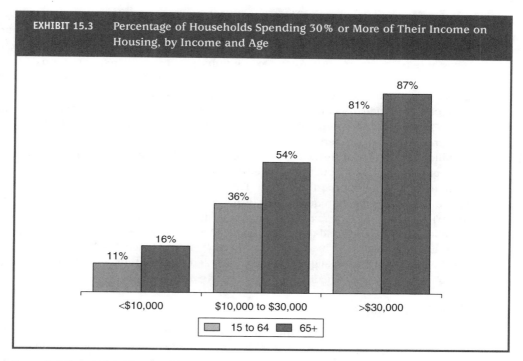

EXHIBIT 15.3 Percentage of Households Spending 30% or More of Their Income on Housing, by Income and Age

Source: U.S. Bureau of the Census (2006c).

a very low outstanding mortgage balance or own their home free and clear, and have received U.S. Department of Housing and Urban Development (HUD)–approved reverse mortgage counseling to learn about the program (U.S. Department of Housing and Urban Development, 2002). There are no restrictions on how the income generated through an equity conversion program can be used. Older adults may choose to use the income for home repairs, health care costs, or living expenses, or as a source of discretionary income. Borrowers may choose one of five payment options (U.S. Department of Housing and Urban Development, 2002):

- *tenure*, which gives the borrower a monthly payment from the lender for as long as the borrower lives and continues to occupy the home as a principal residence;
- *term*, which gives the borrower monthly payments for a fixed period selected by the borrower;
- *line of credit*, which allows the borrower to make withdrawals up to a maximum amount, at times and in amounts of the borrower's choosing;
- *modified tenure*, which combines the tenure option with a line of credit; or
- *modified term*, which combines the term option with a line of credit.

A HECM loan need not be repaid until the borrower moves, sells, or dies.

Although not a home equity program, a *property tax relief* program allows older homeowners to defer property tax payments until they sell their homes or die. There are three types of relief programs: homestead exemptions, property tax credit programs, and property tax deferral programs (Baer, 1998). *Homestead exemptions* are reductions in the amount of assessed property value subject to taxation for owner-occupied housing. Most homestead exemptions provide the same reduction in the assessed property value for all eligible households. *Property tax credit programs* include homestead credit programs that provide the same reductions in property taxes to all eligible households or "circuitbreaker" programs in which tax credits decrease as income increases. *Property tax deferral programs* allow older and disabled homeowners to defer payment of all or a portion of their property taxes until the sale of their property or death. The deferred taxes become a lien against the value of the home. Eligibility requirements (e.g., age, income, homeowner status—owner or renter) for the property tax relief programs differ by state. A survey of 10,000 AARP member households found that households which meet the eligibility criteria of property tax relief programs often are unaware of their existence (Baer, 1998). A lack of awareness was not the main reason eligible households failed to apply for tax relief programs; rather, respondents believed they did not need property tax assistance.

Home Repair Programs

Home repairs and maintenance are a considerable expense for many older adults because the majority have lived in their homes for more than three decades. Although most older homeowners are forced to cut back on cosmetic aspects of home upkeep, findings from the American Housing Survey (Golant & LaGreca, 1994) indicate that they "do not allow vital housing components to deteriorate" (Reschovsky & Newman, 1991, p. 296). Of older households, however, 6% report problems with poorly functioning plumbing, leaky roofs, and inadequate electrical wiring (U.S. Bureau of the Census, 2006c). Physical housing problems are more frequent among older, frail, poor, and minority seniors.

Besides needing specific repairs, many homes do not support frail older adults in conducting daily activities within the home. Older adults who are aging in place may need to modify their homes' structure to accommodate their physical limitations. Modifications in lighting, accessibility, mobility, and bathing facilities can improve functioning and enhance safety (AARP, 2005b).

In response to the increasing demand for assistance with housing upkeep and repairs, a number of home repair programs have emerged across the country. Home repair programs provide assistance with home maintenance or minor repairs. The funding for many of these programs comes from community development block grants or Title III monies from the Older Americans Act (OAA). Programs vary with regard to the type of repairs they subsidize but typically include emergency repairs for plumbing, electricity, heat, and leaking roofs; minor repairs; exterior painting; and the removal of debris.

Two programs that help low-income adults with the costs of heating and cooling their homes are the Department of Energy's Weatherization Assistance Program (WAP) and the Low Income Home Energy Assistance Program (LIHEAP). Under WAP, any household at or below 150% of poverty may be eligible for services. The Department of Energy provides funds to all of the states, which contract with more than 900 local agencies nationwide (United States Department of Energy, 2006). Contractors include community action agencies, other nonprofits, and local governments, who make repairs that improve the energy efficiency of low-income dwellings. The program provides energy-efficiency services to approximately 100,000 homes every year and has weatherized more than 5.6 million homes since its inception in 1976 (United States Department of Energy, 2006). In addition to reducing the utility costs for homeowners, the program help improve health and safety by reducing carbon monoxide emissions and eliminating fire hazards. Funding for the weatherization program in the fiscal year 2006 was $240 million (LIHEAP Clearinghouse, 2006).

Best Practice: Los Angeles Housing Department Handyworker Program

The Handyworker Program of the Los Angeles Housing Department provides free minor repairs to low- and moderate-income homeowners who are senior citizens 62 years and older or physically disabled. Emergency repairs that directly affect the occupants' health and safety are also provided to other low- and moderate-income homeowners. Eligible repairs are limited to work that does not require a city building permit or formal inspection. Typical services include the following:

- emergency repairs, such as repair or replacement of broken doors and windows;
- accessibility improvements for the physically challenged, such as access ramps and hand railings;
- correction of safety hazards, such as repairs to porches, steps, and sidewalks;
- home security improvements, such as fences, security doors, and smoke detectors;
- habitability improvements, such as replacement of sinks, toilets, and floor tiles;
- exterior and interior painting.

For more information, contact the Handyworker Program: phone: 213-808-8803 or 866-557-7368, or visit www.lacity.org/lahd/handyworker.pdf.

LIHEAP provides heating and cooling assistance to low-income families regardless of age either directly, through vendors, or to landlords for home heating and cooling costs, energy crisis intervention, or low-cost weatherization. In 2003, about 36% of the households receiving heating assistance and 47% of households receiving cooling assistance had at least one member 60 years of age or older (United States Department of Health and Human Services, 2003). There is wide variation in states' average household benefit level for various types of fuel assistance. For example, in 2003 the average LIHEAP household benefit for heating costs was $312. Funding for LIHEAP in the fiscal year 2006 was $2.480 million (LIHEAP Clearinghouse, 2006).

Home Sharing

When home expense becomes burdensome, home sharing can be a viable solution to managing those expenses. Shared housing is an arrangement in which two or more unrelated individuals share a home or apartment (AARP, 2005b). "Tenants" often pay modest rent or provide services to the householder in exchange for room and board. For older adults with extra living space in their homes, this housing option can provide financial assistance, companionship in a familiar and comfortable setting, and help with household chores.

According to a recent AARP study (2005b), 7% of people aged 50 and older interviewed found sharing their home with others, whether to help with finances, provide companionship, or for any other reason, to be "very appealing," and another 20% found the idea "somewhat appealing." Those with a household income under $50,000 were more likely to find the idea very or somewhat appealing than those with a household income of $50,000 or more. An earlier study found that older home sharers who are economically secure and active but live alone typically are interested in having someone in their homes at night or someone who will do periodic home maintenance chores (e.g., shoveling snow) but do not expect routine daily assistance or companionship from their "boarder" (Jaffe & Howe, 1988).

Federal Housing Programs

Federal legislation has created a number of housing programs that assist older adults who have limited incomes through Section 8, Section 202, and public housing. In addition, programs under the auspices of the Rural Housing and Community Development Service offer housing assistance for older, low-income individuals living in rural areas.

Section 8

Project-Based Assistance. Under Section 8, rental subsidies are given to landlords who agree to rent to low-income individuals and families. The subsidy covers the difference between the tenants' contribution, an amount that totals 30% of their adjusted income, and fair market rents. Older adults are heads of households in 48% of project-based Section 8 housing (U.S. Government Accounting Office [GOA], 2005).

Housing Choice Voucher Program. In contrast to the Section 8 project assistance component, the participants in the housing choice voucher program find their own housing, including single-family homes, townhouses, and apartments. They are free to choose any housing that meets the requirements of the program (e.g., rent that is not higher than the fair market value) and are not limited to units located in subsidized housing projects. Tenants are responsible for paying 30% of their income for rent. If the rent is higher than the fair market value, the renters are responsible for the difference (USDHUD, 2001). Older adults are heads of households in 16% of tenant-based Section 8 housing (AAHSA, 2001b).

Section 202

Section 202 Supportive Housing for the Elderly Program is the only federally funded housing program designed specifically for older persons. It makes low-cost federal loans to nonprofit sponsors for new construction or rehabilitation of existing structures to provide subsidized rental housing for low- and moderate-income elders 62 years of age and older. Since its inception in 1959, the program has supported the creation of approximately 6,200 housing facilities for older persons, accounting for approximately 250,000 residential units. Beginning in 2002, appropriations have included funding to convert a small number of projects to licensed assisted living facilities. Tenants living in Section 202 units have incomes below 50% of their area's median income. The average Section 202 resident is 79 years old with an annual income of $10,000; about 39% of residents are over age 80 and 90% are women living alone (Bright, 2005). These housing complexes usually offer supportive services, such as transportation, housekeeping, and home-delivered meals.

Public Housing

Public housing is the oldest and largest federal housing program assisting individuals and families with low incomes, including older renters. In 1956, Congress for the first time gave preference to seniors in public housing (The Milbank Memorial Fund, 2006), Throughout the 1960s and 1970s, a large number of developments were built specifically for low-income seniors. With very few exceptions, these were traditional apartments. Older adult renters occupy an estimated 31% of public housing units (GOA, 2005). Local public housing authorities usually operate these housing units, and renters pay rent no more than 30% of their adjusted monthly income. Older residents of public housing are older, poorer, and perhaps frailer than most elderly households. Almost one in five elderly public housing households is headed by someone aged 85 or older, compared with about one in nine nationwide. An estimated 20% of older adults living in public housing experience difficulty with at least one activity of daily living, compared with about 12% of the general population (Brigl, 2001). Older women comprise almost three-fourths of public housing residents and almost one-half of all elderly public housing residents are minorities; approximately 25% of elderly residents are Black and 13% are Hispanic.

Rural Programs

Two housing programs are available to rural elders under the Rural Housing and Community Development Service program. Section 515 offers low-interest construction loans for rental and congregate housing for low-income individuals. Less than one-half of Section 515 housing projects are occupied by older adults (GOA, 2005). Section 504 provides loans and grants to low-income rural residents 62 years of age and older to repair new or existing single-family housing.

Planned and Naturally Occurring Retirement Communities

Although the majority of older adults live in age-integrated communities, almost one-third of all older adults live in a naturally occurring retirement community (NORC) in which, by most definitions, at least half of the residents are 60 years of age or older (Ormond, Black, Tilly, & Thomas, 2004). Naturally occurring retirement communities emerge through long periods as people living in the same location age in place. NORCs evolve in three ways: "aged-left-behind," "aging in place," and "in-migration" (Hunt, 1998). The first two types of NORCs are populated primarily by long-term residents—the first by residents who stayed in a community characterized by out-migration; the second by older residents who gradually became the dominant population in a stable community. The third type is distinguished by the proportion of older residents who are new to the community.

For Your Files: **B'nai B'rith**

B'nai B'rith is the largest Jewish sponsor of nonsectarian, federally subsidized housing for older adults in the United States. B'nai B'rith, through its Senior Citizens Housing Committee, has been involved in a cooperative partnership with the U.S. Department of Housing and Urban Development to make available rental apartments for low-income older adults. It has a network of 35 apartment buildings in 25 communities across the United States, which encompass more than 4,000 apartment units serving more than 6,000 persons. Each project has a volunteer board of directors that makes sure each apartment building is responsive to its residents. Professional staff offer support and assistance to individual apartment building boards of directors.

For more information, contact B'nai B'rith at 2020 K Street, N.W., 7th Floor, Washington, DC 20006; phone: 202-857-6600; www.bnaibrith.org/sservices/index.cfm.

About 6% of households aged 55 or older (approximately 2.4 million households) live in age-restricted communities, such as Leisure World in California and Sun City in Arizona, with owners and renters about evenly split (AARP, 2005b). Such communities are more common in the South and West. Homeowners typically choose age-restricted communities to live in because such communities are easier living, quieter neighborhoods, and maintenance costs are included in fees (National Association of Home Builders Research Center, 2002). As for community attributes, community clubhouse, proximity to shopping, and planned social activities are the most common reasons older adults gave for moving to a planned age-restricted community. It is easy to see that most of these residences support an active lifestyle. For example, the 18,000 residents of Leisure World in Laguna Woods, California, enjoy special-interest activities including fitness, swimming, golf, tennis, arts and crafts, a computer-learning center, and a choice of more than 100 Saddleback College Emeritus courses. Facilities include seven clubhouses, five swimming pools, a performing arts center seating 834, and the community's "living" amenity, the equestrian center. For more information, see www.lagunawoodsvillage.com.

Best Practice: Supportive Services Program—Public–Private Partnerships

Some elderly residents of public and federally subsidized multifamily housing receive supportive services through partnerships between property owners and local organizations, and through programs provided by the Department of Health and Human Services (HHS). For example, property owners can establish relationships with local nonprofit organizations, including churches, to ensure that residents have access to the services they need. At their discretion, property owners may establish relationships that give older adults access to meals, transportation, and housekeeping and personal care services. Examples of such partnerships include

- In Greensboro, North Carolina, Dolan Manor, a Section 202 housing development, has established a relationship with a volunteer group from a local church. The volunteer group provides a variety of services for the residents, such as transportation.
- In Plain City, Ohio, residents of Pleasant Valley Garden, a Section 515 property, receive meals five times a week in the community's senior center (a $2 donation is suggested). A local hospital donates the food and a nursing home facility prepares it. Volunteers, including residents, serve the meals. The senior center uses the funds collected from the lunch for its activities. In addition, local grocery stores donate bread products to the senior center daily. The United Way provides most of the funding for the senior center.
- In Guthrie, Oklahoma, Guthrie Properties, a Section 515 property, has established a relationship with the local Area Agency on Aging. The agency assists residents of Guthrie Properties in obtaining a variety of services, including meals and transportation to a senior center.

Source: United States Government Accountability Office (2005).

Single-Room Occupancy Hotels

Single-room occupancy hotels (SROs) are "cheap hotels and rooming houses located in areas adjacent to the downtown business districts" (Erickson & Eckert, 1977, p. 440). They can be remodeled hotels, tenements, school buildings, hotels that have always served as SROs, or newer buildings built specifically as SROs. Typically, SROs provide inner-city residents with a private room and a shared kitchen, bath, and common area. Some SROs have been built as micro-efficiency units that include a small kitchenette and a bathroom with a shower (Regnier & Culver, 1994). Services provided to tenants range from nothing to highly managed care. Sometimes, SROs will offer limited security, light housekeeping, or an errand service (Rollinson, 1991a). Although perceived to be at the bottom rung of the housing ladder, SROs provide emergency, transitional, and permanent housing for single low-income persons of all ages (Regnier & Culver, 1994).

Most research on older adults living in SROs was published before the mid-1990s. In studies of SROs located in Chicago and New York, the percentage of tenants who were older adults ranges from 15% to 33%. Most of these individuals indicated not only that they were lifelong residents of the city but also that many had lived in the same neighborhood during their childhood (Crystal & Beck, 1992; Rollinson, 1991b).

In contrast to the image of the SRO tenant as primarily male and alcoholic, older adults who live in SROs represent a diverse group with regard to gender, age, health status, marital status, race, and education (Crystal & Beck, 1992; Rollinson, 1990). Approximately 40% of older tenants are women. The age and health profile of tenants creates a picture of an older adult, usually in his or her 70s, coping with chronic conditions such as arthritis and other musculoskeletal problems, diabetes, heart conditions, and sensory losses. Few older SRO residents report a past or current drinking problem. Almost one-half of the older SRO tenants reported never being married; most others were widowed, divorced, or separated. Approximately one-third of the tenants had less than a ninth-grade education, whereas almost one-fourth reported that they had attended or graduated from college. Researchers also report a diverse picture with regard to race of the tenants. Although in the majority of studies, most of the residents were White, the percentage of White residents ranged from 54% to 97% (Bild & Havingurst, 1976; Community Emergency Shelter Organizations, 1985, cited in Rollinson, 1991b; Crystal & Beck, 1992). Residents live on small incomes from SSI and Social Security. The majority of older tenants report average incomes falling below current poverty levels, with their housing costs (i.e., rent and utilities) taking up as much as half of their monthly income. For example, monthly rents at the Ellis Hotel in Los Angeles range from $180 for General Relief recipients to $240 for Social Security recipients (LA4Seniors, 2006).

Researchers and service providers characterize residents of SROs as fiercely independent individuals who are protective of their autonomy and who receive little assistance from relatives, friends, or neighbors (Rollinson, 1990). Rollinson (1990, p. 201) quotes one resident, confined to a wheelchair, as saying, "Some people say, 'Can I help you do this and help you do that,' and being bullheaded as hell I tell them no, except to go to the [grocery] store."

CHALLENGES FOR INDEPENDENT LIVING PROGRAMS

As we discussed at the outset of the chapter, the majority of older adults reside in independent living settings and desire to do so for as long as possible. Many issues need to be addressed, however, to promote independent living in the community.

Removing Barriers to Shared Housing

Several barriers can impede the use of shared housing in later life (Mantell & Gildea, 1989). The most frequently cited barrier is a lack of financial support for programs that help match older individuals with prospective housemates. Limited federal, state, or local support is available for these programs, and the clients served are often unable to pay the actual cost of providing the service. Second, restrictive zoning regulations and building and fire codes prohibit shared housing in many residential neighborhoods (Liebig, Koenig, & Pynoos, 2006). A third barrier is older adults' fear that their income from SSI, food stamps, or fuel subsidies will be reduced if regulatory agencies base decisions on the income of the household. In addition, older adults may be hesitant to share their homes with a stranger. Such attitudes, no doubt, are tied to deep-rooted values of privacy and independence.

Serving Older Adults Living in Public Housing

Several challenges have emerged for older adults living in public housing. While public housing units are adequate for the majority of low-income older residents, the units do not provide the flexibility to allow residents to age in place, nor do they necessarily provide the range of housing options needed to serve the increasing share of frail seniors. In addition, a significant portion of public housing for older adults is rapidly becoming physically and functionally obsolete. Most developments are simply not equipped to meet the residential and supportive service needs of their increasingly frail and diverse residents (The Milbank Memorial Fund, 2006), Furthermore, there are lengthy waiting lists to get into public housing. In some cities, 28 older persons apply for every vacancy that occurs in newer units. The lengthy waiting lists are due in part to the lack of available units and a low turnover rate. In the 2006 fiscal year, Congress appropriated $641 million for new Section 202 construction and project rental assistance; in production terms, this translates to only 5,000 or fewer new units that will be built (National Low Income Housing Coalition [NLIHC], 2006). Finally, as the low turnover rate suggests, many older tenants who move into public housing stay there until they are no longer able to live independently, creating a tremendous need for supportive services to help them age in place. About one-third of Section 202 properties have a service coordinator available to assess residents' needs, identify and link residents to services, and monitor the delivery of services (NLIHC, 2006). In addition, in 2004, HUD completed conversion of seven existing 202 housing units into assisted living facilities. This is one of the first attempts toward developing an affordable continuum of care within public housing complexes for low-income seniors.

Promoting Communities for Older Adults

The future of planned retirement communities is uncertain because many of the original residents are aging in place. In addition, some older individuals who move to a planned community find that they miss interacting with children and younger adults, who typically live within traditional community neighborhoods.

Because naturally occurring retirement communities typically emerge within traditional residential environments, health and other supportive services are not usually available within or close to the immediate neighborhood. Residents therefore must be able to seek out and obtain these services on their own. NORCs that develop within structured environments, such as an apartment complex, are likely to have some form of building management and may also have resident councils or recreation committees. How successful NORC supportive services programs are depends on how successful service providers are in establishing strong relationships with the NORC organizational structure and its residents (Ormond et al., 2004).

Enhancing SROs

Although SROs offer the most vulnerable persons in society a place to live, they provide little in the way of comfort, security, or support. Many buildings are in deteriorating condition and poorly maintained. Many SROs in New York, San Francisco, and Los Angeles were built before or at the turn of the century (Ovrebo, Minkler, & Liljestrand, 1991). The rooms are sparse and small; most cannot easily accommodate wheelchairs. Kitchenettes often consist of a nonworking stove (Rollinson, 1990). Elevators frequently break down, leaving frail residents stranded in their rooms. Lack of adequate heating in the winter and extreme heat in the summer, holes in the wall, and rodents are problems reported by residents (Crystal & Beck, 1992; Rollinson, 1991a).

> **Best Practice: Communities for a Lifetime**
>
> Communities for a Lifetime is a statewide initiative started by former Florida Governor Jeb Bush to assist Florida cities, towns, and counties in planning and implementing improvements benefiting the lives of all residents, youthful or senior. This initiative recognizes the diverse needs of residents and the unique contributions individuals can make to their communities. Participating communities use existing resources and state technical assistance to make crucial civic improvements in such areas as housing, health care, transportation, accessibility, business partnerships, community education, efficient use of natural resources, and volunteer opportunities to the betterment of their communities. A Community for a Lifetime values individuals of all ages and engages communities in a process of continuous self-assessment and improvement. Through this process, communities enhance opportunities for people to age in place, or continue living in their own communities for a lifetime, while also benefiting people of all ages. Once a community commits to creating a Community for a Lifetime, they assemble a team of community partners to gather information about the opportunities, programs, and services that are available to older adults. The information is used by community planners to develop work plan strategies for incorporating universal design for housing, accessibility, health care, transportation, and efficient use of natural resources. As of April 2006, 100 Florida cities, towns, and counties had committed themselves to creating a better place for older adults to live, providing all residents with the opportunity to achieve their full potential and contribute to the betterment of their communities. For more information, go to www.communities foralifetime.org/index.html.

Although SROs are fraught with serious problems, they provide housing to a group of older persons who are at risk of being homeless. However, the SRO as a housing option for low-income older persons is diminishing. Since the 1970s, the number of SRO units has rapidly declined. An estimated 1,111,000 SRO units were eliminated from 1970 to 1980 (Hooper & Hamberg, 1986). The major forces behind the loss of SROs include downtown revitalization, gentrification, and lack of funding to rehabilitate deteriorating buildings (Ovrebo et al., 1991). This loss of housing represents a serious problem for older SRO residents, many of whom reported that they did not know what they would do if they had to move.

SUPPORTIVE LIVING ENVIRONMENTS

Supportive living environments are designed to help older adults who are self-sufficient and are capable of self-care to some extent, but who need some assistance with ADLs. Generally, supportive environments provide older adults varying degrees of assistance and oversight.

Accessory Dwelling Units

Accessory Dwelling Units (ADUs) are residential units that provide independent living facilities for one or more persons, with designated areas for cooking and sanitation, plus space for living, sleeping, and eating (Liebig et al., 2006). Between 65,000 and 300,000 units are created each year (Cobb & Dvorak, 2000).

There are several types of ADUs. Elder Cottage Housing Opportunity (ECHO) housing units (sometimes called "granny flats" or garden suites) are small, self-contained, movable housing units located next to the home of a family member. The units also can be made to fit into the space of an attached garage or to be connected directly to the main house. They have their own electrical system, temperature controls, and plumbing. Meters can be attached to the unit to keep utility costs separate from the main house. Configurations of the units vary; most have a living room, kitchen, bedroom, and bath. Once the units are no longer needed, they are removed. In some cases, where space is available, mobile homes may serve as ECHO housing (Hare, 1990).

To create an accessory or mother-in-law apartment, families remodel an existing room or basement into a living area in which a frail older adult can live. An accessory cottage, also known as guest cottage or carriage house, is a permanent separate structure placed on the same parcel or lot as the single-family dwelling. Garage or barn apartments are similar to accessory cottages because they are not part of the primary dwelling; the latter is more popular in rural areas (Liebig et al., 2006). As with ECHO housing, accessory apartments and cottages provide the same benefits of privacy and support, although the construction is more permanent.

Both ECHO housing and accessory apartments/cottages allow older adults to live with or near their families. They offer families a way to provide assistance to older family members yet allow privacy and independent living. Other benefits include lower housing costs, increased intergenerational interaction, and a possible delay of institutionalization.

In a nationwide study conducted by AARP (1992), 3% of the respondents ($n = 1,505$) indicated that they had purchased or rented a small, removable house on their relative's property. Another 18% said they would consider this alternative living arrangement.

Congregate Housing

Although public housing often is referred to as congregate housing, many congregate facilities are privately owned. Most congregate housing facilities have separate apartments for each resident plus common, shared areas for meals and recreation, including "congregate dining, social lounges, laundry facilities, recreation spaces, and a secure barrier free environment" (Heumann, 1990, p. 46; Monk & Kaye, 1991). These facilities provide services in a residential setting for persons who can no longer independently manage the tasks of everyday living. The typical onsite staff includes a building manager, janitorial services, and social/activity organizer. Medical personnel are not usually onsite in a congregate facility.

Residents in congregate housing receive at least one major meal served congregately per day and have the option of receiving assistance with additional meals, housekeeping, personal care, transportation, and other support services if needed. Residents typically have some limitation that precludes independent living, but that does not require continuous medical or nursing care or full-time personal care.

Continuing Care Retirement Communities

Continuing care retirement communities (CCRCs) provide a full range of housing options for retired adults, from independent living through nursing home care. There are more than 2,200 CCRCs in the United States with more than 725,000 residents (AAHSA, 2006). The average CCRC has been in operation for fewer than 35 years. Religious groups and other nonprofit organizations are frequent sponsors of CCRCs.

CCRCs offer incoming residents a contract that remains in effect for the balance of their lifetime. There are three basic types of CCRC agreements (AAHSA, 2001a).

An *extensive agreement contract* includes shelter, residential services, and amenities as well as long-term nursing care for little or no substantial increase in monthly payments, except for normal operating costs and inflation. They provide for the prepayment of medical expenses, similar to an insurance arrangement, and are sometimes known as "life care" agreements. About 42% of CCRCs offer extensive agreements.

A *modified agreement contract* also includes shelter, residential services, and amenities but offers only a specified amount of long-term nursing care for little or no substantial increase in monthly payments, except for normal operating costs and inflation adjustments. After using the specified amount of nursing care, residents pay either partial or full per-diem rates for the care they require. About 16% of CCRCs offer modified agreements.

A *fee-for-service contract* includes shelter, residential services, amenities, and emergency and infirmary nursing care. Access to long-term nursing care is guaranteed but at full per-diem rates, about 25% of CCRCs offer modified agreements.

Basic continuing care agreements typically require a lump-sum entrance fee, paid on moving into the community, and monthly payments thereafter. Still other CCRCs have periodic fee-only agreements where there is no entry fee and the costs of the living unit, service, and care are covered solely by a monthly fee. Least common are CCRCs with equity agreements that involve the actual purchase of real estate or membership; service and health care package transactions are generally separate from the purchase transaction.

Entry fees and monthly fees vary greatly from one CCRC to another. Average entrance fees can range from lows of $20,000 to highs of $400,000 (AARP, 2004); average monthly expenses per resident for a nonprofit CCRC is $2,672, or $32,064 annually (AAHSA, 2006). In some places, residents own their living space, and in others the space is rented. In some communities, the entrance fee may be partially refundable.

As one might expect from the high contract fees, CCRCs typically attract an affluent older population. The typical CCRC resident is a White, widowed, divorced, or never-married woman in her early 80s (AAHSA, 2001a). They tend to have higher incomes and educational attainments than the general population of older adults. Krout and colleagues (2002) found that a decline in the health of one's spouse or in one's own health and freedom from the burden of home maintenance were motivating factors for those who recently moved to a not-for-profit CCRC designed for people older than 65 in good physical and mental health. Enticing features of the CCRC included the quality of the management of the facility, the size, design, and choice of units, climate, and location near cultural activities.

Attitudes toward CCRCs have changed since this type of retirement housing was introduced in the 1960s. Current and future generations of older adults are looking for retirement communities where they can enjoy an active life, rather than simply shopping for quality health care they hope never to need (High, 2000). CCRCs have responded by adding new housing, health care, and amenities options to their current structures. Examples include fitness centers, casual dining programs, business centers, computer labs, putting greens, expanded libraries, and indoor pool/fitness complexes.

Assisted Living

Assisted living has emerged as a popular choice for people who need supportive and health-related services and help with unscheduled activities of daily living. Nationwide, there are about 33,000 assisted living facilities (ALFs) accommodating more than a million residents (American Association of Homes and Services for the Aging, 2006). Although definitions of assisted living vary across states, the term is generally defined as a residential setting that provides or coordinates personal care services, 24-hour supervision, scheduled and unscheduled assistance, social activities, and some health-related services (Wright, 2004). These settings may include personal care boarding homes with additional services, residential care units owned by and adjacent to nursing homes, congregate housing settings that have added services, purpose-built assisted living programs, or the middle level of CCRCs. Ownership of these facilities may be either nonprofit or for-profit.

The average assisted living community has 58 units (The National Center for Assisted Living, 2006a). Fifty-one percent of assisted living units are studio or efficiency apartments, 39% are one-bedroom apartments, and 6% have two bedrooms. They most often offer private occupancy units with at least full bathrooms, kitchenettes with refrigerators and cooking capacity, and lockable doors; three meals a day in a group dining room; general housekeeping and maintenance services; personal care according to individual needs; onsite delivery or coordination of nursing, health, and social services; and supervision and oversight for persons with cognitive limitations. Facilities use fewer medical staff than nonmedical staff, and the majority of facilities contract services from a variety of consultants, ranging from beauticians to physicians (Wright, 2004).

In 2006, the national average, private-pay monthly rate for a private room with a private bath in an assisted living facility was $2,968, with rents ranging from $1,161 a month to $4,729 a month (Metlife, 2006a). Most facilities charge higher rates for added services. Most of the rates, even at the high end, are substantially less than nursing home care for private-paying residents. Insurance companies are increasingly allowing holders of long-term care policies to use their benefits for assisted living if the services are cost-effective. Public payment for assisted living includes supplemental payments to the facility for services for SSI clients; reimbursement in Medicaid, Medicaid waiver, or state long-term care programs; or some combination of these sources.

The typical assisted living resident is female, aged 85, in need of help with ambulating, in need of medication reminders, forgetful, and in need of help with bathing or dressing. Residents come to assisted living facilities from a variety of settings, including a private home or apartment (60%), a retirement or independent living community (12%), a family residence (such as living with adult children) (10%), another assisted living residence or group home (9%), or from a nursing care facility (8%) (The National Center for Assisted Living, 2006b). Most facilities admit and retain residents with a variety of disabling conditions and physical health care needs, but few residents typically need moderate or heavy care. The average length of stay of residency in an assisted living facility is about 27 months (The National Center for Assisted Living, 2006b). Thirty-four percent of residents will move into a nursing care facility, 30% will pass away, and the remainder will move home or to another location.

Personal Care Boarding Homes

Board and care homes are "non-medical community-based living arrangements that provide shelter (room), board (food), and 24-hour supervision or protective oversight and personal care services to residents" (Hawes, Wildfire, & Lux, 1993, p. 3). The names used to identify board and care homes, and the nature of the homes, vary considerably. Small homes may provide for as few as two residents, whereas some institutions may designate all or a large percentage of their beds for board and care residents. All states license board and care homes, although licensing requirements differ. The variability of the names used to classify board and care homes makes it difficult to get an exact count of the number of these facilities nationwide. It is estimated, however, that as of 1998, there were approximately 34,000 licensed board and care homes and a similar number of unlicensed homes, accommodating 360,000 residents in the United States (Home and Community Based Services, 2002). Unlicensed homes include facilities excluded from mandatory licensure because of size or service criteria established by the state in which they operate as well as homes that meet a state's criteria for obtaining an operating license but avoid securing one.

We know little about the characteristics of board and care residents except that persons seeking this type of housing alternative are likely to need some supervision and personal care. Most residents are characterized as physically or cognitively frail and at risk for further health and functional declines (Hopp, 1999; Morgan, Gruber-Baldini, & Magaziner, 2001; Quinn, Hohnson, Andress, McGinnis, & Ramesh, 1999). Compared to larger facilities, smaller board and care homes (five to six residents) have a higher proportion of Black residents, people with lower incomes and educational levels, residents with higher physical dependency, and more residents with cognitive impairments (Cardner, Morgan, & Eckert, 2006).

The cost of living in a board and care residence ranges from $350 to $3,500 per month, depending on its location, the size of living space, the amount of privacy, and the amenities provided (Helpguide, 2006). Some residents rely on assistance from federal and state programs to pay at least part of the cost of living in a board and care home. For example, the monthly check of a SSI recipient may go toward the payment of the home's charges. Most states also provide some form of additional payment to supplement an older person's SSI payment. In some states, payment for board and care homes comes from Medicaid waiver program funds, block grants, or county funds.

Foster Care

Adult foster care "serves people who, because of physical, mental, or emotional limitations, are unable to continue independent functioning in the community and who need and desire the support and security of family living" (U.S. Department of Health, Education &Welfare, 1964, p. 2). Foster care includes support services, supervision, and personal care provided by a private host family or an individual who takes a small number of older adults and encourages them to participate in the lives of the family and in the community (Sherman & Newman, 1988). Foster care homes are considered to be a social care model in contrast to the medical model of nursing homes. Individuals needing only supervision and assistance, but not continuous medical attention, can benefit from foster care. Elders generally go into foster care because they do not have family who can take care of them or because their family is unable or unwilling to provide daily care.

Research on foster care for older adults is scant. The landmark study of Sherman and Newman (1988) provided an extensive examination of three populations of foster care residents: residents with mental illness, residents with mental retardation, and frail elders. The elder residents in foster care are likely to have one of three histories: they may have been in foster care for many years, they may have been residents of institutions (e.g., a psychiatric hospital) for many years and only recently been placed in foster care, or they may recently have been placed with a foster family from the community. Many elders in foster care will remain with their family until their death. Others will leave the family for a more specialized care center, such as a nursing home, psychiatric hospital, or residence for persons with mental retardation. In Carder, Morgan, and Eckert's (2006) comparison of small care facilities for older adults, they describe Oregon's adult foster care program, which began in the early 1980s. The program requires that facilities provide residents with three meals daily, assistance with personal care, assessment, and care planning. Oregon uses the Medicaid 1915(c) waiver to help finance adult foster care and requires training of both managers and staff, including successful completion of a competency examination. Surveys of resident and family members suggest the family like, home-style setting and the interpersonal relationship between the resident and the provider heavily influenced ratings of satisfaction and quality of care.

Best Practice: Mary Sandoe House

The Mary Sandoe House assisted living project in Boulder, Colorado, is an exemplary housing alternative that has been operational since 1988. Its multiple sponsors include the City of Boulder Housing Authority, the Boulder County Community Action Program, the Boulder Gray Panthers Service Project, Inc., and an interfaith housing group. Funding for the project was leveraged through the Community Development Block Grant program, Colorado Housing and Finance Authority low-interest loans, and local fundraising. Juniper Partners, Inc. provides day-to-day oversight of management and conducts board development training and technical assistance.

A small project built in an existing neighborhood, the Mary Sandoe House accommodates elders in 12 private bedrooms adjacent to shared living and dining areas. The average age of the residents is 86. Many have mobility limitations because of a stroke or arthritis, and some suffer from mild dementia. Support services include some bathing assistance, supervision of medications, personal laundry, social activities, and arrangements for special transit. Meals are served family style.

The underlying philosophy that influenced the design of the house and continues to influence its day-to-day management can be summed up in two words: good neighbor. Residents of Mary Sandoe House are regarded as part of the neighborhood. Neighbors are invited to outdoor barbecues, and neighbor children are encouraged to visit the residents. Typical residential activities, such as tending a garden, picking up the mail, and socializing on the patio, are part of the daily routine of the residents.

Another attractive and unique aspect of the Mary Sandoe House is that half the residents have low to moderate incomes. Rents vary from $900 to $1,650 per month. This price range is comparable with similar but much larger projects.

Often, group living projects in single-family neighborhoods meet with strong resistance. When they do, city planning committees are compelled to deny special use permits for these projects. Mary Sandoe House planners launched a successful proactive approach to allay fears that neighbors might have about building a small assisted living project in their neighborhood of single-family homes. In teams of two, planners visited neighbors close to the proposed project. They discussed the nature of the project and showed them architectural sketches of the house. One of the 20 neighbors who were contacted spoke out against the project at a public meeting. This neighbor was not against the group living project but felt that the land should be retained as open space.

Persons associated with Mary Sandoe House believe it has been successful, in part because many sectors of the community—public and private—were committed to the concept of a small residential program that could blend in with the day-to-day activities of an existing neighborhood.

For more information, contact Mary Sandoe House, 1244 Gillaspie Drive, Boulder, CO 80305; phone: 303-494-7317.

Long-Term Care Facilities

At the most dependent end of the housing continuum are long-term care facilities, known more commonly as nursing homes. In 2004, 3.6% of individuals 65 years of age and older resided in nursing homes (The Lewin Group, 2006a). The typical nursing home resident is female, non-Hispanic White, not married, over the age of 75, and in need of assistance with several activities of daily living (National Center for Health Statistics, 2000). The person requires skilled, 24-hour care because of severe physical or cognitive limitations. Given the unique role of nursing homes in the continuum of care and the broad range of issues to consider, we will consider them separately in Chapter 19.

CHALLENGES FOR SUPPORTIVE LIVING ENVIRONMENTS

Supportive living environments make it possible for many frail elders to continue living in the community. A wide range of supportive living options, including long-term care facilities, is needed to address the physical, psychological, and social needs of older adults. Exhibit 15.4 displays a summary of the different housing options discussed in this chapter

EXHIBIT 15.4   Spectrum of Housing Options

Housing Option	Little or No Assistance	Moderate Assistance	Cannot Perform Without Assistance
Single-family dwelling	■		
Public housing	■		
NORCs—Naturally occurring retirement communities	■		
House sharing	■		
Home with Chore services Nutrition services Home repair Home equity conversion Low-income energy assistance	■	■	
Congregate housing	■		
ECHO housing accessory apartments		■	
Home with Delivered meals Homemaker Home health aide Telephone reassurance Visiting programs		■	
Home with adult day services		■	
Assisted living/personal care boarding homes		■	
Foster care		■	
Long-term care facilities		■	■
Continuing care retirement communities		■	■

Source: Adapted from American Association of Retired Persons (1985).

and the level of assistance appropriate in each option. We now turn to the concerns that will need to be addressed in the future regarding supportive living arrangements for older adults.

Removing Barriers

Although ADUs promise many benefits, there are several barriers facing elders and their families interested in this housing option. In some jurisdictions, zoning laws prohibit the addition of such units, and neighbors often are concerned about ADUs becoming permanent rentals, thereby changing the neighborhoods from single-family to multifamily dwellings and negatively impacting property values, parking, and community services (Cobb & Dvorak, 2000; Liebig et al., 2006). In addition, few manufacturers of ECHO housing exist, limiting the purchasing opportunities for families who are looking for solutions for immediate care needs. A viable alternative may be a mobile version of an ADU used in Canada, Homecare Suite, which can quickly be installed in a garage space (Chapman & Howe, 2001).

Enhancing Services

Almost all the research shows cost savings with congregate housing compared with long-term care facilities. Congregate housing, however, relies on the availability of community-provided services to assist residents in meeting their care needs. Where such services are not readily available, staff at the congregate facility must carefully monitor residents and coordinate their care to appropriately support the residents' independence. Although older adults may prefer to "age in place" with assistance from community programs, the successful linking of housing with services requires a competent, stable, and committed workforce, an issue which currently plagues the long-term care system (Stone, 2006).

Protecting Residents

In the mid-1980s, reform advocates called for increased regulation among CCRCs to protect elderly consumers (Saunders, 1997). In an effort to prevent strong government involvement in the industry and maintain security for older adults without the negative side-effects of regulation, CCRCs formed their own regulating agency, the Continuing Care Accreditation Commission (CCAC). Acquired by the Commission on Accreditation of Rehabilitation Facilities (CARF) in 2003, CARF-CCAC has adopted basic standards that cover critical areas such as the organization's governance structure, financial status, and quality of services provided to residents. In order to qualify for accreditation, CCRCs must perform self-evaluations that focus on these aspects of operation, as well as undergo inspections from the CARF-CCAC; CCRCs go through recertification every five years. As of January 2007, some 340 organizations throughout the United States had achieved CARF-CCAC accreditation (Commission on Accreditation of Rehabilitation Facilities, 2007).

In the past, the financial stability of the CCRC industry was a serious concern, resulting from a number of bankruptcies among various CCRCs. Today, fears are alleviated somewhat as the industry has gained more experience in management and as regulation has taken hold in many states (Saunders, 1997). Concern over possible bankruptcy, however, still exists as opinions on exactly how much of a threat financial failure is varies among those monitoring the industry.

Although there are federal laws that impact assisted living, oversight of assisted living occurs primarily at the state level. The varying laws and regulations affecting these settings have created a diverse and fluid operating environment for providers and a mix of terminology, settings, and available services for consumers (National Center for Assisted Living, 2006c). States vary significantly in their licensing requirements, quality standards, and monitoring and enforcement activities. The Assisted Living Workgroup (ALW) was formed at the request of the U.S. Senate Special Committee on Aging to address quality issues in ALFs. In 2003, the ALW issued a report with recommendations for improving quality in assisted living, including a system to grade the performance of assisted-living facilities and to provide the consumer with all the needed information to determine the quality of any assisted-living facility in the United States (Pettey, 2003).

States face a variety of issues in deciding whether and how to regulate board-and-care settings, including resources, affordability, local culture, quality standards, and consumer demand (Carder et al., 2006). Some states require a license for every residential setting that houses people who need personal care or supervision; most states require licensure only if the home actually provides such services or advertises that it provides care and supervision. Licensure requirements also may depend on the size of the facility and the number of persons receiving care. The content of the licensure standards also varies from state to state, as do minimum staffing levels and training requirements. Needless to say, evaluating the quality of board and care homes is an ongoing challenge.

Enhancing Opportunities for Foster Care Residents

Socialization and social network interactions beyond the immediate household are often low among residents of foster homes (Sherman & Newman, 1988). Thus, although these individuals are physically residing within a neighborhood, their participation in community activities appears to be marginal.

Developing Housing Options for Marginalized Older Adults

The issues and needs of the aging lesbian, gay, bisexual, or transgender (LGBT) population is gaining attention in the gerontology research (Herdt & de Vries, 2004). Housing and supportive services is a critical issue, as older LGBTs often find that they must conceal their sexual identity when they begin to require supportive services (Brotman, Ryan, & Cormier, 2003). De Vries (2006) describes several housing communities designed to openly address the needs of this growing population of elders. For example, RainbowVision, located in Sante Fe, New Mexico (www.rainbowvisionprop.com), is said to be the first retirement and care community developed specifically for LGBT older adults. It offers a range of options from condominiums for purchase to independent living in leased residences to assisted living with access to health care and supportive services.

Expanding Housing Options for Older Adults

In closing, although older adults have a myriad of options regarding their living arrangements, problems in housing availability and affordability continue to exist. As boomers age, the tension between the issues of person–environment fit will become apparent for many more older adults, and a variety of housing options and programs will continue to be in demand. Enhancing the affordability and availability of housing for Older Americans was among the top 50 resolutions put forth by delegates of the 2005 White House Conference on Aging. Strategies for implementing these resolutions include:

- creating new mechanisms at the federal, state, and local level (such as trust funds, tax cuts, and bonds) to increase the supply of accessible housing, and retro-fit or modify existing homes;
- developing housing guidelines for older Americans, which encompass low income/limited assets, support intergenerational communities, and provide incentives to governments (local, state, and federal) to adapt zoning; and
- developing new residential models of housing that meet universal design standards, including new housing that is accessible, adaptable, and affordable for a diverse population.

In addition, delegates put forth resolutions encouraging community designs to promote livable communities that enable aging in place, and expanding opportunities for developing innovative housing designs for seniors' needs.

CASE STUDY

Finding a New Home

Ellen, an active 77-year-old widow, had resided in a triplex rental for eight years. Ellen was happy with her living arrangement and said that she planned to "live here the rest of my life." An outgoing person, she became well acquainted with her neighbors and enjoyed the convenient location of her home. She spent many hours out-of-doors tending her roses and helping with other yard duties voluntarily. Because she had established herself as an excellent renter, the owner considered Ellen's fixed income of $1,000 per month and in eight years had increased her rent by only $75, bringing it to $350 per month. She could cover her living expenses and enjoy recreational activities at a local senior center.

In 1994, the owner notified Ellen that he had turned over his property to his daughter and that she would raise the rent to $700 per month. Ellen reported that "the rent increase devastated" her and that for days she "cried at the drop of a hat" because she had no idea what she was going to do. Ellen did not want to depend on her two children, who lived nearby. She wanted to be independent. If she found another rental, the same thing could happen to her again. Where would she find affordable rent now that this mid-sized community was growing rapidly and rentals were in great demand?

Ultimately, a friend advised her to contact the manager of a small mobile home park in a nearby community of 7,500. Ellen knew nothing about mobile homes and was skeptical but open-minded. She had heard that the manager was "very strict" about whom he accepted into the park. Initially, the manager told her that nothing was available. As the conversation progressed, Ellen won him over with her pleasing personality. He offered that she could look at one unit that was available. Ellen was more than impressed with the well-kept home that was for sale by an older couple.

Her next problem was financial. Her banker advised her to use a certificate of deposit of $35,000, her entire savings, for collateral. This would more than cover the full cost of the mobile home at $28,000 and generate enough interest to pay the interest of the loan. The lot fee was $175 per month and included water and trash rates. Ellen pays on the principal each month in an amount that varies depending on her monthly finances. Ellen has settled into her two-bedroom mobile home with an attached garage and "more storage space" than she has "ever had." Her children like her new home and visit often. Ellen's grandson says, "Grandma, you do not live in a mobile home, you live in a home." Ellen tells her friends, "I love it, I have never been happier in my life. Please God don't do anything to my little house."

Case Study Questions

1. Citing research, explain why Ellen's emotional reaction to having to move from her apartment home of many years could be expected.

2. What factors does Ellen have working in her favor in this situation? What circumstances could be working against her?

3. Ellen has advanced arthritis in her hips and knees. What bearing does this condition have on her future housing choices?

4. On the basis of the person–environment fit model, what housing options would be appropriate for Ellen? Why?

5. Where might Ellen go to find out more about housing options in her community?

Learning Activities

1. Investigate the housing opportunities available for older adults in your community. What types of services, if any, are offered? Do the residents reflect what you have learned about senior housing in this chapter?

2. Interview someone from the public housing authority. What does the person see as the primary issues facing housing for older adults? What policy changes have had to be implemented during the past decade?

3. Conduct a review of recent housing legislation (federal, state, and local) that deals with housing for older adults. What is the focus of legislation or policy? What are its strengths and weaknesses?

4. Interview residents who reside in public or residential housing facilities. What do they like about the facility? What are their primary concerns? What do they like about living in an age-specific environment? What don't they like about it? What do you perceive to be the advantages and disadvantages for residents living there? Would you encourage a family member to live in age-specific housing? Would you consider it as an alternative for yourself?

For More Information

National Resources

1. National Resource Center on Supportive Housing and Home Modification, Andrus Gerontology Center, 3715 McClintock Avenue, University of Southern California, Los Angeles, CA 90089–0191; phone: 213-740-1364; www.homemods.org; e-mail: homemods@usc.edu.

   The purpose of the center is to promote supportive housing that encourages healthy, independent living. The center conducts applied research, evaluation and policy analysis, training and education, policy updates, and national teleconferences. The center also provides reports, guidebooks, newsletters, and fact sheets to make available objective information about housing.

2. National Council on the Aging, 1901 L Street N.W., 4th Floor, Washington, DC 20036; phone: 202-479-1200; www.ncoa.org.

   The National Council on the Aging has resource materials on a wide variety of topics, including senior housing and supportive services available to older adults living in their own homes.

3. National Council of Senior Citizens, 8403 Colesville Road, Suite 1200, Silver Spring, MD 20910; phone: 301-578-8800.

   The council is an advocacy organization of older adults whose primary purpose is to work for legislation to benefit older adults. It is one of the major sponsors of housing for older adults—its Housing Management Corporation manages buildings across the country.

4. Assisted Living Federation of America, 1650 King Street, Suite 602, Alexandria, VA 22314-2747; phone: 703-894-1805; www.alfa.org.

   This is the largest national association exclusively dedicated to professionally operated assisted living communities for seniors. ALFA's member-driven programs promote business and operational excellence through national conferences, research, publications, and executive networks. ALFA works to influence public policy by advocating for informed choice, quality care and accessibility for all Americans seeking assistance with long-term care. ALFA produces numerous publications and reports on the business of assisted living, including its flagship magazine, *Assisted Living Executive*.

5. American Association of Homes and Services for the Aging, 2519 Connecticut Avenue N.W., Washington, DC 20008; phone: 202-783-2242; www.aahsa.org.

   This national association of nonprofit organizations represents 5,000 nonprofit nursing homes, continuing care retirement communities, assisted living residences, senior housing facilities, and community service organizations for older adults. This group also sponsors the Continuing Care Accreditation Commission that accredits continuing care retirement communities. Free information on long-term care and housing for older adults is available on its website, along with links that explore different housing options.

6. *Journal of Housing for the Elderly*, The Haworth Press Inc., 10 Alice St., Binghamton, NY 13904; phone: 800-429-6784; www.haworthpressinc.com/store/product.asp?sku = J081.

   This journal covers the latest efforts of housing researchers and policy experts—from research on energy conservation or privacy needs to policy implications of home equity conversion. It also examines management issues, housing-related service delivery innovations, case histories of successful housing alternatives, and financing strategies.

Web Resources

1. *Manitoba Senior Citizens' Handbook*: www.gov.mb.ca/shas/counciloaging.html.

   Our friends up north have put together a great page that explains all the types of living accommodations available to older adults. Take a look at the different housing options available for older adults in Manitoba.

2. U.S. Department of Housing and Urban Development: www.hud.gov.
   This is the place to start to look for information about housing policy or programs. Visitors can search USDHUD's database and gain access to housing reports, program information, and a variety of housing data. The site also has consumer information about housing.

3. HomeStore.com—Senior Living: www.springstreet.com/seniors/index.jhtml?source = a1rnftjt597.
   This website displays buildings, grounds, and interiors of retirement communities, assisted living facilities, and nursing homes in color photographs. Detailed information on each property may also be found, as well as names of moving companies, self-storage, financing, and retirement-planning books.

4. Mature Market Resource Center: www.seniorprograms.com.
   The Mature Market Resource Center has two web-based organizations. First, the Association of Marketing and Sales Executives in Senior Housing is a web-based national membership organization dedicated exclusively to the needs of marketing, sales, and communications executives in senior housing. Second, the National Association of Senior Health Professionals is a web-based membership organization specifically designed to address the unique needs and special interests of professionals in the rapidly growing field of senior health.

5. Assisted Living Federation of America (ALFA): www.alfa.org.
   ALFA's website provides information to consumers, including a sample resident agreement, videotapes to help consumers and families ease the transition to senior housing, and a directory of ALFA members.

6. Consumer Consortium on Assisted Living (CCAL): www.ccal.org.
   The Consumer Consortium on Assisted Living is the only national consumer education and advocacy organization focused on the needs, rights, and protection of assisted, living consumers and their caregivers. CCAL educates consumers, trains professionals, and advocates for assisted, living issues.

NOTE

1. Unless otherwise noted, the statistical information is on single-family dwelling characteristics.

16

Care Management

Ruby, 86, suffers from Parkinson's disease. Widowed for five years, Ruby lives in a small house one block from the main street of the town in which she has lived for 25 years. Ruby is becoming quite frail and must always use a walker. She has wonderful neighbors who are helpful, a 76-year-old sister-in-law who lives 5 miles away, and two nieces who are caring and attentive but live out of state. To help her remain independent and to enable her to continue living in her own home, Ruby's care manager recommended a variety of service options, including Meals on Wheels, home health care, and the use of the senior bus for visits to the doctor when her neighbors are not available to take her.

$C$are management is central to the integrative delivery of services for older adults. Without it, many older adults such as Ruby become frustrated when seeking help from an often fragmented, complex, and costly service system. Care managers serve as navigators, guiding older persons in their pursuit of services that will foster their independence. The National Advisory Committee of Long-Term Care Case Management defines care management as "coordinating services that helps frail elders and others with functional impairments and their families identify and secure cost-effectively administered services appropriate to the consumers' needs" (Connecticut Continuing Care, Inc., 1994, p. 5). This dual mission of planning and individualizing services to promote client independence while controlling costs makes care management a cornerstone of community-based service provision for older adults (Rife, 1992).

Known by a variety of names (e.g., case management, case coordination, and service management), care management occurs in a diverse range of long-term care programs for older adults. Although programs differ in how they implement, access, and monitor their services, they do agree on the core elements of care management (Austin, 1996; National Chronic Care Consortium, 1997; Quinn, 1993; Urv-Wong & McDowell, 1994).

The care management process begins with *case finding* (see Exhibit 16.1). The purpose of case finding is to locate individuals who might benefit from services. Care managers often rely on referrals from other professional service providers to help them in identifying viable clients. Gatekeepers, or individuals who by the nature of their day-to-day work come into routine contact with many people, can be trained to successfully identify isolated older individuals with functional limitations and refer them to care management programs (Emlet & Hall, 1991). Once these individuals are identified, care managers begin the *intake and*

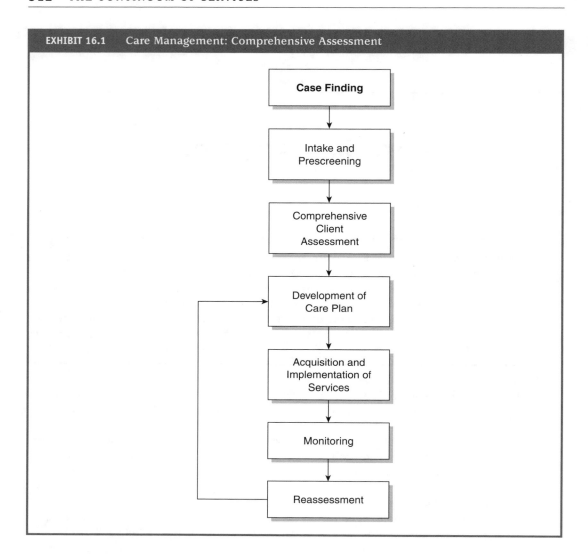

EXHIBIT 16.1   Care Management: Comprehensive Assessment

prescreening process by obtaining basic information about them (e.g., presenting problem, age, income, living arrangements, current level of both formal and informal service use, and type of disability). Care managers also evaluate potential clients according to program criteria (i.e., income and level of frailty) to determine eligibility for particular services.

After a client is accepted via the prescreening, the care manager continues the process by conducting a more *comprehensive client assessment*. Using a multidimensional assessment tool (see Exhibit 16.2), the care manager gathers in-depth information about the person's physical wellbeing and medical history, psychological and mental functioning,

> **EXHIBIT 16.2   Care Management—Comprehensive Assessment**
>
> When the care manager determines that a client is eligible for care management services, he or she conducts a multidimensional assessment that profiles details of the client's needs and support systems. Although the specific assessment tool used varies across programs, during the assessment process, care managers typically address the following questions:
>
> - What are the present state and history of the client's illness?
> - What medications are being taken?
> - What is the client's perception of his/her health?
> - How is the client coping with his/her situation?
> - How good is the client's short- and long-term memory?
> - How well is the client able to dress, feed, bath, walk, toilet him or herself?
> - Who, if anyone, helps support the client among family, friends, church, neighbors?
> - What physical barriers in the client's dwelling help or hinder his/her mobility?
> - What financial resources are available to the client to pay for services?

Source: Quinn (1993).

functional ability (i.e., activities of daily living [ADLs] and instrumental activities of daily living [IADLs]), social activities, formal and informal service use, economic and financial status, in-home safety, and family relationships (Krout, 1993a; Quinn, 1993). From the assessment, the *development of the care plan* occurs. The care plan describes the type of problem the client has and the planned outcomes of the services. The care manager describes the needs of the individual in conjunction with a client's values and preferences to set desired outcome goals and to design a care plan of informal and formal services to best meet the needs of the individual. The care manager then identifies, coordinates, and negotiates service provision and funding. How the care manager handles the *acquisition and implementation of services* depends on which care management model is being used (the different models will be described later in the chapter).

Monitoring is also a function of the care manager. After arranging for services, the care manager continues to periodically monitor client satisfaction with the plan and the appropriateness and implementation of the plan (e.g., quality, timeliness, and duration). After a specified time, the care manager conducts a *reassessment* of the client and care plan to detect changes in the client's needs and to evaluate the effectiveness of the care plan in meeting the client's goals. On the basis of this evaluation, the care manager revises or adjusts the care plan as appropriate to reflect the client's current needs, or the client may be discharged from the program.

In the remainder of this chapter, we focus our attention on the rapidly developing field of care management. We begin by examining the political influence on and support for care management services. This section is followed by a profile of care management users and providers. We end the narrative portion of the chapter with a discussion of the challenges facing care management programs now and in the future.

POLICY BACKGROUND

Federal support has been critical to the development of care management programs serving older adults. With the passing of the Comprehensive Health Planning and Public Health Service Amendments of 1966, care management began to surface as a method for helping individuals overcome the federal bureaucracy and improve their access to federal health care programs (Spitz & Abramson, 1987). In the 1970s, when the government began to allocate significant dollars for the development of community-based services, many programs incorporated care management as a key service (Quinn, 1993). By 1979, 333 care management programs for older adults existed throughout the United States (Downing, 1985).

Federal initiatives supporting the development of community-based services continued through the 1980s, but with greater focus on cost containment. With the Omnibus Budget Reconciliation Act of 1981, Congress attempted to reform the Medicaid program by allowing states to modify Medicaid regulations. States could apply for waivers that limited the services offered from a statewide program, allowed reimbursements to provider organizations for services not ordinarily part of the state's Medicaid plan, or allowed modifications of the existing eligibility criteria for the client applying to the Medicaid program. This was a significant policy change because public programs could now include a range of both health and personal care services and care management services through one funding source (Quinn, 1993). Although an optional service in all state waiver program plans, the majority of states allow reimbursement for care management as part of their specialized home and community-based services.

The Older Americans Act (OAA) began supporting care management demonstration and research projects with the Act's 1978 revisions. The 1985 reauthorization of the OAA identified care management as a basic service. This legislation authorized Area Agencies on Aging to "support services designed to avoid institutionalization including care management" (§ 321 [5]). The reauthorization of the OAA in 2006 once again directed funding under Title III, Part B for care management services, and identified care management as an important component of in-home services for frail older adults under Title III, Part D.

USERS AND PROGRAMS

Public and private care management services have proliferated during the past decade in response to demographic changes, increased concern about the cost of services, and the complexity of the health care and service systems. In this section, we describe the general characteristics of individuals using care management and the persons and programs providing care management services. In addition, we briefly present evaluation outcomes from several long-term care demonstration programs built around the provision of care management.

Characteristics of Care Management Clients

It is difficult to profile the typical care management client because most authors describe the consumers of care management in descriptive (e.g., frail or nursing home–eligible) rather than in empirical terms. Typically, publicly funded programs require a predetermined level of client frailty to qualify for care management services (Quinn, 1993). Private care management services often are available to any individual who has the resources to pay for the service. The following examples show the similarity and diversity of clients found among and within care management programs.

Like Ruby, whom we met at the beginning of the chapter, many care management clients are White, older, female, and widowed. A national study of 553 rural, primarily community-based care management providers found that most clients were women, over 75 years of age, and widowed (Krout, 1993a). Most of the clients lived alone and had yearly incomes below $15,000. Approximately one-half of the individuals receiving services were Medicaid eligible. The agencies retained the older adults as care management clients for an average of 32 months. The most frequently noted reasons for termination of services were the client's recovery, death, institutionalization, relocation, or need for a higher level of care.

The 864 clients referred to hospital-based care management programs located primarily in urban areas of New Mexico and Arizona ranged in age from 60 to 106, with an average age of 78.7 years (Warrick, Netting, Christianson, & Williams, 1992). Two-thirds of all clients were female; the greatest proportion of clients were White (80%), followed by Hispanics (13%). They reported having an average of 11 years of formal education and a yearly income of approximately $9,600. Overall, 41% of the clients said that they had experienced major health deterioration within the previous six months of receiving care management services, and 13% had undergone major surgery. Clients enrolled in the program immediately following hospitalization presented care management needs different from those of individuals referred from other community service programs. Many hospital-referred clients needed intensive, immediate assistance as they exited the hospital. They did not need long-term intensive care management services as required by community-referred clients, who, in comparison, were older, less likely to have informal caregivers, and more likely to be functionally dependent. Approximately 36% of all clients continued in care management for at least one year. Clients terminated from the program because of death, nursing home admission, self-sufficiency, referral to another care management agency, or relocation outside the hospital service area.

Best Practice: Kaiser Permanente's Care Management Institute

Kaiser Permanente's Care Management Institute (CMI) is a unique, pioneering institution with a mandate to drive, fund, and catalyze care management activities throughout its nonprofit HMO. Created in 1997 for the express purpose of helping Kaiser Permanente improve the quality of care and health outcomes for its members, CMI draws on the extensive clinical experience, research, and data of an integrated health care system with more than 8 million members. CMI synthesizes knowledge about the best clinical approaches in order to create, implement, and evaluate effective and efficient care management programs.

Kaiser Permanente currently cares for over 920,000 members who are aged 65 or older. To meet the diverse needs of their aging members, care management strategies for elder care are multifaceted and highly flexible. CMI's population-based approach has focused primarily on those with the greatest care needs, emphasizing clinically proven techniques for managing the most serious health challenges. Its integrative approach facilitates awareness of successful practices. Tools and guidelines developed and used by CMI include

- *Evidence-Based Dementia Guidelines and the Dementia Care Program*—an outline of the information needed for clinicians to make an early diagnosis of dementia. The guidelines and program also describe successful models of managing dementia over time.
- *Palliative Care Source Book*—describes models of care for those with advanced, life-limiting illnesses in different settings, including hospital, clinic, home, and skilled nursing facilities.
- *Integration Into KP HealthConnect*—provides point-of-service decision-support around geriatric issues in KP's electronic medical record system and will promote optimal information transfer across care settings to improve continuity.

For more information, contact CMI at One Kaiser Plaza, 16th Floor, Oakland, CA 94612; phone: 510-271-6424; www.kpcmi.org.

Older clients of the Community Care Services Program (CCSP), a care management program funded through the Medicaid waiver program in Georgia, ranged in age from 65 to 103 years; the majority of clients are White women (Diwan, 1999). An examination of the time spent with clients identified four variables predictive of higher use of care manager time: problematic client behaviors, greater difficulties in performing activities of daily living, problematic informal support, and problematic formal services. A comparison of high-end users of the care management services with the rest of program's clients revealed that these clients had a higher prevalence of dementia and mental illness, multiple health conditions, and more problematic client, caregiver, and service provider situations.

In the private sector, geriatric care managers (GCM) serve as consultants for families with dependent older adults or as contracted agent representatives for corporate employee benefit services. Results of a national survey completed by 712 members of the National Association of Professional Geriatric Care Managers suggest that, although the focus of geriatric care managers' work is on the needs of an older person, it is often family members who seek and pay for the GCM's services (Stone, Reinhard, Machemer, & Rudin, 2002). In fact, the primary contact is often not the older person. Only 21% of respondents said they usually communicated with the elderly client. The GCMs reported serving an average of 17 clients per month. Hourly fees for care management services averaged $74 an hour; they charged an average of $168 to develop a care plan and $175 for initial consultations. The most common services provided by the GCMs were assessing clients' functional abilities (90%), assessing family and social support (94%), developing a care plan (93%), finding and arranging appropriate services for the client (95%), and providing ongoing management of the care plan (90%). About two-thirds of the GCMs were licensed professionals (e.g., nurses, social workers). Of the 615 GCMs employed at the time of the survey, slightly more than half (57%) were working full time. More than two-thirds (68%) were self-employed, and 28% were working for an organization.

For Your Files:	**National Association of Professional Geriatric Care Managers**

The National Association of Professional Geriatric Care Managers (GCM) is an organization of practitioners whose goal is the advancement of gentle and dignified care for the elderly and their families. In 2006, the GCM membership was comprised of approximately 2,000 individuals representing themselves or a company, who were doing business in the field of geriatric care management. GCM members assist older persons and their families to cope with the challenges of aging. Most GCM's members have master's degree level training in gerontology, social work, nursing, or counseling. Member benefits include quarterly publications, *Inside GCM* and the *GCM Journal,* an annual conference, a membership directory, and professional development opportunities. For more information, contact GCM at 1604 N. Country ClubRoad, Tucson, AZ, 85716-3102; phone: 520-881-8008; www.caremanager.org.

CARE MANAGEMENT PROGRAMS

Program staff composition, qualifications, and numbers vary depending on the size and mission of the organization providing care management services. Typically, care management programs set minimum qualifications for their care managers, usually expressed in varying combinations of academic and work experience in human services (e.g., gerontology, nursing, and social work). Besides the primary care managers, some organizations employ care manager assistants to work with clients, families, service providers, and other internal agency staff to help the care manager in the day-to-day management of the client careload (Quinn, 1993; Schraeder, Fraser, Bruno, & Dworak, 1990). There also may be a care manager supervisor who maintains a supportive and consultative environment for the care managers by helping them with clinical and stress management issues (Applebaum & Wilson, 1988). The supervisor typically is responsible for managing program staff and supervising the care managers, negotiating service provider contracts, maintaining and analyzing data for program evaluation, and implementing quality assurance protocol (Schraeder et al., 1990).

Agencies and organizations use various approaches to carrying out care management, ranging from simple referral services to the actual delivery of comprehensive services. Each model varies both organizationally and operationally. The main differences between models are the level of authority directly controlling service use, the types and systems of service provision, and the method of payment. No evaluation data exist demonstrating that any one approach to care management is better than another (National Chronic Care Consortium, 1997).

In the *broker model,* care managers act as brokers for clients and service providers by linking the two through a referral system (Howe, 1994; Quinn, 1993). The purpose of broker care management is to match the target population with appropriate services on the basis of predefined agreements and standards of practice. The broker model supplies individuals with objective information from which to make decisions, a care plan with options and recommendations to help guide them, and a neutral party to help with the process of securing services. They have no service dollars to spend on the clients' behalf; thus, they cannot guarantee their clients that services are delivered as prescribed. This model works particularly in "service-rich" communities in which the client has many service options and the care manager has no direct conflict of interest with the various providers. Care management provided under this model is usually a freestanding service provided by both public and private organizations (Milne, 1994).

For Your Files: Connecticut Community Care, Inc.

Connecticut Community Care, Inc. (CCCI) is a statewide, private, nonprofit organization. Since its inception in 1974, CCCI has helped thousands of individuals to stay at home through the use of care management strategies. Services provided by CCCI include simplifying the health and home care maze, providing professional objectivity, relieving caregiver stress by linking appropriate services and respite support with the individual's needs, identifying cost-effective home care services and solutions, and advocating for the elder's needs. The Case Management Institute (CMI), founded in 1985, provides training, consultation, and education services to CCCI and to organizations and individuals nationwide.

For more information, contact Connecticut Community Care, Inc at 43 Enterprise Drive, Bristol, Connecticut 06010-7472; phone: 860-589-6226; www.ctcommunitycare.org.

Schraeder et al. (1990) describe four variations of the broker model. *Simple broker models* of care management inform and arrange needed services. Care managers under this model do not authorize or purchase services, nor are they directly responsible for the delivery of services. In the *combined broker model,* the organization providing care management furnishes some services for the client and coordinates the remainder with external agencies. The *complex broker model* authorizes types and levels of services provided with certain financial controls or capped expenditures. The *consolidated broker model* consists of a single or merged provider system delivering a full range of services through directed provisions or contracts. This care management model exists within a prepaid, capitated funding structure housed under one administrative umbrella.

Under the *service management model,* used by many of the Medicaid waiver programs, care managers have funds available for services. The care management agency contracts with area providers to deliver the services authorized in each client's care plan. Most states have policies that limit the total cost of services that can be authorized by care managers. "Cost caps" usually are 60–80% of a state's comparable Medicaid nursing home rate (Quinn, 1993). Under this model, the care manager is fiscally accountable, and the care manager's authority to purchase services is constrained by the range of services offered and the supply of those services in the local delivery system (Austin, 1996).

Based on prospective financing, whereby programs receive a specific dollar amount for each client they serve, regardless of whether it costs more or less to deliver the care that is needed, the *managed care model* operates much like a health maintenance organization (U.S. General Accounting Office [GAO], 1993; Quinn, 1993). Clients pay a predetermined fee, and care managers are responsible for providing all needed services to clients. The care managers have control over a pool of funds to purchase services for clients. Providers are prepaid, so that the liability for excess costs is placed on the care managers. Often, the managed care agency will control cost by providing services directly or by selectively contracting with outside providers to offer services to clients at a discounted price.

The *medical group model* provides a direct link between primary care physicians, nurse or social work care managers, and older patients (Shelton, Schraeder, Britt, & Kirby, 1994; White, Gundrum, Shearer, & Simmons, 1994). This model emphasizes a collaborative team approach under the leadership of the primary care physician. It stresses patient targeting, comprehensive multidisciplinary office-based and in-home assessment, individualized care planning, arrangement and coordination of needed services, continuing care management, follow-up, monitoring, and patient/caregiver education. The care manager helps facilitate the person's medical care by addressing the psychosocial and environmental influences affecting care. The use of care management in this setting complements and enhances the medical group's practice by providing a direct link between clients/caregivers in their homes and primary care physicians (Schraeder et al., 1990).

Best Practice: Professional Care Management Institute

The Professional Care Management Institute (PCMI) is a nonprofit organization that specializes in designing and delivering training programs to professionals in the field of community-based long-term care. PCMI's mission is to enhance the quality of care management services to clients, support the professional development of care management staff, and promote the utilization of care management concepts and skills in the provision of human services. It comprises a core staff, a Board of Directors, Training Advisory Committee, Accreditation Committee, and Independent Consultants/Trainers that all work to help reach PCMI's mission.

Since the institute was founded in 1987, PCMI has provided over 10,000 units of training (1 day of training + 1 person = 1 training unit) to 12,000 professionals from over 250 different organizations in Pennsylvania, New Jersey, Delaware, and Ohio. Offering more than 30 programs ranging from clinical programs for care managers to leadership programs for supervisors, managers, and administrators, PCMI programs combine up-to-date information and current theory with a practice orientation. In addition, PCMI provides a range of consultation services to public and private agencies. The institute works with organizations interested in developing or modifying service delivery programs, strategic planning, executive coaching, managing organizational culture, program evaluation, needs assessments, employment development programs, and a variety of other issues and topics.

Care managers who want to improve their professional status may become certified through PCMI's Care Management Accreditation Program. The certification is verification that the care manager has completed a comprehensive series of training courses and has attained a level of competency and experience in the practice of care management.

For more information, contact Professional Care Management Institute, 2605 Egypt Road, Norristown, PA 19403-2317; phone: 610-650-0496; www.p-c-m-i.org.

Under the auspices of the *acute care hospital-based model*, there is a linking of previously disconnected disciplines and departments within the hospital (e.g., finance, patient care delivery, and administration). This model organizes patient care from a team approach, which in turn results in better quality of care for the patient (Cohen & Cesta, 1994). Most hospitals view care management as a cost-effective means of shortening the patient's length of hospital stay while reducing the use of unnecessary tests, treatments, procedures, and other hospital resources (Rethinking an Old Notion, 1996; Sinnen & Schifalacqua, 1991; Trella, 1993).

Episodic care management occurs only when called for by providers in any of the other models of care management (Howe, 1994). The key feature of this model is that it can only be reactionary. It occurs in reaction to admission, consultation, or a phone call. The objective of this approach is to provide, during periods of stress, specialized diagnostic services and intervention services that are beyond the capabilities of the client and the primary care provider. The suppliers of episodic care management services include hospitals, specialized treatment centers, and health care specialists (e.g., physical therapist).

Evaluation of Care Management Programs

Does care management prevent or delay institutionalization? Is it cost-effective? To answer these questions, the federal government and several private foundations have funded numerous community-based long-term care demonstration projects that have included care management services. The fundamental hypothesis tested by these projects is whether community care can be a cost-effective substitute for institutional care. Some of the evaluations indicate that the use of home- and community-based services is not cost-effective when compared with nursing home costs. The findings also suggest, however, that the use of care management is an effective and successful way to control the total cost of home and community-based care programs.

Probably the most notable care management demonstration project was the National Long-Term Care Channeling Project. This federally funded program, started in 1980, examined the effects of care-managed, community-based long-term care on increasing older adults' use of home care, reducing their unmet health care needs, increasing their confidence in receipt of care and satisfaction with arrangements for it, and enhancing their satisfaction with life while not resulting in large reductions in informal caregiving (Kemper, 1988). Contrary to its original intent, however, the project increased costs of care. The evaluators suggested that one reason for increased costs was that although the population served was extremely frail, its members were not at high risk for nursing home placement. Thus the costs of the additional home care were not offset by reductions in nursing home placements.

In 1985, the Social/Health Maintenance Organization Demonstration Project began at four sites across the country (Abrahams, Nonnenkamp, Dunn, Mehta, & Woodard, 1988) and continues to be evaluated. Each federally funded site has a care management unit responsible for allocation of long-term care services. Individuals enrolled in the organizations pay premiums to receive services. The project sites consolidate services and providers to provide a full range of medical, personal care, and social services. They pool funding resources (e.g., Medicare, Medicaid, private insurance premiums, and client out-of-pocket fees) to provide members with acute health care plus expanded long-term care services. The care manager must administer service dollars judiciously because payments for services are capitated and prospective (Quinn, 1993). With the introduction of "provider risk" in the care management process, the project provider organizations can remain financially sound only if they keep their costs below the negotiated capitation rate.

Support from private organizations stimulated hospitals' interest in the use of care management services. The Robert Wood Johnson Foundation provided four-year demonstration grants to 24 hospitals throughout the country under its 1983 program for Hospital Initiatives in Long-Term Care (MacAdam et al., 1989). The purpose of the program was to encourage hospitals to develop new programs to better meet the needs of older persons. The participating public and not-for-profit hospitals set up unique projects. Each program initiated organizational changes; administrative improvements; educational activities for clinicians, staff, and consumers; care management programs; and community-oriented long-term care services. Care management was the only service that the foundation required all grantees to implement. Although most of the hospitals viewed care management as a valuable, relatively low-cost addition to the widening range of services they provided older adults, on completion of the demonstration period, most were unable to document changes in outcomes because of the provision of care management. Twenty-two hospitals reported, however, that they planned to continue some level of care management activities; one hospital ended the service; and one hospital was unable to report the future course of the service.

The Flinn Foundation sponsored the Hospital-Based Coordinated Care demonstration project at six sites in Arizona and New Mexico from 1986 to 1989 (Christianson et al., 1991; Warrick et al., 1992). The purpose of this project was to encourage private, not-for-profit hospitals to provide care management services to older adults at risk of rehospitalization after discharge. The clients and the community network of long-term care service providers had a positive view of the care management program. It delivered quality services to older individuals who met conventional eligibility criteria related to need. In contrast, the care management programs encountered several obstacles when trying to integrate into their own hospitals. For example, top administrators often lacked a strategy for blending long-term care with acute care service delivery in their organizations. Internal conflicts with hospital social workers, discharge planners, and home health agency staff about "ownership" of the patients in the hospital emerged during the implementation period and persisted throughout the project. In addition, most physicians had limited contact with the program care managers. They were not frequent users of, or effective advocates for, the program. After the grant funding ended, most hospital administrators chose not to continue the program primarily because of the inability of care management to pay for itself (Christianson et al., 1991).

The Program of All-Inclusive Care (PACE) developed through a combination of private and public funding. PACE projects seek to replicate On Lok, an innovative community-based model of capitated acute and chronic care for nursing home–eligible seniors in San Francisco's Chinatown. The On Lok program emphasizes the use of day health care and reliance on an extensive multidisciplinary team to manage and deliver services for frail, older participants (Wells, 2002). The program sites receive support from CMS, which provides waivers that allow capitated contracts using Medicare and Medicaid funds, and private foundations and sponsoring organizations largely support the initial start-up costs (i.e., site support, staff development, and service expansion). As of 2006, there were 34 approved PACE organizations serving 11,000 participants in 22 states (National Pace Association, 2006). The typical PACE participant is an 80-year-old woman who has 7.9 medical conditions and is limited in three activities of daily living. Approximately 49% of PACE participants have dementia. Several critical pieces need to be in place for the successful development of a PACE program (Kane, Illston, & Miller, 1992; Trice, 2006). The first is the necessity for sites to obtain sufficient start-up funds. Without such funds, the financial viability of the program is a constant source of concern. Another issue is the importance of building and maintaining staff with the skills and abilities to work in a multidisciplinary setting. Finally, care managers must develop the right patient mix in both acuity and dementia to accommodate the needs of all clients in a capitated system. These lessons learned will be valuable to the 13 states receiving awards from CMS in 2006 to support the development of 15 PACE models in rural areas (National Pace Association, 2006).

As described by Grabowski (2006), the STAR + PLUS program is designed to integrate the delivery of acute and long-term care Medicaid services through a managed care system within Harris County, Texas. Begun in 1998, the program had enrolled 57,000 aged and disabled Medicaid recipients by June 2002. The primary emphasis of the program is care coordination provided by a health maintenance organization employee who coordinates all the enrollee's services; develops an individual plan of care with the enrollee, family members, and providers; and authorizes all long-term care services. Evaluations of the program found lower program costs under capitation. STAR + PLUS was estimated to generate a 17 percent increase in savings relative to traditional FFS Medicaid. However, the evaluations do not adjust for covariates that may confound observed differences across the treatment and comparison groups.

In 2001, in response to the landmark Olmstead decision that required state and local governments to administer services, programs, and activities in the most integrated setting appropriate to the needs of qualified individuals with disabilities, the Centers for Medicare and Medicaid Services (CMS) began offering "Real Choice Systems Change" grants to encourage states to examine and improve the services provided through waivers and other programs to assist these individuals. In Colorado, for example, all Medicaid clients who receive non-developmental disabilities-related long-term care services are entitled to services from a care manager at one of 23 Single Entry Point (SEP) care management agencies. Responses to a client satisfaction survey from 1,281 randomly selected clients from all SEP agencies revealed that 80% of respondents were "very satisfied" with their current care managers (Colorado Department of Health Care Policy and Financing, 2006). Nearly all SEP clients (93%) said they knew the names of their care managers and approximately 88% reported that they felt comfortable calling their care managers with questions or concerns. Communication between care managers and clients was generally rated very positively. Most of the respondents indicated that they were always involved in their care planning (71%) and were offered choices among different providers. However, less than half of the respondents reported receiving accurate, useful information about consumer directed care, and only about one-third said that their care managers had discussed consumer directed care with them and encouraged them to participate.

Care management also is an important component of the Aging and Disability Resource Centers (ADRC), a federally funded initiative launched in 2003. Administered through the Administration on Aging and the CMS, ADRCs provide a coordinated system for providing (a) comprehensive information on available public and private long-term care programs, options, and resources; (b) personal counseling to assist individuals in assessing their existing or anticipated long-term care needs, and developing and implementing a plan for long-term care designed to meet their specific needs and circumstances; and (c) consumer access to the range of publicly supported long-term care programs for which consumers may be eligible, thus serving as a convenient point of entry for such programs. Forty-three states and territories have received three-year competitive grants since the program was launched (The Lewin Group, 2006b). Although the operational configuration of the ADRCs varies from state to state, all grantees must serve older adults and at least one disability target population. Preliminary evaluation found that the ADRCs provided information and long-term support to more than 750,000 contacts in the first two years of operation. Although much of the role of the ADRC involves information and referrals, most ADRCs engaged in short-term care management (STCM), characterized as intensive assistance to stabilize a consumer's situation to enable the individual to remain in the community and follow-up to ensure that consumers' needs were met. Forty-seven percent of the programs have care workers on staff (average of 5.8 per program), and 33% have nurse care workers (average of 2.7 per program). These workers are responsible for providing clinical consultation and/or health promotion services, performing assessments, determining level of care, conducting options counseling, interacting with Medicaid eligibility workers, and confirming eligibility approval for consumers. For additional information on the ADRC initiative, visit the ADRC Technical Assistance Exchange website at www.adrctae.org.

CHALLENGES FOR CARE MANAGEMENT PROGRAMS

Care management provides the entry into the community-based long-term care system. It plays a significant role in the coordination of services and resources for many older adults. However, some providers suggest that the scope of geriatric care management must be expanded from the existing primary focus on service coordination to include theoretically driven interventions that hold more promise for influencing long-term change in health-related behaviors and improving outcomes (Enguidanos et al., 2003). We end this chapter by addressing several current and future challenges facing care management programs.

Providing Care Management Services

Considerable debate has emerged about where in the structure of services care management should reside, whether agencies that provide home care services should be allowed also to be care managers, and how care managers should interact with other agencies and individuals who are authorized to bill for services (Kane & Frytak, 1994). To address these issues, two criteria need to be considered: the client's wellbeing and the interest of the organization paying for services. As Kane and Frytak point out, the care provided should meet unmet needs and result in improved or maintained physical, social, and emotional functioning of the individual. Service should be provided in a courteous and respectful manner and should be perceived as satisfactory. From a payer's perspective, the program should make efficient and effective expenditures. Kane and Frytak report that proponents of care managers in the provider role say that using independently employed care managers to authorize and monitor service is inefficient and redundant and does not lead to allocation in the patient's best interest. Proponents of nonprovider care management argue that publicly funded long-term care programs are efficient and effective only to the extent that they are under the authority of care managers who are not providers of care. Given these opposing positions, policy makers and researchers must explore more specifically what care management means operationally to home care agencies, nonprovider care management agencies, and state programs that fund both types of programs.

Ensuring the Effectiveness of Care Management Programs

How effective programs are in delivering care management services rests with several critical elements. First, care managers must receive proper training. Interviews with 95 care managers from six states in the GAO (1993) study identified the following as key practices essential for effective care management: the ability and skills to comprehensively assess client needs, time to have adequate contact with clients, knowledge of resources available in the community, and continual training to maintain and improve skills. Second, large caseloads limit the ability of care managers to give clients sufficient attention to ensure that clients' needs are met and that services are provided adequately. Other effects of large caseload sizes include limited time available to spend with each client and increased risk of burnout for care managers. Third, some barriers to effective care management outcomes are outside the control of local care management agencies. These include a lack of financial resources, inadequate availability of services in the local area, and extensive administrative requirements imposed by state administering agencies. In rural areas, the vast geographical areas for which many rural care managers are responsible often limit their ability to see their more "low-risk" clients regularly (Urv-Wong & McDowell, 1994).

To increase the effectiveness of care management programs, there also is a need for greater evidence-based design of care management programs (Cudney, 2002). However, collecting adequate data is an ongoing challenge for agencies (Schneider, Landon, Tobias, & Epstein, 2004). As noted by Horvath and colleagues (2006), available data do not always measure the goals of the program or they may capture outcomes, but do not allow researchers to link outcomes to program strategies.

Providing Quality Care Management Services

Although most publicly funded care management programs have some requirements concerning qualifications, training, and timely completion of activities (Justice, 1993), there are no uniform state or federal guidelines for the practice of care management. Geron and Chassler (1995) have called for guidelines that reflect changing practice and legislative realities; that promote flexibility in practice according to consumer values, preferences, and needs; that foster the efficient use of resources; and that ensure the equitable provision of quality services to those who are in need.

Diversifying Careloads

Care managers can increasingly expect to manage a more diverse careload as the number of minority and ethnic elders continues to grow. To successfully work with minority populations, it is vital for care managers to develop cultural competencies (Administration on Aging [AoA], 2001a, 2004c; Arnsberger, 2005). Greater understanding, sensitivity, respect, and appreciation of diverse cultural norms (i.e., history, lifestyles, experiences, and beliefs) will be needed if care managers are to effectively serve older clients and their families in cross-cultural situations.

Addressing Ethical Issues Facing Care Managers

Sometimes, care managers find their personal and professional ethics in conflict (Kane & Caplan, 1993; Galambos, 1997; National Chronic Care Consortium, 1997). For example, many care managers have control over the services used by their clients by virtue of the funding for the services and the contracts or agreements that the care management agency has with other organizations to provide services. This controversial issue raises questions about care managers' control of the use of particular services by their older clients. Care management firms that also provide direct services in addition to care management services may restrict client access to a greater variety or less costly selection of services.

The increasing medicalization of aging also jeopardizes the capacity of care managers to provide the social services critical to meeting the needs of older persons and their family caregivers (Binney, Estes, & Ingman, 1990). The problem stems from public policy decisions that often define long-term care as a need for medical services. This either makes the need for medical services an absolute condition for access to "free" social services or makes the medical services "free" and charges for social services. Consequently, care managers sometimes provide unnecessary medical services to make individuals eligible for social services (Shapiro, 1995).

Promoting Care Management in the Future

Delegates of the 2005 White House Conference on Aging promoted care management as part of several resolutions made for policy recommendations. For example, care management was identified as a strategy for

- improving state- and local-based integrated delivery systems to meet twenty-first century needs of seniors;
- supporting informal caregivers of seniors to enable adequate quality and supply of services; and
- promoting economic development policies that respond to the unique needs of rural seniors.

Care management services will continue to evolve along with the health care system in this country, and will undoubtedly become even more important as the number of Medicare and Medicaid recipients enrolled in managed care programs increases. Thus it is critical to continue to evaluate the effectiveness and efficiency of both public and private care management services.

CASE STUDY

When Information and Referral are Not Enough

Five years ago, Helen, 83, was diagnosed with a benign brain tumor that is causing partial memory loss. The tumor also may be the cause of several other physical symptoms such as excessive tearing in one eye, constant postnasal drip, imbalance, and difficulty swallowing. Because Helen no longer drives or arranges appointments, and is unable to keep house or cook, Ross, her husband of 55 years, has taken over most of the household duties. Helen taught high school English for many years and was an avid reader. She continues to read with encouragement, but she loses her concentration quickly. Her math skills are completely intact, and she is an avid cribbage player. Helen's social skills are appropriate but repetitive. She offers visitors coffee and sweets often during the visit and forgets that they previously discussed subjects. She has a keen memory for some aspects of her past and has completely lost her memory of other past events. Within a year of diagnosis, she lost the memory that her parents were killed in an automobile accident when she was 19 years old.

Ross is a retired electrical engineer. An organized person, he keeps lists and has an established routine for everything he does. These habits carry over into his approach to caregiving. He reads constantly, writes letters to the editor and to his elected representatives, and keeps abreast of local, state, and national events. He is interested in the status of the educational system and the future of children. Ross has suffered from periods of depression throughout his life. He has sought professional counseling several times, once within the past year after becoming depressed about Helen's memory loss and overwhelmed with the caregiving responsibilities. Meal preparation was especially worrisome to Ross. He was placed on an antidepressant, but had serious physical and psychological reactions to the drug. As a result, their two daughters, who live 100 miles away, encouraged and helped their parents to move into an alternative care facility. They stayed at the facility for two months. After Ross stabilized, he arranged to return home.

Home is a small, modest house near a midsize university. Although hardly considered wealthy, Ross and Helen receive retirement pensions from their engineering and teaching professions and Social Security totaling $2,225 per month. Ross speaks of investment savings as well. They have excellent health insurance coverage. In short, they can purchase most items that they want, but they want little.

Once, they were moderately involved in the community. Ross volunteered for a congregate meal program and was an advisory board member for several human service agencies. Because of Helen's condition, however, they have withdrawn from all their social activities. They continue to go for daily drives in the country when the weather is pleasant. They no longer go out to eat. Recently, Helen was hospitalized for a blood clot in her leg. This has added to Ross's worries, and a friend who visits the couple weekly fears that Ross is headed for another bout of depression that could destabilize the couple's situation.

Case Study Questions

1. Care finding—that is, locating individuals who might benefit from care management services—is the first step in the care management process. Who might be possible referral sources for this care? What elements make this care an appropriate referral?

2. What information provided in this case study would be the most critical for a care manager to consider in the prescreening process? Do you believe that Helen and/or Ross may be in danger of institutionalization? Why or why not?

3. The comprehensive assessment is a detailed step in care management. The following are only a few of the many questions to consider:
   a. Who is the client in this care scenario?
   b. What is the central problem?
   c. What additional information would you want to know about Helen and Ross?
   d. What outcomes would you as a care manager like to see achieved for Helen and Ross?
   e. What strengths and/or resources do they already have in place?

4. If you were to develop a plan of community services for Helen and Ross, what would you include and why?

5. Considering the outcome(s) and the community resources you have determined for Helen and Ross, what would be considerations in monitoring the progress of this care?

Learning Activities

1. Interview an Area Agency on Aging director or staff member who works closely with care management. What are perceived to be the benefits of and issues related to care management? Does the staff member want to see amendments to the OAA to address concerns? What type of direction does the agency receive from the AoA and the state Office on Aging?

2. Interview the director of a care management program or a care manager. What are the requirements (education and experience) to be a care manager? What are the responsibilities of a care manager? What are primary concerns with the program? What does the individual believe are the benefits of care management (to older adults, caregivers, service providers, and the community)?

3. Interview a caregiver or client receiving care management. How has this service affected the lives of the caregiver and client? How would they manage without it? What changes would they like to see in the program?

For More Information

National Resources

1. National Long-Term Care Resource Center, University of Minnesota, Institute for Health Services Research, School of Public Health, 420 Delaware Street SE, Minneapolis, MN 55455; phone: 612-624-5171; www.hpm.umn.edu/ltcresourcecenter.

   The resource center has issued reports on care management in long-term care, including *Models for Care Management in Long Term Care: Interactions of Care Managers and Home Care Providers*. Contact the center for a list of publications about care management.

2. National Association of Professional Geriatric Care Managers, 1604 North Country Club Road, Tucson, AZ 85716; phone: 520-881-8008; www.caremanager.org.

   The National Association of Professional Geriatric Care Managers is an organization of practitioners whose goal is the advancement of dignified care for older adults. Association members assist older adults and their families in coping with the challenges of aging. The association publishes a national referral directory as well as the *Geriatric Care Management Journal*, which is published four times a year.

3. Aging Network Services, 4400 East-West Highway, Suite 907, Bethesda, MD 20814; phone: 301-657-4329; www.agingnets.com.

   Aging Network Services is a nationwide, for-profit organization of private practice geriatric social workers who serve as care managers for older adults by providing a comprehensive assessment of older adults in their own homes and assisting in arranging the delivery of home care services.

4. *Care Management Journals*, Springer Publishing Company: 11 West 42nd Street, 15th Floor, New York, NY 10036; phone: 877-687-7476; www.springerpub.com/journal.aspx?jid = 1521–0987

   Created from two well-established and authoritative journals in the field, this new publication offers a digest of contemporary expertise in the home care field. The *Journal of Care Management* contributes readily applicable professional-style articles about care/care management in many practice settings. It is complemented by the *Journal of Long Term Home Health Care*, which presents a creative, interdisciplinary approach to program and policy analysis as it affects frail homebound older adults.

5. *Professional Care Management*, Lippincott Williams & Wilkins, 530 Walnut Street, Philadelphia, PA 19106-3621; phone: 888-291-4242; www.lippincottscaremanagement.com/pt/re/lippcaremgmt/home.htm;jsessionid = Fq7LMq0yXnGlJCh5R2s58yLTDZbTLhGkhyD1bZqjkkvpMpv8yDTF!2118075020!-949856145!8091!-1.

   This journal features best practices and industry benchmarks for the professional care manager. It is focused on coordination of patient care, efficient use of resources, improving the quality of care, data and outcomes analysis, and patient advocacy.

Web Resources

1. Numerous private care management agencies describe their services on the web. Take a look at how this growing field is advertising its services (we do not endorse these programs; we list them only as a source of information):
   - Florida Health Consultants: www.flahealth.com.
   - Elder Care Solutions: www.eldercaresolutions.com.
   - Cresscare: Care Management Agency for Elders: www.cresscare.com.
   - Senior Care Management: www.seniorcaremgt.com.
   - Care + Plus—Geriatrix Senior Care Management: www.geriatrix.net.

2. The American Society on Aging: Healthcare and Aging Network: www.asaging.org/networks/index.cfm?cg = HAN.

   Multiple articles on managed care for older adults are located within the archives section of this website. One is specifically related to care management and Latino elders; another focuses on Medicare-managed care.

17

Home Care Services

Margaret, 72 years old, has had multiple sclerosis for 20 years. For approximately 15 of those years, she and her husband, Wilbert, have lived a relatively normal life. The disease, however, has progressed to the point that Margaret needs assistance with most of her daily living activities. Wilbert has been a model caregiver, but the last five years have taken their toll on him. Wilbert never thought that he could afford regular home health care for Margaret. He was relieved to learn that she qualified for home health care under Medicare because she is totally confined at home. The home health agency schedules aides early in the morning. This allows Wilbert to attend his weekly Lions Club breakfast meeting. Wilbert would never complain about his caregiving responsibilities, but he does admit that he really enjoys the weekly breakfast outing.

Home care is a continuum of comprehensive care, providing individuals services that allow for maximum health, comfort, function, and independence in a home setting (Harper, 1991). Older adults such as Wilbert and Margaret choose to use home care services for several reasons, including the hope of avoiding institutionalization, familiarity of the home environment and sense of independence associated with this familiarity, lower perceived costs, and the continuity of family life and care (Mollica, 2003).

In the United States, there are three primary types of home care: skilled home health care, nonmedical home care, and hospice care. More than 20,000 providers deliver home care services to some 7.6 million individuals who require services because of acute illness, long-term health conditions, permanent disability, or terminal illness. Annual expenditures for these services are estimated at about $38.3 billion (National Association for Home Care & Hospice [NAHC], 2004). Skilled home health care represents the largest segment of public expenditure for home care. Nonmedical home care services are care services of a nontechnical nature that emphasize the daily needs of individual users. The services include home aides, homemaker services, respite care, and home-delivered meals. The intent of hospice care is to provide supportive and palliative care for persons who are terminally ill and their families but not to treat the underlying conditions.

Research on home care often combines skilled and nonskilled services without specifying which services are being analyzed. This makes it difficult to profile the users and providers of these services. Because specific chapters in this book are devoted to services that fall under the rubric of nonmedical home care (e.g., care management, nutrition services, and respite care), our primary focus in this chapter is on home health services and related nonmedical services (i.e., home health aide and homemaker services) that provide personal assistance to older persons confined to their homes. The latter part of the chapter focuses on hospice care.

HOME CARE

Policy Background

The first home care agencies were established in the 1880s to serve individuals who otherwise would not have access to medical care (Arneson, 1994). From that time until the mid-1960s, the industry grew slowly. With the passage of Medicare and Medicaid in 1965, however, the use of formal home care services increased dramatically.

To be eligible for home health coverage under Medicare, a person must meet five qualifying criteria (Medicare Rights Center, 2006). First, a physician must certify the need for services. Second, the individual must remain under the care of a physician. Third, the person must be homebound, meaning that he or she is unable to leave the home because of illness or injury without the assistance of a person or device and without a considerable and taxing effort. Fourth, the individual must need part-time or intermittent skilled nursing care (defined as up to and including 28 hours of skilled nursing and home health aide services combined provided on a less than daily basis)[1] or physical therapy or speech therapy. If the older adult meets these conditions, he or she may also receive occupational therapy, medical social services, and home health aide services. Fifth, Medicare must certify the home health agency providing services.

If a person meets all five of the above qualifying criteria, Medicare will pay for the types and amounts of home health services covered if the services are "medically reasonable and necessary." Services are covered in full with no deductible or co-payment from the beneficiary. The passage of the 1980 Omnibus Budget Reconciliation Act (OBRA) greatly expanded Medicare's home care benefit. Specifically, it removed the 100-visit limit, and an acute care hospitalization was no longer necessary to receive home care services. Because one must need skilled nursing or therapeutic care to obtain home care services from Medicare, typical coverage averages two to three months. Thus services normally do not address chronic needs for home care.

The introduction of Medicare's prospective payment system in 1983 also contributed to the growth of the home care industry, particularly with respect to home health care services. The cost-containment strategy promoted earlier hospital discharges, thereby sending patients home "quicker and sicker" with initiation and maintenance of treatments formerly performed only within the hospital now provided in the home. As a result, the acuity of illness, types of therapeutic care administered, and the amount of direct care to persons in their homes increased dramatically. The Balanced Budget Act of 1997 reduced growth in Medicare home health expenditures by introducing a new per-beneficiary limit, requiring reimbursement limits to be held to a below-inflation rate of growth, and restricting agency payments to the lowest of its allowable costs, per-visit cost limits, or per-beneficiary costs limits. As a result, home health care payments declined from about 9% of total Medicare spending in 1997 to 4% in 2004 (NAHC, 2004).

States may also provide home care services under three provisions of the federal Medicaid statute: (a) state plan home health services, (b) state plan optional services, and (c) 1915c waiver programs. In 2003, all states operated the Medicaid home health benefit and multiple home and community-based services (HCBS) waivers; 30 states offered the optional state plan (Kaiser Commission, 2006). Federal law sets forth minimum mandated benefits and allows states the option of providing other services. States must provide the following home health services for all individuals eligible for Medicaid and entitled to nursing facility placement: part-time or intermittent nursing, home health aide, and medical equipment and supplies. Although all states require the provision of these particular home health services, federal law does not set the amount of service provided. The optional home care services that states may provide to individuals include personal care services, home- and community-based care for functionally disabled elders, private-duty nursing, and respiratory therapy for ventilator-dependent individuals. Both mandatory and optional services offered under the Medicaid state plan must meet the following federal requirements: (a) Services must be uniformly offered throughout the state, (b) the recipient must have free choice of providers, (c) comparable services must be available to all individuals, and (d) any limits placed on the amount of services must be sufficient in amount, duration, and scope to achieve the purposes of the Medicaid program.

In 2002, the Centers for Medicare and Medicaid Services (CMS) developed the Independence Plus waiver to promote the use of consumer-directed (CD) care in Medicaid. These waivers encourage person-centered planning, individualized budgeting, and self-directed services and supports (Kassner, 2006a). Under this program, persons eligible for services can hire family members, friends, or neighbors to provide home care. According to Kassner (2006a), not only does CD HCBS meet consumers' preferences, it also helps address worker shortages, the need for culturally appropriate workers, and the availability of services in rural and other hard-to-reach areas, by expanding the pool of available workers. In 2004, 62 CD care programs serving older adults were available in 40 states.

If states want to provide services without complying with mandated and optional state plan requirements, they may obtain a waiver of one or more of them under certain federal provisions (Rosenzwieg, 1995). OBRA 1981 revised Medicaid's funding to allow states to cover HCBSs for individuals who would otherwise require institutional care. The Section 2176 waiver program permits states to provide a comprehensive range of HCBSs to individuals who, but for the provisions of such services, would be institutionalized. Services that states may cover include care management, homemaker, home health aide, personal care, adult day care, health care, habilitation, respite care, and other services approved by the state Medicaid agency and CMS as cost-effective. Section 1396 legislation, enacted in 1987, waives the same rules but applies only to persons aged 65 and older. As of 1999, all 50 states and the District of Columbia had waiver programs serving older adults (Harrington, Carrillo, Wellin, Miller, & LeBlanc, 2000).

Three other federal programs also authorize home-based services: Title III of the Older Americans Act (OAA), the Social Services Block Grant Program under Title XX of the Social Security Act, and the Department of Veterans Affairs. Area Agencies on Aging have the option of funding home health care services under Title III-B. In 1987, legislators added Title III-D to the OAA, which provided additional financial support for nonmedical in-home services for frail older persons (e.g., case management, lifeline systems, and deep cleaning). The intent was that they provide new and additional services, not just increase already existing services.

Although states have broad authority to spend their Title XX allocations on a wide array of social services, most states use some portion of their funds to support home services (e.g., homemaker and chore aide) for frail elders.

The Department of Veterans Affairs provides limited home care to qualifying veterans living within a 30-mile radius of Veterans Administration medical centers with a home care unit. The services covered are similar to those provided by Medicare. There is a co-payment for services based on eligibility category, secondary insurance status, and ability to pay.

Funding of home care can also come from private sources. Almost 18% of home care services are covered through out-of-pocket payments (NAHC, 2004); private insurance also constitutes about 18% of home care payments. Most policies cover skilled nursing and therapist services; fewer cover the costs of nonmedical home care services such as home health aides or homemakers.

Users and Programs

Characteristics of Home Health Care Clients

According to the 2000 National Home and Hospice Care Survey, of the nearly 7.2 million Americans receiving formal home health services, 70.5% were 65 years of age and older (National Center for Health Statistics, 2002). Among these older home care users, 17% were aged 65 to 74, 31% were aged 75 to 84, and 22% were aged 85 and older. Seventy percent of home care users were women aged 65 and older. Approximately 79% of the older home care users were White and 12% were Black. About 15% of older home care users live in non-metropolitan areas.

One consistent predictor of home care service use is functional disability. Of all elderly home care users, 59% reported receiving help with at least one activity of daily living (ADL). Bathing and dressing are ADLs with which older clients most frequently need assistance, followed by transferring to or from a bed or chair and walking (Exhibit 17.1).

About 60% of older home care users receive help with at least one instrumental activity of daily living (IADL). The most frequent IADL with which older home health clients received help was with light housework (37%) (Exhibit 17.2). In addition, 22% of older home health clients received assistance with preparing meals, and 19% needed help taking medications.

Approximately 74% of older home health patients received skilled nursing services, whereas 28% received homemaker services. Thirty-six percent of older clients received therapeutic services (e.g., physical therapy, occupational therapy, nutritional therapy) and 11% received psychosocial services. In 2000, the average length of service among older patients was 304 days; the median length of services was 77 days.

Family status also influences the use of home care services. Most older adults rely on family members, particularly their spouse, daughters, and daughters-in-law, for daily support and assistance. Approximately 38% of older home health care users are married (National Center for Health Statistics, 2002). When family members are not available or unable to provide care, reliance on formal home services increases.

Mixed evidence exists regarding the relationship between other personal background characteristics and the use of home care by older adults. One such variable is cognitive status. Some researchers suggest that individuals with fewer cognitive limitations are more likely to be using home care services (Borrayo, Salmon, Polivka, & Dunlap, 2002), whereas

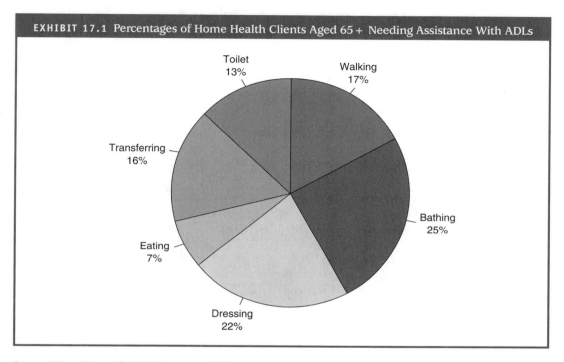

EXHIBIT 17.1 Percentages of Home Health Clients Aged 65 + Needing Assistance With ADLs

Toilet
13%

Walking
17%

Transferring
16%

Bathing
25%

Eating
7%

Dressing
22%

Source: National Center for Health Statistics (2002).

others report no relationship between cognitive abilities and home care use (Grabbe et al., 1995). Still others report higher use of home care among older adults with cognitive impairments than those without such problems. For example, a study of effect of cognitive status on the use of in-home services (i.e., homemaking, nursing, personal care, and home delivered meals) by 380 caregivers and care receivers in Canada found that care recipients with dementia were more likely to use personal care services and use two or more in-home services than caregivers and their care recipients with no cognitive impairment and those with cognitive impairment but no dementia (Hawranik, 2002). Part of this confusion in use-age patterns comes from the use of different definitions of home care in these studies.

Race rarely is a significant predictor of the use of home care, although older Whites are the predominant users of home care services (National Center for Health Statistics, 2002). However, Peng, Navaie-Waliser, & Feldman, (2003) found differences in the type of home health care use among older adults from racial and ethnic minority groups and their White counterparts. On average, all home health care recipients received at least two different types of home health services. White and Asian recipients had a greater variety of services and were more likely to have received multiple services than Black or Hispanic recipients. Regardless of race or ethnicity, having a greater number of comorbid conditions was the strongest predictor of increased use of home health services. Other variables associated with higher service use included pain, more ADL dependencies, being female, and being eligible for both Medicare and Medicaid (i.e., dually eligible).

EXHIBIT 17.2 Percentages of Home Health Clients Aged 65 + Needing Assistance With IADLs

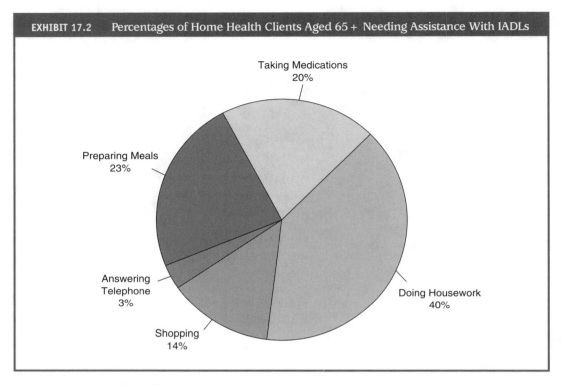

Source: National Center for Health Statistics (2002).

Differences in home heath service use between rural and urban residents are often attributed to access issues rather than individual characteristics of users. Rural areas are less likely to have a home health agency; when they do, the agency is likely to be smaller and to provide fewer services than agencies in urban areas. Dansky, Brannon, Shea, Vasey, and Dirani (1998) found, however, that even after availability of services was controlled for, older residents living in completely rural areas received approximately 3.5 times the number of home health visits that residents in rural counties with urbanized areas received. They suggested that home health services provide a "safety net" in remote rural areas, substituting for both informal support and other formal services.

Home Health Care Programs

In 2000, there were 1,355,300 home health agencies in the United States (National Center for Health Statistics, 2002). Of these, 93% were certified by Medicare or Medicaid. Approximately 43% of the agencies were proprietary, 57% were nonprofit, and 9% were government and some other type of ownership. Ten states had over 200 Medicare-certified home health agencies: California, Florida, Illinois, Louisiana, Minnesota, New York, Ohio, Oklahoma, Pennsylvania, and Texas. Texas, with 1,087 home health agencies, had the highest number of Medicare-certified agencies, whereas Vermont reported the fewest such agencies, with 13.

It is relatively easy for new home care agencies to establish themselves, especially if they are not providing Medicare-certified home health care. Nonmedical home care services are not subject to federal regulation. States put forth their own definitions of and regulations for home care; both vary from state to state (Arneson, 1994). Although most states require state licensure for nonmedical home care services, standards are minimal and not difficult for most agencies to meet.

According to the U.S. Department of Labor, in 2002 there were 675,100 home health workers employed by private, freestanding home care organizations (this figure excluded hospital-based and public home care agency employees) (NAHC, 2004). Home care staff consisted of both skilled professionals (e.g., doctors, nurses, physical, occupational, and speech therapists, lab technicians, and social workers) and paraprofessional members (e.g., homemakers, home health aides, and companions). The largest numbers of employees were home care aides (317,888) and nurses (111,324 RNs; 48,542 LPNs). Licensed Practical Nurses and Licensed Vocational Nurses provided a greater mean number of home health visits per eight-hour day than any other group of staff members (NAHCH, 2004).

For Your Files: National Association for Home Care & Hospice

The National Association for Home Care & Hospice is a trade association that represents the interests of more than 6,000 home care agencies, hospices, and home care aide organizations. NAHC is the premier clearinghouse for home care and hospice information. Its research department compiles and reports the data for use in policy analysis and educational campaigns to policy makers and the general public. Publications include *Caring Magazine* and other informational and newsletters and periodic reports providing basic statistics about home care and hospice.

For more information, call 202-547-7424; www.nahc.org.

Source: National Association for Home Care & Hospice (2007).

The majority of home health aides are middle-aged women, disproportionately minority, who provide personal care and assistance with daily living to frail elders (Yamada, 2002).These workers are the least skilled and lowest paid workers in the home care industry. As a group, they do not belong to unions and have little job security, few fringe benefits, limited training, and little opportunity for advancement. On a positive note, most aides report that their positions afford them time and schedule flexibility, autonomy, independence, and an opportunity to provide concrete help. They find their work intrinsically satisfying because they are committed to their older clients and the clients' families, and feel that they accomplish something worthwhile (Harris-Kojetin, Lipson, Fielding, Kiefer, & Stone, 2004).

For Your Files: **Caring for Lesbian and Gay Older Adults**

The Center for Applied Gerontology at the Council for Jewish Elderly (CJE) in Chicago has produced *Understanding and Caring for Lesbian and Gay Older Adults: Frontline Worker Sensitivity Training System*, an interactive one-hour curriculum tailored to direct-care staff who work with elders living at home and in institutional settings. It consists of a 76-page trainer's guide and a CD-ROM with PowerPoint slides and masters of handouts. The materials equip providers to offer their own in-service training to enhance cultural competence regarding lesbian and gay older adults. For more information or to order a copy of the curriculum, contact CJE at 777-508-1006 or visit their website at www.cje.net.

Source: ASA Connection: The Monthly e-Newsletter of the American Society on Aging (June 2005).

Challenges for Home Health Care

As the health care delivery system continues its evolution, receiving health and supportive care at home will be part of the normal pathway of care. For many older adults, receiving medical care and nonmedical services in their home is less expensive than institutional care. It is the most preferred care modality among older adults. We end our discussion of home health care by addressing several current and future challenges facing home health care agencies.

Working With New Clients

The majority of new home health care clients are recent hospital discharges (NAHCH, 2004) who are likely to be in a state of partial recovery from the conditions that first precipitated their acute care stay. These older individuals may encounter overwhelming stress as they attempt to adapt not only to the illness and hospitalization but also to the continuing need for physical care and emotional support. In addition, cognitive limitations are prevalent in new admissions, which can seriously impair the older person's ability to absorb and retain discharge information or acclimate to the home environment (Dellasega & Stricklin, 1993). Four major types of stressors face the home care patient: (a) inadequate patient teaching and insufficient discharge planning; (b) acute illness at discharge, resulting in having home care demands, high use of complex and sophisticated technology in providing care, and client dependency; (c) a home setting poorly adapted for client care, resulting in an unsafe environment; and (d) inadequate or inappropriate resources, including informal caregivers, insufficient finances, and inability to access the service system (Wagnild & Grupp, 1991). Agencies need to work with older patients to reduce the impact of these stressors because older persons unable to manage them will not achieve optimal care outcomes.

Serving Older Adults in Rural Communities

Many rural communities have a greater need for in-home medical and nonmedical services than they can meet. A recent study found that nearly 24% of rural residents received home health care services from an urban agency or a branch office of an urban agency (Franco, 2004). These home health care users tended to be younger and less frail than those receiving care in agencies in rural areas, suggesting that the limited supply of home care services are targeted to those most in need. In addition, rural Medicare beneficiaries are less likely than urban beneficiaries to obtain specialty services such as therapy services or medical social services (Kenney, 1993). More research is needed to further explore the home care needs of rural elders and the degree to which the more limited supply of specialized in-home services impacts their health and overall wellbeing. Federal health and human services policies also need further scrutiny to ensure their viability for promoting and supporting adequate and effective programs for rural older adults.

Financing and Paying for Services

Although public funds pay for a large amount of home care, many older adults also must pay for some of their care. More than 1,000 companies now offer coverage through long-term care insurance (America's Health Insurance Plans, 2004a). The cost of long-term care insurance varies widely, depending on the options selected. Persons aged 65 years old and in good health can expect to pay between $2,000 and $3,000 a year for a policy that covers nursing home care and home care, with premiums adjusted for inflation (AARP, n.d.). As new strategies are considered to improve the financing available for home care services, a key policy decision that legislators must address is determining an appropriate balance between public- and private-sector financing that meets the needs of frail older adults, does not undermine the efforts of informal caregivers, and is equitable and politically viable (Stone, 2000).

Recruiting and Retaining Staff

Given the growth and diversity in the health care system, there often is competition for employees among home care agencies, hospitals, and nursing homes as well as from other service sectors (e.g., discount stores). This competition, along with minimal wages and benefits, the lack of job security, and limited opportunity for career development, contributes to high turnover rates, particularly among nonmedical health care staff. These personnel issues present concerns about the quality of care to recipients. In addition, there is an impending decline in the supply of RNs and LPNs (Decker & Dollard, 2001), due to fewer young workers entering the health care workforce, the aging of the nursing workforce, increased options for women, and increased dissatisfaction with the health care workplace (Kimball & O'Neill, 2002). With the predicted future increase in the demand for home health care services, the home health industry will need to develop and implement creative strategies for the recruitment and retention of all of its employees.

Ensuring Quality Care

Home health care agencies must continually address the issue of quality assurance. CMS (2003) developed and published a set of home health quality measures on every Medicare-certified home health agency in the United States. The quality measures are intended to help consumers compare the quality of care provided by home health agencies as well as to motivate home health agencies to improve care and to inform discussions about quality between consumers and clinicians. The challenge for communities is to continually promote consumers' use of these measures when making decisions about home care. More information about the measures is available at www.cms.hhs.gov/quality/hhqi.

A staple of state quality assurance systems has been the consumer satisfaction survey (Folkemer, 2006). Consumers typically are asked whether they are satisfied with their case workers, their care plans, and their personal care workers. These surveys have often failed, however, to provide any depth of information about consumer preferences in service delivery or desired outcomes, as there is a well-known reluctance of many older people to criticize those providing care, both because of inherent courtesy and because of dependence on providers (Kane, 2000). Clearly, alternative approaches to assessing client satisfaction need to be developed. There also is a lack of consistency in home care research as to the definition of client outcomes, which makes it difficult to generalize the findings beyond the specific study population. The lack of use of a consistent set of measures makes it difficult for state officials to examine the association between various programs, practices, and outcomes (Kane, 2000).

In the wake of health care reform, enrollment in Medicare HMOs has increased (see Chapter 11). The outcomes for HMO patients compared with fee-for-service patients, however, have come into question. A national sample of 1,260 patients receiving home health care for 12 weeks revealed that, although the cost for HMO patients was about two-thirds as much as for the fee-for-service patients, patients in fee-for-service programs had better outcomes (Schlenker, Shaughnessy, & Crisler, 1995). Approximately 57% of fee-for-service patients improved in their ability to perform ADLs, compared with 43% of HMO patients. Schlenker et al. suggest that HMOs provide too few home health care visits to patients and attribute the difference in care, in part, to the capitation payments provided to HMOs by Medicare. Conversely, Porell and Miltiades (2001) found that, among older people who were functionally impaired, neither HMO enrollment nor having private supplementary insurance affected the risk of further functional decline or functional improvement. With the trend toward more managed care, agencies must continually evaluate their services as related to client outcomes.

Supporting the Future of Home Health Care

Several of the top 50 resolutions put forth by delegates of the 2005 White House Conference on Aging gave support for home health care services by proposing resolutions that expand and enhance delivery and payment for these services. These include

- developing a coordinated, comprehensive, long-term care strategy by supporting public and private sector initiatives that address financing, choice, quality, service delivery, and the paid and unpaid workforce;
- promoting innovative models of non-institutional long-term care; and
- fostering innovations in financing long-term care to increase options available to consumers.

The numerous strategies outlined for implementing the resolutions included the following:

- End the institutional bias in Medicaid long-term care by opening eligibility to any and all long-term care options.
- Provide permanent Medicaid funding for home- and community-based services.

- Increase the use of technology to facilitate non-institutionalized care and enhance communication among care providers.
- Attract and retain new health care providers with advanced training in geriatric medicine, mental health, social work, nursing, dentistry, allied health professions, and direct care workers by establishing geriatrics as an underserved profession.
- Implement a national and state tax credit to encourage the purchase of long-term care and health savings plans that allow individuals a choice of services.
- Provide regulatory and reimbursement flexibility and incentives for existing LTC providers to retool diversity and to provide fuller array of aging services in rural areas.
- Explore fiscally responsible approaches to combining social insurance, private insurance, individual saving, and social welfare in new and innovative ways.

Whether the federal government and the private sector are able to meet the challenges facing home health care remains to be seen.

Best Practice: Visiting Nurse Association of the Treasure Coast

Health Care on Wheels, operated by the Visiting Nurse Association (VNA) of the Treasure Coast in Indian River County, Florida, is a unique program addressing the needs of residents who do not have a primary care physician or health insurance. A mobile medical unit, staffed with a nurse practitioner and basic screening and testing equipment, operates 70 hours per week in neighborhoods with high concentrations of residents lacking access to primary health care. The van also carries a computer that allows staff to quickly and easily manage demographic data associated with the program. Services include screening for issues such as blood pressure and blood sugar, physicals, flu shots, and a few diagnostic activities. Colds, ear infections, and urinary tract infections are examples of illnesses that the nurse practitioner is prepared to diagnose and treat.

Since 1992, the program has processed 5,000 visits to the mobile unit, with clients divided almost equally between children and adults. Older adults represent about 10% of the caseload. Most of the older clients are without a primary health care provider. Through collaborative agreements with a number of programs in the area, the VNA also provides vouchers to help its low-income outreach clients pay for prescription medications. Financial support for the VNA Health Care on Wheels Program comes from a special tax district set up within Indian River County. The tax district governing board provides direction to the VNA by designating the areas in which the mobile medical unit can best meet community needs. Once an area has developed needed medical services such as access to a medical clinic and primary care providers, the mobile unit is assigned to another area.

For further information, contact Program Director for Health Services, VNA of the Treasure Coast, 1110 35th Street, Vero Beach, FL 32960; phone: 772-567-5551 or 800-749-5760; www.vnatc.com.

HOSPICE

Hospice is a philosophy of caring for individuals who are terminally ill and their family members. It is a comprehensive approach providing palliative medical, social, emotional, and spiritual support. As of 2005, there were approximately 4,000 hospice programs in the United States (National Hospice and Palliative Care Organization, 2006); 2,844 of these programs were Medicare-certified (Hospice Association of American, 2006). Although most hospice patients are older adults, persons of any age may receive hospice care.

Policy Background

The Tax Equity and Fiscal Responsibility Act enacted in 1982 created the Medicare hospice program. Originally, reimbursement for coverage was limited to 210 days. The passing of OBRA (1990) removed this limitation. Medicare now provides for unlimited days of coverage for hospice care when provided by a Medicare-certified hospice program for as long as the doctor certifies that there is a need. To be eligible for hospice care, a person must be certified as terminally ill, with only about six months to live, by the patient's physician or a hospice staff physician, and the hospice care must be part of the written plan of treatment established by the attending professionals.

Medicare entitles the person to the following services: physician services; nursing care; medical social services; home health aides; counseling for the patient, family, and other caregivers; short-term inpatient care; physical, speech, and occupational therapy; homemaker services; and medical supplies, appliances, and equipment. When a patient receives these services from a Medicare-certified hospice, Medicare pays providers one of four fixed prospective per-diem rates, based on service level and setting, for every day of hospice benefit coverage. Medicare hospital insurance (Part A) pays almost the entire cost of care. Hospice can charge the patient $5 for each prescription drug or other similar products for pain relief and symptom control provided on an outpatient basis by the hospice program. Hospice also can charge 5% of the Medicare payment amount for inpatient respite care (about $135 per day in 2007). Patients can stay in a Medicare-approved hospital or nursing home for up to five days each time they get respite care. There is no limit to the number of times patients can get respite care (Centers for Medicare & Medicaid Services, 2007). In 2004, Medicare expenditures for hospice services were 6.7 billion (Hospice Association of America, 2006).

Although Medicare is the most common source of funding for hospice services, other entities also cover the cost of participation in hospice. Medicaid provides hospice coverage in 48 states plus the District of Columbia. Medicaid hospice expenditures totaled $706 million in 2002 (Hospice Association of America, 2006). Hospices also receive reimbursement from private health insurance, HMOs, preferred provider organizations, and private pay, and to a lesser extent from local (e.g., United Way), state, and federal sources. More than 80% of employees in medium and large businesses have coverage for hospice services, and 82% of managed care plans offer hospice services (National Hospice and Palliative Care Organization, 2001).

There is currently no mandatory nationwide accreditation or "seal of approval" for hospice programs. To be eligible for Medicare or Medicaid reimbursement, programs undergo a certification process to ensure that appropriate care is provided to clients and that all employee and clinical records are in compliance with licensure requirements (Hospice Association of America, 2006). Some hospices voluntarily seek accreditation from the Joint Commission on Accreditation of Healthcare Organizations or the Community Health Accreditation Program. Less is known about hospices that do not participate in Medicare or Medicaid or national accreditation programs, as rules and regulations for licensure vary by state.

Users and Programs

Characteristics of Hospice Clients

The National Hospice and Palliative Care Organization (2006) estimated that in 2005, 1.2 million patients were served by hospice programs in the United States. Although the average length of stay in hospice was 59 days, approximately one-third of hospice patients received care for seven days or less. The balance between hospice patients with cancer diagnoses and those with noncancer diagnoses has shifted dramatically in recent years. In 1992, 76% of hospice patients had a primary diagnoses of cancer; in 2000, 51% of hospice patients had a cancer diagnosis (Hospice Association of America, 2006).

The 2000 National Home and Hospice Care Survey (National Center for Health Statistics, 2002) found that 81% of hospice patients were aged 65 or older; 33% of patients were at least 85 years of age. Of the older patients, 58% were women. Approximately 86% of older hospice patients were White and 7% were Black. The average time older patients received care from hospice was 101 days; the median length of service was 52 days. Most (77%) hospice patients died at their own personal residence; 19% died in institutional facilities such as a hospital or nursing home; 4% died in other settings (National Hospice and Palliative Care Organization, 2006).

In 2000, 89% of the hospice programs in the United States were certified by Medicare and 85% were Medicaid-certified (National Center for Health Statistics, 2002). A variety of organizations provide hospice services. Approximately 40% of hospices are independent community-based organizations; 44% are part of a group or chain, 25% are divisions of hospitals, and 4% are operated by a health maintenance organization. Freestanding hospices serve the majority of hospice patients; skilled nursing facility-based hospices served the fewest number of patients. Approximately 73% of hospices are nonprofit, 22% are for-profit, and 5% are government or other organizations. The majority of hospices are located in metropolitan areas (73%).

The numbers of Medicare-certified hospices range from just 3 in Alaska and the District of Columbia to 168 in California (The Kaiser Foundation, 2003). The majority of states (92%) provide hospice care for more than a thousand Medicare recipients annually; only four states served fewer than 1,000 patients in 2003. Almost 95% of the population lives within 25 miles of a hospice program (Harper, 1995).

Hospice patients receive individualized services, depending on their personal needs. In 2005, Medicare-certified hospices employed more than 73,000 paid professionals (Hospice Association of America, 2006). These individuals included medical personnel such as physicians and nurses, home health aides, social workers, clergy, and pastoral counselors. The largest numbers of employees were registered nurses (23,416) and home health aides (14,755). In addition, 42,000 volunteers provided assistance and support to patients and their caregivers. The largest numbers of volunteers were homemakers (2,186) and counselors (1,327). All Medicare hospice volunteers must participate in intensive volunteer training programs.

Hospices also offer bereavement groups and services for families and caregivers to help them with their grief. Most hospices offer these programs and services to the community at large, not just those families served directly by hospices. Bereavement services include follow-up phone calls and visits, information regarding meetings or group offerings, and literature and material on grief. A survey completed by 260 hospice providers indicated that either nurses or individuals with human services backgrounds (e.g., social work, clergy, and counseling) coordinate bereavement services (Demmer, 2003). Because of a lack of time and too few bereavement staff, programs tend to focus on less time-intensive services such as mailing of letters and literature on grief versus phone calls and home visits.

For Your Files: **Hospice of the Florida Suncoast**

The Hospice of the Florida Suncoast, located in Largo, Florida, received funding from the Administration on Aging to examine end-of-life issues affecting family caregivers and to develop a curriculum and train experts from around the country. One of the products developed was a 900-page tool kit entitled *Caregiving Near Life's End*. In addition, the hospice also conducted and published the results of a national survey, the Caregiving at Life's End National Needs Assessment. Ordering information for the manual and information on state trainers who have completed the course as well as other useful information for caregivers and providers on end-of-life issues can be found on the hospice's website: www.thehospice .org/caregiv/index.html.

Challenges for Hospice

Hospice programs in the United States focus on home care and dehospitalization (Mor & Allen, 1995). Family members, along with the hospice staff, provide care to their terminally ill loved ones. Hospice, along with other health care providers, will be affected by the ever-changing nature of health care and the graying of the population. We end this section with a discussion of the challenges facing hospice programs now and in the future.

Serving a Greater Diversity of Patients

White, middle-class patients are the predominant users of hospice programs. For hospices to respond to the needs of ethnic minority patients, workers need to be sensitive to culture-specific issues and practices. Challenges to overcome in providing hospice services across cultures include language differences, family values, lack of trust, and the hospice patient's feelings of discrimination or inequality (Noggle, 1995). To successfully expand services into minority communities, hospices must establish a pattern of education and communication appropriate to consumers, volunteers, and professionals of all races, ethnicities, and cultural groups (Bowman & Singer, 2001; Harper, 1995; Stein & Bonuck, 2001).

Supporting Patients Without Families

By design, the hospice home care model supports the efforts of families caring for terminally ill patients at home. An increasing number of hospice candidates, however, do not have home support available, or the support that is available is inadequate or unreliable (MacDonald, 1992). Thus hospice programs face either not serving this group of individuals or providing care for patients whose needs far exceed available resources. To address this issue, hospices need to develop creative approaches to serving patients without primary caregivers. Without strong community support (e.g., donations and volunteers) and supportive legislative action, most hospices will continue to struggle with how to provide care to individuals who are for the most part alone.

Assessing Hospice Care

Hospices vary considerably in their performance and in the services they provide. Although the National Hospice and Palliative Care Organization (NHPCO) developed and promotes standards of care for hospice programs, there is no means of enforcement; thus a problem in the U.S. hospice community is the lack of consistency among hospices as to compliance with standards (Connor, Tecca, LundPerson, & Teno, 2004). To address this issue, the NHPCO established a national database to be used to establish benchmarks for hospice practice throughout the country. This database provides a critical tool for furthering the use of consistent operations and performance measurement in hospice.

Enhancing Bereavement Programs

Bereavement programs are often the most underdeveloped component of the hospice program. Program staff indicate a desire to provide more group and educational programs, as well as more home visits to families, but cite lack of sufficient staff time, lack of personnel, and funding pressures as barriers to increasing the delivery of bereavement services (Demmer, 2003). Thus the lack of resources for bereavement services is an issue facing most hospice programs.

Educating Americans on End-of-Life Issues

Delegates to the 2005 White House Conference on Aging included educating Americans on end-of-life issues as one of their top 50 resolutions. Strategies proposed to implement this resolution included

- educating people about hospice and palliative care;
- developing health care and community collaborations with faith-based communities, aging service, and other community providers to promote advance care planning and completion of advance directives for all individuals;
- adopting the Physician Orders for Life Sustaining Treatment (POLST) recommendation as a nationwide end-of-life planning document; and
- simplifying advance directive laws to ensure that any authentic expression of a patient's wishes is respected and followed.

Will Home Health Care Work for Harriet?

Harriet is a 79-year-old woman who has never married. She lives in a small mobile home situated on land several miles from a rural town of 2,500 persons. Until three years ago, she lived with her bachelor brother who had been at the center of her life. His sudden death left Harriet confused and depressed because her life had revolved around the companionship and care of her brother. Her health has deteriorated steadily since his death. People in her community describe Harriet as a colorful character. She dropped out of school when she was 16 years old and took a job as a ranch cook's assistant. Her interest in ranching led to several years of traveling the rodeo circuit, assisting well-known bronco riders. Eventually, Harriet ended up owning a small grocery store in the town where she now lives. Her independent spirit became well known by her customers and business acquaintances. Harriet made no time for other social contacts beyond work and her brother. Harriet is not a religious woman and has little patience for "frivolous" socializing. Until recently, she devoted her spare time to raising and showing an exotic breed of house cat.

Although she accumulated considerable savings, she spent most of it supporting her brother, who had an alcohol problem. She does receive a monthly Social Security check of $524. Because she owns her mobile home and the acre of land on which it is situated, her monthly expenses average only $225. She has Medicare and a small supplemental health insurance policy. Harriet has a history of diabetes and high blood pressure, which have gone untreated. She has fallen several times, and it is becoming difficult for her to get in and out of her bathtub. This, combined with some incontinence, has made it difficult for her to maintain her personal hygiene. She recently was discharged from the hospital after gallbladder surgery. Her wound is not healing quickly.

Case Study Questions

1. The chapter discusses several predictors of use for home health services. Describe these predictors. Which apply to Harriet?

2. What are the social and environmental dynamics of Harriet's situation that a home health agency would take into consideration when assigning a worker to this case?

3. What criteria would Harriet have to meet to qualify for Medicare home health services? What other payment sources might be available to Harriet?

4. Harriet is likely to resist the idea of home health care. What arguments could best make the case to Harriet that this is a good option for her?

Learning Activities

1. Review current Medicare, Medicaid, or Older Americans Act legislation that pertains to home care services. What do the various laws mandate? How do they differ, and where do they overlap? What areas do you believe legislation needs to address in preparation for future growth of the aging population?

2. Interview a home health care provider or hospice staff member. What situations does the provider encounter? What types of on-the-job or in-service training do workers receive? What are the education and experience requirements for staff positions? What are some of the obstacles as well as benefits of the service? What changes would the staff like to see?

3. Interview someone who receives or is the caregiver of someone who receives home health or home care services. What does the recipient or caregiver feel are the benefits of the program? Where are the gaps? How would the individual change the program or services, if at all? What would the individual do without the program or services? How did the household find out about the program and select the provider?

4. Check local newspapers, television, radio, and magazines for home care service and hospice ads. Who are they trying to reach? How would you respond to the ads?

5. Design a new home care or hospice program. What elements would be primary? Who would you serve? How would you market your program?

For More Information

National Resources

1. National Association for Home Care, 228 7th Street SE, Washington, DC 20003; phone: 202-547-7424; www.nahc.org.

   The National Association for Home Care represents home health agencies, hospice programs, and homemaker/home health aid agencies. *Caring Magazine* and *Home Care News* are published by the association. Contact it for a list of publications.

2. National Hospice Organization, 1700 Diagonal Road, Suite 625, Alexandria, VA 22314; phone: 703-837-1500 or 800-646-6460; www.nhpco.org.

   The national office offers technical assistance and training to local hospice organizations. It operates a toll-free referral line to local hospice programs. Numerous free publications are available.

3. Visiting Nurse Association of America, 8403 Colesville Road, Suite 1550, Silver Spring, MD 20910-6374; phone: 240-485-1856; www.vnaa.org.

   The VNA is the parent organization of local VNAs that provide personal care; speech, physical, and occupational therapies; and nutritional counseling. A fact sheet is available.

4. National Hospice Foundation, 1700 Diagonal Rd. Suite 300, Alexandria, VA 22314; phone: 703-243-5900 or 800-854-3402; www.hospicefoundation.org.

   The foundation promotes home care and hospice care through the establishment of standards of care, educational programs, and research. Free consumer guides about home care and hospice are available.

5. Catholic Charities, 1731 King Street, Suite 200, Alexandria, VA 22314; phone: 703-549-1390; www.catholiccharitiesusa.org.

   Catholic Charities is a social service agency that offers assistance to people of all ages and has extensive support services, including homemaker services, through its local offices.

6. *Home Health Care Services Quarterly*, The Haworth Press Inc., 10 Alice St., Binghamton, NY 13904; phone: 800-429-6784; www.haworthpress.com/store/product.asp?sku = J027.

   The journal publishes creative and scholarly articles that provide new insights into the delivery and management of home health and related community services. It is aimed toward service providers and health care specialists involved with health care financing, evaluation of services, organization of services, and public policy issues.

7. *American Journal of Hospice and Palliative Medicine*®, Sage Publications, Inc., 2455 Teller Rd., Thousand Oaks, CA 91320; phone: 805-410-7763; www.sagepub.com/journalsProdDesc .nav?prodId = Journa1201797.

   Provides physicians, nurses, psychologists/psychiatrists, pastoral care professionals, hospice administrators, and related health care professionals with high-quality, practical, and multidisciplinary information on the medical, administrative, and psychosocial aspects of hospice and palliative care.

Web Resources

1. GriefNet: www.griefnet.org.

   GriefNet is a web page that can connect visitors with a variety of resources related to death, dying, bereavement, and major emotional and physical losses. It offers interactive discussion and support groups—all for bereaved persons and those working with the bereaved, both professional and laypersons. The support and discussion groups are accessed by e-mail. Groups include grief-chat, a general discussion list for any topic related to death, dying, bereavement, or other major loss; and grief-widowed, a support group for anyone who has lost a partner or a spouse at any age, at any time, of any sexual orientation. This is a great site. Be sure to stop by for a visit.

2. National Hospice and Palliative Care Organization: www.nhpco.org/templates/1/homepage.cfm.

   The National Hospice and Palliative Care Organization site offers a wide range of links, including How to Find a Hospice, Basics of Hospice, Discussion Groups, Publications and Resources, and Specific Diseases. This well-designed site furnishes much useful information.

3. HomeCare On Line: http://www.nahc.org.

   This website of the National Association for Home Care offers information about state associations, consumer information, news updates, and legislative information. Visitors can search the database for information.

4. ElderCare Locator: www.eldercare.gov/Eldercare/Public/Home.asp.

   ElderCare Locator is a free national service of the Administration on Aging. Just one phone call or website visit provides an instant connection to resources that enable older persons to live independently in their communities. Support services for caregivers are also available.

NOTE

1. Additional hours and days of services may be provided subject to review by fiscal intermediaries on a case-by-case basis, on the basis of documentation justifying the need for and reasonableness of such additional care.

18

Respite Services

William, 78 years old, was at the end of his rope when he called the Area Agency on Aging. He had resisted making the call for months, but a close friend urged him to get help. William had watched his wife's memory fade year by year, but he couldn't completely accept that she had Alzheimer's disease. His doctor was advising him that the stress and continuous physical exertion were aggravating his arthritis. The case manager suggested that William consider having a trained respite worker come into his home twice a week. Reluctantly, William agreed. After a month of respite help, he is beginning to appreciate the six hours per week when he can concentrate on other things.

Respite care is temporary, short-term supervisory, personal, and nursing care provided to older adults with physical and/or mental impairments (George, 1987). Programs provide respite services in the older person's home or at a specific site in the community (e.g., adult day services, nursing home, or hospital). Although older adults are the recipients of care, these dual-purpose programs also provide temporary periods of relief or rest for caregivers. Like William, the primary caregiver tends to be a spouse who has assumed the role of caregiver because of the failing physical or mental health of his or her partner. The role of spousal caregiver often comes at a time in the couple's lives when they may be experiencing health problems or the reduction of functional capacities associated with aging. When a spouse is not available or is unable to provide care, adult children assume the caregiving responsibilities for their aging parents. It is usually a daughter or daughter-in-law who takes on the major responsibility. These women often face the competing demands of caring for an aging parent, managing a household, parenting their own children, and working outside the home (Center on an Aging Society, 2005a; International Longevity Center-Schmieding Center Health and Education Task Force, 2006; MetLife Mature Market Institute, 2006b; National Alliance for Caregiving/AARP, 2004).

Although family caregivers experience a sense of pride and emotional gratification when they perceive themselves as successfully fulfilling their caregiving responsibilities (Rapp & Chao, 2000; Roff et al., 2004), the demands of providing daily care for an older family member are not without physical, psychological, and social liabilities. Caregivers often experience poor physical health and emotional distress. Fulfilling the role of primary caregiver often restricts the use of personal time, interferes with employment responsibilities and obligations, and strains family relationships (Blieszner, Roberto, Wilcox, Barham, & Winston, 2007; Center on an Aging Society, 2005b; Marks, 1998). To help alleviate the burden and stress of caregiving, respite services have become an integral part of the continuum of support services for older adults. They provide relief for caregivers from the constant responsibilities of caring for dependent older adults and allow both the caregivers and care receivers time for independent relationships and activities (Gaugler et al., 2003).

In this chapter, we present information about the types of respite programs available for older adults and their caregivers. The chapter begins with an overview of federal support for respite services, followed by a presentation of the general characteristics of older adults who participate in respite programs and a description of the primary types of respite services. We end the chapter with a discussion of the challenges facing providers of respite services now and in the future.

POLICY BACKGROUND

Some of the first support for respite care for older adults came from the Older Women's League. In the early 1980s, the league sponsored model legislation in several states to encourage the development of statewide respite programs for caregivers of frail older adults. As a result, several states mandated respite care as part of their state-sponsored programs for older adults and their families (e.g., Illinois's Alzheimer's Disease Program, New York State's Expanded In-Home Services for the Elderly Program, California's Alzheimer's Disease Institute; Petty, 1990).

In its 1987 report, *Losing a Million Minds*, the U.S. Congress, Office of Technology Assessment, firmly established the need for respite care, particularly for persons with dementia. Of the top 10 services rated by caregivers of persons with dementia as essential or most important, six related to respite care: (a) a paid companion who can come to the home for a few hours each week to give caregivers a rest, (b) a paid companion for overnight care, (c) personal care for the older person, (d) short-term respite outside the home in nursing homes or hospitals, (e) adult day care, and (f) nursing visits at home. In addition, the OTA report suggested that the provision of respite services postpones the need for nursing home placement.

Despite these findings and other research documenting the need for and effectiveness of respite services, the federal government provides limited financial support for respite services. Because the government defines respite care for the older individual as "personal care," it is not a reimbursable service under Medicare. Medicaid allows for such care through its waiver programs and can cover both in-home respite and adult day services. A 2003 study of state-funded home and community-based care programs reported that 14 states had single-service programs (i.e., provided a single service to older people only) that supported respite care or adult day services programs with funds ranging from $124,557 in Delaware for respite services to $2.2 million in California for that state's Alzheimer's Day Care Resource Center Program (Summer & Ihara, 2004). In addition, 42 states reported multiservice home- and community-based care programs (i.e., primarily targeting older people and providing two or more services) that supported respite care or adult day services.

Some respite programs receive support through OAA funds under Title III-D, which authorizes the support of in-home services, including in-home respite and adult day care.

In addition, the Act provides funds for educational programs that teach caregivers about Alzheimer's disease, how to cope with the disease process, and how to use behavior management techniques. As part of the OAA amendments of 2000, Congress created the National Family Caregiver Support Program (NFCSP), representing the largest new support program under the OAA since 1972. NFCSP funds may be used to support services that provide information about services, assist with access to services, provide individual counseling or organize support groups and caregiver training, provide respite care, and provide supplemental services. States and Area Agencies on Aging have the flexibility to determine the funding allocated to these services. In 2006, $156 million was appropriated in support of caregivers through the NFCSP (Kassner, 2006b).

In December 2006, Congress passed legislation establishing new respite care programs to help families who are taking care of persons with serious illnesses. The Lifespan Respite Care Act (S 1283/HR 3248) provides grants to state agencies, public and private nonprofit groups, and other organizations to make respite care available and accessible to family caregivers, regardless of age, condition, or special need. Individuals with Alzheimer's disease, including those with early onset Alzheimer's, are eligible for services. The Bill directs the Secretary to work in cooperation with the National Family Caregiver Support Program, the Administration on Aging (AoA), and other respite care programs within the Department of Health and Human Services to ensure coordination of respite care services. The Bill also establishes a National Respite Resource Center to maintain a national database on lifespan respite care, provide training and technical assistance, and provide information, referral, and educational programs to the public on lifespan respite care.

Family caregivers who work and must pay for respite services for their care receivers may benefit from federal and state dependent care assistance plans (Coleman, 2000; National Governors' Association, 2004). If employers offer this benefit option, authorized under Section 129 of the Internal Revenue Code, dependent care assistance plans provide reimbursement of up to $5,000 per year for out-of-the-home dependent care expenses. Qualifying individuals include spouses or dependents who are unable to care for themselves, regardless of age, and who regularly spend at least eight hours each day in the employee's household. This time requirement makes such plans less useful for adult children and other individuals with elder care responsibilities because many of these employees do not share a household with the older person whom they are helping (Johnson & Weiner, 2006). In addition to dependent care assistance plans, the dependent care tax credit (DCTC) assists families in meeting the cost of care by allowing taxpayers to offset a portion of their employment-related dependent care expenses against their federal income tax liability. An expense is "employment related" for the purpose of claiming the DCTC if it is a dependent care expense that is necessary to enable the family member to be gainfully employed. The federal dependent care tax credit reduces the amount of income tax the employee owes by a percentage of the expenses the employee has incurred because of dependent care responsibilities. The amount ranges from 20% to 30% of qualified expenses, depending on a taxpayer's adjusted gross income. Individuals eligible to receive care and the types of expenditures allowed are the same as those that apply to the dependent care assistance plan. Thus employees with children are the primary users of federal dependent care tax credits. State tax credit programs build on the federal tax credit, using the federal eligibility rules, and defining the state credit as a percentage of the federal credit. Twenty-six states and the District of Columbia provide tax deductions or tax credits to provide some financial relief to caregivers (National Governors' Association, 2004). Some states offer a deduction for expenses, usually up to $2,400, but most offer tax credits of $500 to $1,000. Unlike deductions, tax credits generally benefit lower income taxpayers and are often viewed as a more equitable way of providing tax incentives to family caregivers.

USERS AND PROGRAMS

Respite programs typically provide care for older adults with a wide range of physical and mental disabilities. Some programs, however, provide services for specific subgroups of older adults such as persons with Alzheimer's disease (Cox, 1997; Lawton, Brody, & Saperstein, 1991) or developmental disabilities (Factor, 1993). The small number of reports that include data on client and family characteristics makes it difficult to develop an accurate profile of respite care users. Thus we begin this section by providing a general profile of older adults who use respite services. We then focus our attention on the three most common types of respite programs: in-home respite care, adult day care, and institutional respite care. Where data are available, we provide information about the older adults and caregivers using each type of respite care.

Characteristics of Older Adults Using Respite Services

Drawing on the limited research literature, Montgomery (1992) profiled older adults participating in respite programs. Typically, these elders are around 80 years of age. Male participants tend to be younger than their female counterparts. They also are overrepresented in the client population in comparison with the gender distribution of this age group in the general population—about 40% of the clients are male and 60% are female. More than 85% of the older adults live with their caregivers, who are either spouses or adult children. Most older respite users have multiple impairments that limit their ability to perform activities of daily living.

Respite Programs

A variety of agencies, including both for-profit and nonprofit organizations, operate respite programs. Programs differ with respect to their definitions of respite, target populations, eligibility criteria, and the amount and type of respite offered. Costs for respite services vary, depending on the type and level of care provided to the participants. Most programs rely on contributions from their clients, who pay either a preset amount or contribute on a sliding scale according to their financial resources.

In-Home Respite Care

In-home respite care takes place in the home in which the older person lives. Depending on the needs of the caregiver, in-home respite can occur on a regular or occasional basis and can take place during the day or evening hours. Some programs provide personal and instrumental care for the older person, whereas others provide only companionship or supervisory services (Lawton et al., 1991; Montgomery, Marquis, Schaefer, & Kosloski, 2002). Professionals and nonprofessionals, employed by community-based agencies that offer respite services (e.g., home health agencies, senior support programs, and church-affiliated organizations) typically provide the care. Several communities have developed programs that rely on family members, friends, and trained volunteers to provide in-home respite care (Administration on Aging [AoA], 2004d). For example, Alaska offers a consumer-directed respite program whereby caregivers can hire family members to provide respite for a care recipient as long as they do not live in the same residence. In Minnesota, the Normandale Ministry for Healing and Wholeness program uses a Care Team Model, matching caregivers with a team of two to three trained volunteers who provide in-home respite and other care-related services as needed.

Data from a seven-state study of respite care (Montgomery et al., 2002) that included 1,143 in-home term respite users suggest that the typical older adult using in-home respite care is 80 years old, White (63.8%), female (64.5%), married (49.3%), lives in a rural area (62.3%), has been diagnosed with Alzheimer's disease, and has an average of 4.7 ADL limitations and 13.2 IADL limitations. Caregivers of in-home respite users have a mean age of 63.6 years. Most are female (70.0%), either a spouse (42.1%) or adult child/child-in-law (41.7%), married (71.2%), and either working at least part time (30.6%), or retired (41.2%). They have been providing care for an average of 44.5 months.

For Your Files: Alzheimer's Association

The Alzheimer's Association, the world leader in Alzheimer's research and support, is the first and largest voluntary health organization dedicated to finding prevention methods, treatments, and an eventual cure for Alzheimer's disease. The Association offers a wide range of materials containing information and advice for persons afflicted with Alzheimer's disease, caregivers, and professionals. Its 24/7 Helpline provides reliable information, referrals, and support in 140 languages. Alzheimer's Association chapters are located nationwide; chapter programs are tailored to the communities they serve, so the range and type of programs varies from chapter to ch apter. The national office of the Alzheimer's Association is located at 225 N. Michigan Ave., Fl. 17, Chicago, IL 60601–7633; phone: 800-272-3900; www.alz.org.

Older adults who receive in-home care typically exhibit more frequent social and behavioral problems than do participants in other types of respite programs (Cox, 1997; Gaugler et al., 2003). Their caregivers report a higher degree of burden and provide more intense care compared with caregivers using other types of respite. Caregivers using in-home respite services also spend fewer hours per day away from their care receivers than those using adult day services (Berry, Zarit, & Rabatin, 1991). These caregivers, however, spend less time on caregiving activities on days on which they use in-home services compared with caregivers using adult day programs, perhaps because of the amount of time consumed preparing the older adult for the out-of-home program.

An alternative type of in-home respite is called Video RespiteTM (Lund, Hill, Caserta, & Wright, 1995). This series of 20 to 50 minute video tapes was designed to capture and maintain the attention of persons with dementia. While the person with dementia watches and participates with the visitor on television, caregivers have opportunities for respite breaks in their own homes.

In-home respite is the type of respite most acceptable to family caregivers (Conlin, Caranasos, & Davidson, 1992; Lawton et al., 1991). It typically is more flexible than other forms of respite because it most easily accommodates to the specific day and time that the caregiver wants. Caregivers also view in-home respite as more acceptable than other types of programs because they do not have to take the older adult out of the environment in which he or she is most comfortable. But in-home respite has its limitations because in-home respite services can be expensive, particularly if frequently used for several hours per day. Families also may be reluctant to use in-home respite services because they do not like having strangers in their homes or taking care of their loved ones (Miller & Goldman, 1989).

Adult Day Care

The National Adult Day Services Association (NADSA, 2006) defines adult day care as a community-based group program designed to meet the needs of adults with functional impairments through an individual care plan. It is a structured, comprehensive program that provides a variety of health, social, and related support services in a protective setting during any part of a day but less than 24-hour care.

Since 1974, the number of adult day care centers operating nationwide has grown from 18 (Weissert, 1977) to more than 3,500 (NADSA, 2006). The adult day care industry promotes two models of care, the medical model and the social model. Adult Day Services (ADS) programs typically follow a social model, focusing on the socialization needs of the participants through the provision of individual and group activities, meals, and health maintenance programs. In addition to meeting the socialization and support needs of participants, Adult Day Health Care (ADHC) programs offer intensive health and therapeutic services prescribed in individual plans for each participant (Lucas, Scotto, Andrew, & Howell-White, 2002). It is difficult to identify any given center as falling into either category, however, because all centers provide varying degrees of social programs and health services. A national survey of 3,407 adult day centers conducted in 2001–2002 found that 21% of centers are based on the medical model of care, 37% are based on the social model of care, and 42% are a combination of the two (Wake Forest University School of Medicine, 2002). Although there are some special-purpose centers (e.g., for Alzheimer's family care and rehabilitation), distinctions between centers tend to be based on the intensity of services and activities provided rather than on the philosophical orientation of the centers. Whatever a program's primary emphasis, NADSA (2006) recommends that all adult day care programs provide eight essential services: personal care, nursing services, social services, therapeutic activities, nutrition and therapeutic diets, transportation, emergency care for participants, and family education.

Approximately three-fourths of all adult day care centers are in urban settings (Wake Forest University School of Medicine, 2002). Although some adult day centers are freestanding agencies, 74% are affiliated with larger organizations, such as churches, senior centers, nursing homes, medical centers, or the Veterans Administration (NADSA, 2006). Most centers are not-for-profit or public agencies (78%); 22% are private for-profit agencies. Regardless of the hosting agency, most centers are small, averaging 20 participants per day. Typical staff members for adult day centers include an administrator (or executive director), a program director, and one or more of the following: program assistants/aides, recreation or activity aides, nurse and nurse aides, therapist, social workers, custodial workers, van drivers, administrative personnel, and office staff (O'Keeffe & Siebenaler, 2006). Volunteers, including students, also play an essential role in the staffing of many adult day care programs. The average daily fee for adult day care is $56, but this can vary depending upon the services provided. Funding comes from participant fees, third-party payers as well as public and charitable sources.

According to NADSA (2006), the average age of the typical day care participant is 72; the majority of participants are White and approximately 66% are women. Some 75% of participants live with a spouse, adult children, or other family and friends. More than one-half of the day care participants suffer cognitive limitations, and about 40% are functionally dependent (Wake Forest University School of Medicine, 2002; see Exhibit 18.1). Caregivers of adult day service users have a mean age of 58.7 years (Montgomery et al., 2002). The majority of these caregivers are female (73.0%), an adult child/child-in-law (52.5%), married (66.4%), and working at least part time (44.2%). They have been providing care for an average of 39.1 months.

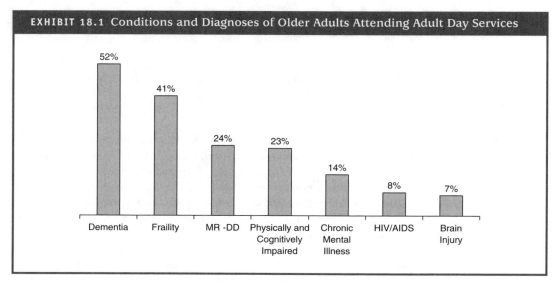

EXHIBIT 18.1 Conditions and Diagnoses of Older Adults Attending Adult Day Services

Source: Wake Forest University School of Medicine (2002).

Best Practice: Parker Jewish Institute for Health Care and Rehabilitation

The Parker Jewish Institute for Health Care and Rehabilitation in New Hyde Park, New York, offers short-term rehabilitation/sub-acute care, long-term care/skilled nursing, adult day health care, Alzheimer's day care, home health care, and hospice care. The extensive network of inpatient and outpatient/community health care and rehabilitation services for older adults serves more than 7,000 patients each year. Parker has been successful due to flexible hours, a drop-in service, and a six-day-a-week operation. With the center open from 7:00 a.m. to 7:00 p.m. Monday through Friday, and on Saturdays and holidays from 9:00 a.m. to 5:00 p.m., families have greater flexibility in arranging their schedules.

Another customer-driven service that has been popular with caregivers is an à la carte approach to purchasing services. Instead of one daily or hourly rate, caregivers may purchase meals, shaves, bathing, transportation, and other special services separately. This type of customer choice is unique in the adult day care business. Parker works closely with the New York and Long Island chapters of the Alzheimer's Association and the Long Island Alzheimer's Foundation to provide training programs, support groups, and other professional skills.

According to a 2006 survey of Parker's caregivers, 93.0% believed the program benefited the quality of life of loved ones. They indicated the program provided participants with opportunities to socialize with peers and pursue previous leisure activities. In addition, 40% of the caregivers believed the program had delayed the need for nursing home care. Approximately 88% of the caregivers reported that they also personally benefited from the program. Having their loved one attend the Institute gave them time to socialize with friends, complete tasks or run errands, and an opportunity to rest.

The center also provides fieldwork for students in gerontology and recreation therapy. For more information, contact Parker Jewish Institute, 271–11 76th Avenue, New Hyde Park, NY 11040; phone: 718-289-2105; www.parkerinstitute.org.

An advantage of day care over in-home respite care for the care receiver is that it provides important peer group support and greater opportunities for social interaction. For the caregiver, adult day care offers freedom from caregiving responsibilities for potentially long, continuous blocks of time at a lesser cost than in-home services (Lawton et al., 1991). A disadvantage of using adult day care is the physical and emotional effort required to prepare care receivers to attend a day program. For example, transportation to and from the center is a major issue that caregivers and programs must resolve (Wake Forest University School of Medicine, 2002). Caregivers often view getting the care receiver ready to leave home as more time-consuming and exhausting than providing the usual care. In addition, many caregivers and their care receivers have an adverse emotional reaction to the term "day care," which they perceive is a program for children, not an appropriate setting for older adults (Bane, 1992).

Institutional Respite Care

Institutional settings such as nursing homes, Veterans Administration hospital-based nursing homes, and hospitals provide temporary respite services (TIR). In most situations, caregivers pay out of pocket for institutional respite care. This type of respite care differs from in-home and day programs in that it provides overnight and/or extended services. Beds may be available for both emergency respite care (e.g., illness of a caregiver) and planned respite stays, such as when a caregiver plans an extended vacation or a short weekend of relaxation (Adler, Kuskowksi, & Mortimer, 1995; Lawton et al., 1991). They also may use this type of respite service on a trial basis before permanent nursing home placement (Larkin & Hopcroft, 1993; Miller & Goldman, 1989; Scharlach & Frenzel, 1986).

A comparative study of 1,911 temporary institutional respite users and nonusers (Gräsell, 1997) revealed that more TIR users were likely to be females (75.8%) and had more ADL limitations (M = 6.0) than nonusers (65.6%, M = 5.5, respectively). Both TIR users and nonusers were approximately 80 years of age and had had a diagnosis of Alzheimer's disease for five years. The caregivers of TIR users compared to nonusers were more likely to be female (90.9% vs. 83.3%) and to have significantly higher levels of subjective burden (44.5 vs. 41.0). No differences were found between caregivers of TIR users and nonusers with respect to average age (56.4 vs. 58.1), employment status (21.4% vs. 27.0%), average number of hours per day they provided care (6.0 vs. 6.0), and the average length of time they had provided care (4.0 vs. 3.0).

Institutional respite programs have their advantages and disadvantages with respect to cost, caregivers' perceptions of care and the facility's ability to provide care, and the additional burden of preparation required of the caregiver (Gonyea, 1988; Harper, McDowell, Turner, & Sharma, 1988; Lawton et al., 1991; Rosenheimer & Francis, 1992). Although institutional programs offer respite care at the cost of comparable amounts of in-home respite, caregivers still view it as a costly care alternative. Nursing homes and hospitals usually provide a supervised, professional setting equipped to handle emergencies, which seems to alleviate family anxiety about care. Caregivers, however, often try so hard to avoid nursing home placements that even a temporary placement evokes fear and guilt about future placement possibilities. In addition, although institutions typically can accept older individuals with a range of behavioral problems and functional disabilities, caregivers often fear that their elders will not receive proper, individual attention and care. The preparation required for a nursing home or hospital stay (e.g., filling out forms, preparing personal effects, explaining the situation to the care receiver, and transportation to and from the facility) and limitations on the number of days a person can stay in the program also discourage some caregivers from using this type of respite care.

Best Practice: Social Day Care and Respite Program

The Georgia Mobile Day Care Program provides social day care and respite services in rural Georgia. Program staff travel up to 50 miles one way each day to a program site—generally a senior center in the community. Program staffing varies but typically includes a registered nurse supervising the program, an activity director, an aide, and community volunteers. With a staff-to-client ratio of one to four, most sites maintain a capacity of up to eight clients per site. On a typical day, clients participate in exercises, cognitive activities, movies, crafts, and reminiscing. Lunch and snacks are provided at each site. One-on-one time is set aside at the start and end of each day to allow caregivers and the staff to discuss concerns regarding the client. Caregivers indicated that the program provides them with relief and peace of mind. For more information, contact the Georgia Division of Aging Services, Two Peachtree Street N.W., Suite 9.398, Atlanta GA 30303–3142; phone: (404) 657-5336; www.aging.dhr.georgia.gov.

CHALLENGES FOR RESPITE PROGRAMS

Respite programs play an important role in maintaining and enhancing the psychological and physical wellbeing of older adults and their caregivers. We discuss a number of policy and programmatic challenges that must be addressed in the future.

Increasing the Use of Respite Services

Researchers report that, as a result of using respite services, caregivers enhance their wellbeing (Gaugler et al., 2003; Zarit, Stephens, Townsend, et al., 1998), reduce their feelings of burden and stress (Conlin et al., 1992; Kosloski & Montgomery, 1993), and delay placing their loved one in a nursing home (Kosloski & Montgomery, 1995; Lawton et al., 1991). In addition, most caregivers who use respite services report being highly satisfied with the program and the care their family member receives (Buelow & Conrad, 1992; Henry & Capitman, 1995; Jarrott, Zarit, Stephens, Townsend & Greene, 1999). Yet, despite the potential for positive outcomes, and the growing availability of respite programs throughout the United States, caregivers are still reluctant to use any type of respite service (Cox, 1997; Kosloski, Montgomery, & Youngbauer, 2001). When caregivers do seek respite services, it is often at a time of crisis; their family situation escalates to a point at which they cannot continue providing care without some assistance. Even then, caregivers use respite services only in modest amounts.

To increase program use by family caregivers, providers must address both family-related and system-related variables. Family-related variables include caregivers' lack of awareness, apprehension, and attitudes about using respite services and the reactions of care receivers (Schmall & Webb, 1994). Many caregiving families have little or no contact with formal services, and thus are often unaware of the availability of respite care in their communities. Even when caregivers are aware of such services, their fierce independence and personal beliefs about caregiving may hinder their use. It is not uncommon to hear caregivers say such things as, "She's my mother, I am responsible for her care," or "No one can care for my wife better than I can." Just like William, whom we introduced at the beginning of the chapter, caregivers often feel guilty about leaving their care receivers and believe that using formal services is a sign of failure. They may be even more reluctant to use respite services if they see it as benefiting themselves rather than their care receivers.

In addition, some care receivers respond negatively to and resist respite care, thus reinforcing feelings of guilt often harbored by many caregivers. Karner and Hall (2002) note the importance of describing and emphasizing to caregivers—particularly those from minority and rural communities where family values and traditions are strong influences on service utilization—that community care programs are designed to complement and supplement, not replace, family care.

System barriers related to the use of respite care services include lack of service availability when wanted or needed most and lack of control over who provides services (MaloneBeach, Zarit, & Shore, 1992; Townsend & Kosloski, 2002). For in-home respite users, having different workers every time they request help is a deterrent to the use of such services. Caregivers generally want to have more control over which respite care workers provide care for their loved ones. The limited availability (e.g., only weekdays) and time schedules (e.g., 8:00 a.m. to 5:00 p.m.) of many respite programs prohibit their use by some caregivers, particularly those who are working outside the home. Transportation is another major barrier to the use of respite services, particularly for adult day care. Many family caregivers find it difficult to get their care receivers to a center, and many centers have limited means of providing transportation for their participants. Finally, the lack of reimbursement from Medicare and most private insurance carriers for respite care also is a significant barrier for many families who may otherwise wish to use this service.

Expanding Community Awareness and Education

The limited use experienced by some respite programs suggests the need for agencies and organizations to continually inform and educate people about their services. Caregivers are often unaware that respite services exist and do not understand the concept. They often see respite programs as a "last resort" or "end of the road" solution, rather than a preventive service. Respite services will be more effective in alleviating the stress and strains of caregiving if providers can get caregivers to enroll in their programs earlier in their caregiving career. Strategies for increasing program awareness and use include identifying key members within the community who can work as liaisons for the programs, actively recruiting families through personal contacts with programs already serving majority and minority families, and having bilingual and culturally competent staff members delivering the programs (Gallagher-Thompson et al., 2000).

Providing Flexible and Alternate Formats

Greater flexibility and expanded hours and days are needed for all types of respite programs. Successful programs will adapt to the time needs of caregivers, particularly those who work outside the home. In recent years, the idea of the adult day center as the hub for an all-inclusive system of respite (e.g., weekend programs and overnight services) has emerged. Support for more inclusive programming has received strong endorsement, as evidenced by programs such as the Robert Wood Johnson Foundation's Dementia/Respite Services Program (1988–1992) and Partners in Caregiving Program (1993–1995). Advocates for providers of these programs assert the effectiveness and efficiency of delivering more comprehensive day programs ("The Extra Mile," 1996).

The idea of intergenerational day care centers deserves further consideration (Steinig & Simon, 2005). For example, TLC Health Network in New York has operated an intergenerational child and adult day care program for employees and members of the surrounding community at its Lake Shore campus since 1990. Virginia Polytechnic Institute and State University's *Neighbors Growing Together* program is the oldest university-based shared site intergenerational program in the United States (www.intergenerational.clahs.vt.edu/neighbors). The program, co-located since 1994, consists of the Adult Day Services (ADS) and Child Development Center for Learning and Research (CDCLR). Affiliated ADS and CDCLR faculty and staff have worked to craft an intergenerational community that takes a strengths-based approach to supporting the wellbeing of its members (participants, families, staff, and students) through positive intergenerational contact (Jarrott, Gigliotti, & Smock, 2006). Although there are several intuitively positive sociocultural, organizational, and delivery aspects of providing care across generations, researchers need to evaluate the outcomes for both the children and older adults (Jarrott, 2005).

Reaching Underserved Populations

A frequent criticism of respite services is the lack of programs targeted to minority families. Cultural and attitudinal influences and preferences of agency careworkers determining eligibility for respite services can significantly sway the prescription of respite services (Chumbler, Dobbs-Kepper, Beverly, & Beck, 2000; Degenholtz, Kane, & Kivnick, 1997). Senior programs must be marketed to all groups of individuals. They must employ professionals and volunteers who speak languages other than English and have knowledge of and experience working with individuals from diverse backgrounds.

Providing respite services in rural areas can be especially challenging. Traveling distance for in-home respite providers and transportation for participants to attend out-of-home programs can prohibit the use of services in sparsely populated areas. Programs must consider nontraditional means of program delivery and develop public–private linkages to help expand services.

Enhancing the Quality of Care

Few systematic studies reported in the literature evaluate the outcomes of respite services. We have derived most of what we know about effectiveness of respite services from anecdotal or descriptive reports of small programs. In addition, few studies provide a comparison of respite users with nonusers, or include baseline measures of caregivers' and care receivers' physical and emotional status before using respite care. Researchers need to consider these limitations and work with respite service providers in the development of more rigorous program evaluations (Kennet, Burgio, & Schulz, 2000; Sörenson, Pinquart, & Duberstein, 2002).

Supporting the Future of Respite Programs

The 2005 White House Conference on Aging gave specific support for caregivers by passing resolutions to promote innovative models of non-institutional long-term care and develop a national strategy for supporting informal caregivers of seniors to enable adequate quality and supply of services. As with home care services discussed in the previous chapter, there will be an increased demand for respite services in the next 20 years. Sheer numbers of older adults, especially those over 85 years of age, will force the public and private sector to respond to the respite needs of older adults and their families.

Respite for a Devoted Caregiver

Ben and Ethel have been married for 60 years. Both are 85 years old. They reside in a small apartment that is about the size of an average high school classroom. They partially subsidize their rent through a Section 8 rental voucher program. Ben was a tenant farmer all his adult life. Ethel worked in the home. Both worked hard, but Ben's income was low, and he and Ethel were not able to accumulate any savings. Their only income is Ben's Social Security check of $475 per month. They can barely make ends meet.

Ben has some hearing loss and suffers from gout, which interferes with his mobility. Ethel is bedridden with Parkinson's disease. She is totally incontinent, and someone must turn her three times per day to keep her from getting bedsores. Ethel communicates only by using eye signals and is on a liquid diet. Her condition warrants full-time, skilled nursing care. Ben's devotion to his wife of 60 years prohibits him from placing her in a nursing home. One of his few happy moments is when he is showing off their wedding picture.

Ben and Ethel have one daughter who is employed full time. Their daughter does help her father prepare meals when she has time. The daughter is concerned about the tremendous caregiving load her father has assumed. Ben used to frequent the local senior center a couple days per week to play pool with "the guys." Occasionally, he would take a day trip on the senior center van. The daughter would like her father to "give in" and place Ethel in a nursing home so that he can have some time to himself. Her father simply will not consider it.

Case Study Questions

1. On the basis of the information provided, what barriers are presented that would make it difficult to work with Ben to develop a respite care plan?

2. Despite the barriers that you have identified in the first question, what aspects of this situation lend itself to convincing Ben that respite care is an option for him to consider?

3. Given the financial situation of this couple, what type of respite options would you be looking for in this community?

4. Short of skilled nursing home care, what other community-based services might be appropriate for this couple to improve their quality of life?

5. Do you think the daughter should use legal means to force her father to place her mother in a nursing home? Why or why not?

Learning Activities

1. Interview a director or staff member of a respite program. What services does the program provide and to whom? What is the cost of the services? What does the individual perceive to be the primary obstacles for caregivers in requesting or receiving respite services? What changes would the staff member like to make to the legislative policy as it relates to respite care and to the program?

2. Interview someone who has received or is receiving respite services. How did the caregiver find out about the service? Why did the caregiver decide to use it? What does the caregiver see as the benefits to the service as well as what type of changes would be desirable? How has respite care affected the person's life? How has it affected the life of the care receiver?

3. Design a respite program that encompasses what you believe is necessary for an effective program. Include to whom the program would be directed and how you would fund it.

For More Information

National Resources

1. Alzheimer's Disease and Education and Referral Center (ADEAR), P.O. Box 8250, Silver Spring, MD 20907–8250; phone: 800-438-4380; www.nia.nih.gov/Alzheimers.
   This center, a service of the National Institute on Aging, offers information about diagnosis and treatment, research, and services available to patients and their families.

2. American Health Assistance Foundation, 22512 Gateway Center Drive, Clarksburg, Maryland 20871; phone: 301-948-3244 or 800-437-2423; www.ahaf.org.
   The American Health Assistance Foundation's Alzheimer's Family Relief Program was created to help ease the often-unbearable financial burdens faced by Alzheimer's patients and their families. Since 1988, the program has given more than $2.3 million in emergency financial assistance to families in need.

3. National Adult Day Services Association, Inc., 2519 Connecticut Ave, N.W., Washington, DC 20008; phone: 800-558-5301; www.nadsa.org.
   The National Adult Day Services Association (NADSA) is the leading voice of the rapidly growing adult day services industry in the United States. NADSA is an independent national organization dedicated to raising public and government awareness of the value of adult day services. Adult day services provide community-based care for frail elders as well as persons of all ages with multiple and special needs associated with conditions such as Alzheimer's disease, developmental disabilities, traumatic brain injury, mental illness, HIV/AIDS, vision and hearing impairments, and more.

Web Resources

1. At least two adult day care programs are affiliated with universities. The Virginia Tech Adult Day Services is in Blacksburg, Virginia: www.humandevelopment.vt.edu/ads.html. The Eldercare Center, University of Missouri at Columbia, is located within the School of Health Related Professions: www.umshp.org/eldecare.

2. Administration on Aging, Family Caregiver Options: www.aoa.gov/eldfam/For_Caregivers/For_Caregivers.asp.

This is a great place to start when looking for information about respite and caregiver support services. The Family Caregiver Options page is continually updated with links to national resources. Definitely worth a visit.

3. *Caregiver's Handbook*: www.acsu.buffalo.edu/ ~ drstall/hndbk0.html.

   This site contains a complete version of a handbook for caregivers originally published by the San Diego County Mental Health Services. In addition to 47 chapters that cover every aspect of caregiving, there is also a guide for choosing a residential facility.

4. Caregiver Network, Inc: www.caregiver.on.ca.

   The Caregiver Network is a site maintained by Canadian Karen Henderson, who dedicates her work to her mother. There are numerous links to information about financial and legal issues, social issues, care for the caregiver, day care programs, and other resources of interest to anyone who is a caregiver.

5. Eldercare WEB: www.elderweb.com/home/

   This site is similar to the Caregiver Network but is based in the United States. We think this is one of the first sites on caregiving to be established. It has lots of great information of value to caregivers and older adults. There are links to a library, a forum, and information about health (nutrition was the highlight topic when we visited last), aging, legal, and social issues.

6. Family Caregiver Alliance: www.caregiver.org/caregiver/jsp/home.jsp.

   The Family Caregiver Alliance, a nonprofit organization with caregiver centers throughout California, provides assistance to caregivers of individuals with Alzheimer's, Parkinson's, and other brain disorders. The home page has links to resource centers, information about work and family, a newsletter published by the alliance, publications and fact sheets, and information on events.

7. The Administration on Aging: Caregiver Information: www.aoa.gov/prof/aoaprog/caregiver/caregiver.asp.

   A caregiver information link is available from the Administration on Aging. This website offers a large number of links for caregivers to access various supporting sites, including sites on respite care.

8. CareGuide: www.careguide.com.

   CareGuide is a care management company that works to help people at every stage of the aging process to live comfortable, secure, and independent lives. Its site lists over 170,000 elder care facilities and is endorsed by the American Society on Aging, the Assisted Living Federation of America, and Children of Aging Parents. It also offers information on services available for care recipients and caregivers.

19

Long-Term Care Services

As she approached her mother's room at Prairie View Manor, Sharon thought about the day she had had to come to grips with the reality that Eleanor, then 84 years old, needed nursing home care. She had promised her mother that she would never put her in a nursing home. This promise would nearly break Sharon mentally and physically, jeopardize her marriage, and drive a wedge between her and her children. At first, the extra work cleaning Grandma's house, caring for the yard, and taking her shopping and to the doctor was welcomed. The whole family pitched in to make it work. Eleanor went to the adult day program every day where the family knew she was safe while they were at work and at school. When Eleanor became more frail, her falls more frequent, and the incontinency too difficult to manage, Sharon brought her mother to live with her. Even with a leave of absence from her job, Sharon became exhausted trying to manage her mother's care. Her husband became more and more angry about all the time Sharon was spending caring for her mother, and her children resented having to give up some of their activities to help care for Grandma. Why, thought Sharon, had it taken her so long to seek nursing home care? Eleanor was content. She loved her little room with a view across the countryside. Most happily for Sharon, her mother was still able to participate in limited activities and enjoy the company of a few new friends.

The words "nursing home" conjure up negative images, and most older adults and their families dread the thought of moving to one. Sharon, like many other family members, goes to great lengths to avoid nursing home placement—even when such placement would be physically and psychologically beneficial for everyone. Despite the negative image nursing homes have, they are a critical part of the long-term care continuum in our communities and provide a wide range of vital services to those who live there. Because nursing homes are a part of the long-term care continuum, many refer to nursing homes as long-term care facilities. Indeed, these facilities have evolved into more than "nursing" homes—they are places in which a wide range of restorative, rehabilitative, and medical services are delivered. The term "nursing home," however, is still frequently used in the literature. Therefore, we will use the terms "long-term care facilities" and "nursing homes" interchangeably in our discussion. In this chapter, we review policies that have been instrumental in creating the existence of long-term care facilities and present a profile of users and programs. The chapter ends with a presentation of the many challenges that lie ahead for long-term care facilities.

POLICY BACKGROUND

The growth of the nursing home industry parallels the passage of federal policy that evolved in the first half of the twentieth century (Waldman, 1985). Prior to the enactment of Social Security, Medicare, and Medicaid, many older adults had few options if they needed medical and personal care. In some communities, older adults were boarded out to families which agreed to provide care in their homes; many of these were the homes of retired nurses—thus the basis for the term "nursing home" (Crandall, 1991). In the early part of the century, almshouses or "poor farms" cared for many frail older adults, persons with mental illnesses, and those who were chronically ill. An estimated 60–90% of the persons living in almshouses were over the age of 65 (Fischer, 1978). Almshouses were deplorable places, and the few states that had old age assistance payments and, later, Social Security would not send payments to almshouse residents (Small, 1988). Older adults who were financially well off had the option of living in old age homes run by ethnic or religious groups: German and Scandinavian immigrants built Lutheran Homes, and Jews and Methodists built their own facilities (Waldman, 1985). The 1950 amendments to the Social Security Act of 1935, allowing residents of institutions to receive benefits and health providers to directly receive payments for services, helped expand the creation of nursing homes. But the real impetus to the creation of the nursing home industry came with the enactment of Medicare and Medicaid. Both Medicare and Medicaid provide payments to nursing homes—Medicare for acute care and Medicaid for long-term care for those with low incomes (Crandall, 1991; Small, 1988). Since the enactment of Medicare and Medicaid, the percentage of adults aged 65 and older living in nursing homes doubled from 2.5% in 1963 to 5.1% in 1990 and 4.5% in 2000 (Small, 1988; Hetzel & Smith, 2001; Hooyman & Kiyak, 2002). In 2003, there were 16,323 nursing facilities in the country (National Center for Health Statistics, 2005).

PAYMENT FOR NURSING HOME CARE

The cost of nursing home care in 2005 was $64,240 per year for a semi-private room and $74,095 a year for a private room (MetLife, 2005b). Thus, because of the high cost of nursing home care, many older adults and their families are concerned about having the resources to pay for care or are concerned about becoming impoverished while paying for care. Currently, there are four sources of payment of nursing home costs: Medicaid, Medicare, out of pocket, and long-term care insurance.

Most nursing homes are certified by the Centers for Medicare and Medicaid Services (formally known as Health Care Financing Administration, or HCFA) and are eligible to receive reimbursement for their services to persons qualified for Medicaid and Medicare. Annually, Medicaid pays approximately 39%, or $53.1 billion, of nursing home care for eligible individuals (Congressional Budget Office (CBO), 2004; Centers for Medicare and Medicaid Services, 2004). Medicaid offers nursing home coverage to low-income individuals who meet income, asset, and medical guidelines. Medicare plays a limited role in covering nursing home costs because it pays only for *skilled nursing* services that are needed following a hospitalization (24-hour care provided by a registered nurse, under a physician's supervision) and does not cover custodial care. Medicare pays 17% of nursing home costs (CBO, 2004).

Out-of-pocket payments made by older adults and their families amount to approximately 41% of nursing home care expenses (CBO, 2004). Because of the limited sources that help pay for long-term nursing home care costs, a small but growing number of adults have purchased long-term care insurance policies. Long-term care insurance policy sales have risen an average of 18% a year from 1987 to 2002, and over 9 million policies have been sold since the inception of the market to the end of 2002 (America's Health Insurance Plans, 2004b). Private insurance pays approximately 3% of nursing home costs (CBO, 2004). Older adults have been slow to purchase such policies because of the availability, the cost, the limited benefits, and a belief that Medicare or Medicaid will cover long-term care costs. The extent to which long-term care insurance will play a role in paying for long-term care costs in the future is unknown (see Zedlewski, Barnes, Burt, McBride, & Meyer, 1990; Johnson & Uccello, 2005).

USERS AND PROGRAMS

Resident Characteristics

The decision to place an older adult in a nursing home is a difficult one for family and friends. Contrary to popular perception, families do not "dump" their older members in nursing homes at the first available opportunity. Like Sharon at the beginning of the chapter, they go to great lengths exploring other alternatives and often insist on providing caregiving activities at the expense of their personal wellbeing (Brody, 1985; Smallegan, 1985). Families provide an estimated 80–90% of long-term care to older adults while they are living in the community and continue providing assistance even after nursing home placement (Bowers, 1988; Stone et al., 1987). Nursing home placement is a community resource that is most often the last alternative used by families.

Because of increased longevity and the increase in the number of baby boomers entering later life, the nursing home population is projected to increase considerably over the next 20 years (Sahyoun, Pratt, Lentzner, Dey, & Robinson, 2001; Spillman & Lubitz, 2002). Spillman and Lubitz (2002) estimate that 44% of those turning 65 in the year 2000 will use nursing home care at some point in their lifetimes. Moreover, the number of 65-year-olds who will use nursing home care in their lifetimes will more than double in the next 20 years, and 37% of men turning 65 in 2000 and 50% of women turning 65 in 2000 are projected to receive nursing home care. The increase in the percentage of oldest-old adults in nursing homes, however, is less than the increase in the size of the oldest-old population, suggesting that the rate of institutionalization of oldest-old persons might not increase as rapidly as the oldest-old population itself. For example, the decline in the percentage of older adults living in nursing homes from 5.1% in 1990 to 4.5% in 2000 is attributed in part to the drop in the percentage of those aged 85 and older residing in a nursing home from 24.5% in 1990 to 18.2% in 2000 (Hetzel & Smith, 2001).

For Your Files: **Long-Term Care Insurance**

The America's Health Insurance Plans (AHIP) is an organization representing companies that provide health insurance. AHIP has posted on its website a consumers' guide to long-term care insurance. Here is a summary of some key points. Visit their site (www.ahip.org) to read the entire guide. Most long-term care insurance policies are indemnity policies that pay a fixed amount for each day of care received, once the individual reaches specified disability levels. Fixed amounts range from $50 to $500 per day, depending on the terms of the policy. Good policies will adjust the benefit amount each year (about 5%) to keep up with inflation. The cost of long-term care insurance depends on the age of the beneficiary and the level of benefits and deductibles. For example, a policy offering $150 per day for four years, with a 90-day waiting period, costs a 40-year-old approximately $422 per year, a 50-year-old about $564 per year, a 65-year-old $1,337, and a 70-year-old $5,330. Therefore, the younger the age at purchase, the lower the cost.

Most policies cover skilled, intermediate, and custodial care as well as skilled and non-skilled home care, physical therapy, and care provided by homemaker home health aides. Some policies also cover adult day care and respite care. There are, however, exclusions for pre-existing conditions and some types of disorders. Policies generally limit benefits to a maximum dollar amount or days of care and some pay benefits for a limited number of years. In February 2006, Congress passed legislation giving states the permission to coordinate the purchase and payment of long-term care insurance with Medicaid. The law permits Medicaid to cover long-term care needs beyond the terms of the policy and policy holders would not be required to "spend down" their assets to meet the Medicaid eligibility guidelines (Capretta, 2007).

Those interested in purchasing long-term care insurance should compare policies before they buy. Also check out Consumer Reports, which conducted in-depth reviews of long-term care insurance policies in 1988, 1991, and 1995. The American Association of Retired Persons also has resource materials available.

The length of stay in a nursing home has varied little over the past 20 years, as approximately 30% of residents stay three or more years and 30% stay one year to less than three years (Decker, 2005). However, length of stay does vary among different subpopulations. For example, length of stay for persons aged 65 years of age and older is longer for women than for men—30 months and 25 months, respectively (Gabrel, 2000a). The most common reasons for discharge from a nursing home are admission to a hospital, death, and stabilized health status. Researchers have discovered several personal characteristics associated with the likelihood of living in a nursing home.

Age

Not surprisingly, the majority of nursing home residents are over age 75. In 2005, 34.8% of nursing home residents were between the ages of 75 and 84, 31.7% were between the ages of 85 and 94, and 5.2% were aged 95 or older (Centers for Medicare and Medicaid Services, 2006).

Sex

Mirroring the demographic characteristics of the older adult population, more nursing home residents are women. In 2005, approximately two-thirds of residents were women; 41% of persons living in nursing homes were women over 85 (Gabrel, 2000a; Centers for Medicare and Medicaid Services, 2006). As shown in Exhibit 19.1, there are more long-term care residents who are women than are men at every age category over the age of 65 (National Center for Health Statistics, 2006).

Race

Older adults who are non-White are underrepresented in nursing homes. As shown in Exhibit 19.2, smaller percentages of Blacks, Hispanics, Asian American, and American

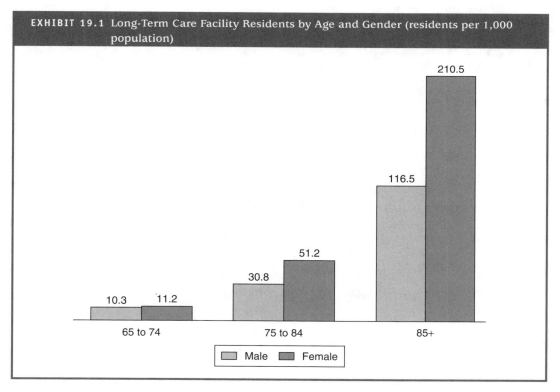

EXHIBIT 19.1 Long-Term Care Facility Residents by Age and Gender (residents per 1,000 population)

Source: National Center for Health Statistics (2005).

Indians aged 65 and older live in nursing homes compared with White elders. The differential use in nursing home care has been attributed to cost, discrimination, personal choice, and social and cultural differences (Moss & Halamandaris, 1977, cited in Yeo, 1993). From testimony given by family members and professionals, Moss and Halamandaris (1977) conclude that all four reasons may be operating to different degrees in keeping older adults of color from receiving nursing home care. For example, among Pacific Asian elders, language differences and cultural differences were the most predominant explanations; among older Blacks, cost and discrimination were the most important factors; Native American elders cited cost and personal choice as the most important; and older Hispanic adults identified more barriers to use than other groups—language and cultural differences, discrimination, and cost.

Marital Status and the Availability of a Caregiver

Widowed older adults represent the majority of those who live in nursing homes, followed by those who have never married. Not surprisingly, the lack of an available caregiver, such as a spouse, adult child, or other relative, increases the likelihood of nursing home placement (Wingard, Jones, & Kaplan, 1987).

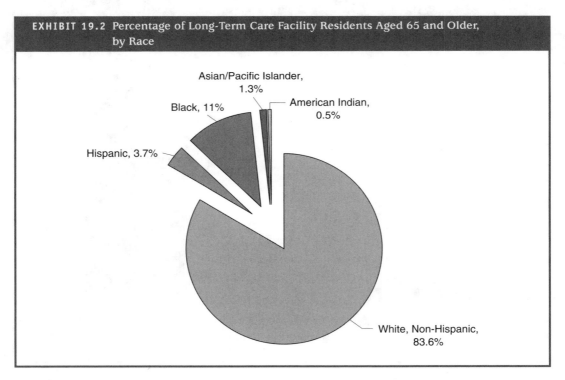

EXHIBIT 19.2 Percentage of Long-Term Care Facility Residents Aged 65 and Older, by Race

Asian/Pacific Islander, 1.3%

American Indian, 0.5%

Black, 11%

Hispanic, 3.7%

White, Non-Hispanic, 83.6%

Source: Centers on Medicare and Medicaid (2006).

Functional Status

A majority of residents of nursing homes have multiple impairments in activities of daily living (ADLs) for which they need assistance. Exhibit 19.3 shows the percentage of nursing home residents who have ADL and cognitive impairments. Forty-two percent of residents have impairments in four or more ADLs, and almost one-quarter are reported to have a moderate level of cognitive impairment. Exhibit 19.4 presents the percentage of residents who have difficulty with their mobility, continence, eating, and those who have difficulty with all three activities. Mobility is the most problematic activity for all residents regardless of age. The percentage of residents needing assistance with ADLs increases with age. Those aged 85 + are more likely than younger residents to need assistance with mobility, continence, and eating, and with all three activities combined. Thus the majority of nursing home residents are quite old and in need of personal care assistance in a number of ADLs.

LONG-TERM CARE FACILITIES

Nursing home care is provided predominantly by for-profit enterprises. Some 56% are affiliated with a nursing home chain (Gabrel, 2000b). Nonprofit nursing homes have an average of 101 beds, and for-profit homes average 87 beds; occupancy rates are, on average, around 95% (Sirrocco, 1988). The American Association of Homes and Services for the Aging (1988) reported that 2,108 of the more than 4,000 member agencies are associated with ethnic or denominational organizations. Such homes are sponsored by religious organizations, including those that are Baptist, Catholic, Mennonite, Jewish, and United Church of Christ. Others are under national sponsorships, such as the British American Home; a few are racially specific, such as the Eliza Bryant Center in Cleveland, which serves only older Blacks (Kaplan & Shore, 1993).

Levels of Care

Prior to federal legislation passed in 1987, nursing homes had two levels of care on which reimbursement was based. Nursing homes were categorized as skilled nursing facilities or as intermediate care facilities. Skilled nursing facilities were designed to care for residents who needed skilled nursing care that was more medically oriented. Residents in intermediate care facilities required custodial, rather than skilled nursing, care. These classifications were based on Medicare and Medicaid payment criteria for nursing home care. Because the two levels of classification did not accurately reflect the variations in the functional abilities of nursing home residents, the federal government replaced the dichotomous classification with one designation: the nursing facility (Boondas, 1991). Centers for Medicare and Medicaid Services (CMS), which administers Medicare and Medicaid, designed a different classification system in 1998 called the Resource Utilization Groups: Version III (RUG-III). Instead of paying facilities retrospectively

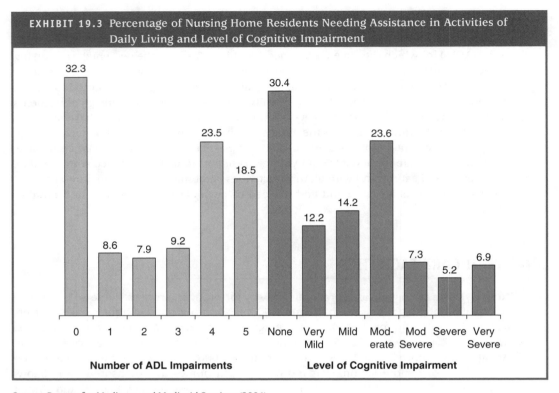

EXHIBIT 19.3 Percentage of Nursing Home Residents Needing Assistance in Activities of Daily Living and Level of Cognitive Impairment

Source: Centers for Medicare and Medicaid Services (2006).

after services were delivered based on "reasonable costs," facilities are now paid prospectively based on a patient's care needs and classification. Under the 1998 RUG-III classification system, nursing homes began to use seven major classification groups for cost reimbursement: rehabilitation, extensive services, special care, clinically complex, impaired cognition, behavior problems, and reduced physical functions (Zbylot, Job, McCormick, Boulter, & Moore, 1995). The seven major groups were further divided into 44 case mix groups based on intensity of ADL needs. Such classification reflected the many types of residents in need of nursing home care. However recent changes enacted in 2006 refined the 44 RUGS-III groups by adding nine new Rehabilitation plus Extensive Services, thus increasing the classification types to 53 RUGS (Leavitt, 2006). Changes in the RUGS were driven in part by of the increase in the number of residents with diverse health care needs, and the fact that nursing homes are expanding the range of services they offer.

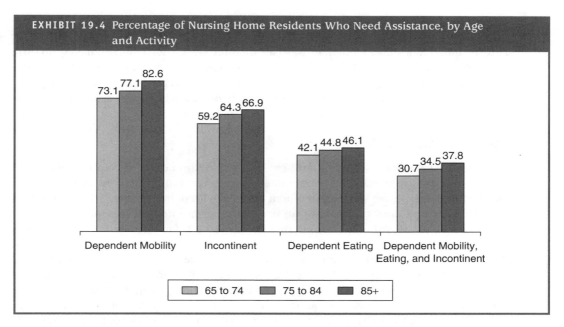

EXHIBIT 19.4 Percentage of Nursing Home Residents Who Need Assistance, by Age and Activity

Source: Gabrel (2000a).

Post-Acute Care

When patients need medical and rehabilitative care services after a hospitalization of at least three days, the care patients receive is referred to as "post-acute care". Older adults needing medical or rehabilitative care provided in an institution are frequently discharged to either an Inpatient Rehabilitation Facility (IRF) or a Skilled Nursing Facility (SNF). Patients in IRFs must be able to withstand a more intensive rehabilitation care schedule (e.g., tolerate a minimum of three hours of rehabilitation per day) and show consistent functional improvement (Kramer, 2006). In contrast, patients who receive post-acute care (often referred to as subacute care) in SNFs have different guidelines that allow for a less intensive rehabilitative protocol to occur over a longer timeframe (Gage et al., 2007).

Many long-term care facilities now offer a wide range of rehabilitative services that cater to a specific target population. For example, they may specialize in serving rehabilitation patients who need help recovering from hip replacement or spinal cord injuries. Other subacute units are considered to be "medical subacute" units and serve patients who need intensive medical care, such as ventilator care, wound care, or IV therapy. Typically, subacute units require staff to be more highly trained, require more physician involvement, and use interdisciplinary teams to plan and monitor care. The growth of subacute care has been encouraged by Medicare's prospective payment system, which pays hospitals a flat rate for care, resulting in a shorter length of stay (see Chapter 11). A shorter length of stay, in turn, encourages patient care in these "stepdown" or subacute units. Studies of the effectiveness and efficiency of subacute care units are being conducted; it is generally thought that postacute care is a cost-effective alternative to inpatient acute hospital care (Office of the Assistant Secretary, 1995).

Specialized Alzheimer's Unit

In the past decade, increasing numbers of nursing homes have created specialized services to care for persons with Alzheimer's disease and other dementias. Included in these efforts are cluster settings, in which persons with dementia are grouped together on a floor or unit, and special care units (SCUs) that are housed in separate wings or buildings. In a national review of nursing homes, 19.2% facilities had at least one distinct special care unit, and 65.7% of these units were for Alzheimer's disease (Freiman & Brown, 1999). SCUs have increased in part because of the special care needs of persons with various types of dementias. For example, persons with dementia are more likely to need assistance with ADLs, to need help remaining continent, to have psychiatric symptoms (delusions and hallucinations), and to have behavioral problems (e.g., wandering and physically hurting self or others) than those without dementia (U.S. Congress, Office of Technology Assessment [OTA], 1992; U.S. Department of Health and Human Services, 1991). In response to a congressional request, the OTA conducted a comprehensive review of the available research on SCUs. Their best estimate, based on national data, was that 8–10% of nursing homes had SCUs for persons with Alzheimer's disease or dementia, and that more facilities reported having plans to create such units. Not surprisingly, larger nursing homes were more likely than smaller ones to have SCUs, and nursing homes in the West were more likely to report having SCUs than were homes located in other geographical areas. The majority of nursing homes indicated that residents of SCUs were charged more for their care than were residents of non-SCUs. Descriptive studies showed that units varied greatly in their patient-care philosophy, number of residents, physical design, staffing patterns and ratios, activity programs, and patient-care practices. Patient-care philosophies included goals such as to provide a safe, secure, and supportive environment for residents; reduce feelings of anxiety; maintain optimal levels of physical and cognitive functioning; and provide holistic care. The number of residents living in SCUs ranged from less than 10 to more than 40. Studies showed that, on average, SCU residents were younger, White, and male, and were more likely to have a specific diagnosis, such as Alzheimer's disease, than other residents with or without dementia. SCU residents also were less likely than other nursing home residents with dementia to have impairments in ADLs but were more likely to exhibit behavioral problems.

According to the OTA (1992) report, most SCUs had some special environmental adaptations for residents, including alarm or locking systems, secured areas for wandering, and color coding of rooms and personal markers to help residents find their way around the unit.

Many of the SCUs provided some type of specialized training for staff; these units had a higher staff-to-resident ratio than did non-SCUs. In addition, studies indicated that SCUs had activities designed to increase stimulation and reduce resident stress. Activities offered to residents in SCUs included singing, exercises, games, painting, field trips, reality orientation, and reminiscence therapy. A review conducted in 1996 found that 19.2% of nursing homes had at least one distinct special care unit, and 65.7% of these units were specifically for Alzheimer's disease (Freiman & Brown, 1999).

Some argue that segregating persons with dementias from other nursing home residents improves resident wellbeing, enhances family interaction and satisfaction, increases staff satisfaction, and improves the nursing home experience for residents who do not have dementia (Maas, 1988; Ronch, 1987). For example, Buchanan, Choi, Wang, Hysunsu, and Graber (2005) examined national data of all Medicaid and Medicare-certified nursing homes to examine the differences between residents with Alzheimer's disease in SCUs and those residents with Alzheimer's who were not in SCUs. They found that SCU residents had more structured activities and received better management of mood, behavioral problems, and cognitive losses. Others argue that there are no discernible differences in resident outcomes for those living in SCUs (Rabins, 1986; Ronch, 1987). Slone, Lindeman, Phillips, Moritz, and Koch (1995) evaluated studies of effectiveness of SCUs and concluded that existing studies were inconclusive because some investigators reported improvements in residents' ADL performance, mood, behavior, and cognition, whereas others found no differences in these outcomes. Chappell and Reid (2000) conducted one of the most comprehensive examinations to date of resident outcomes in SCU and non-SCUs in Canadian nursing homes. When examining changes in resident outcomes in six different areas (e.g., physical functioning, social skills, agitation) over a one-year period, they found that residing in a SCU was unrelated to any of the changes in these areas. They concluded that many non-SCUs were implementing a similar quality of care to SCUs. These seemingly contradictory findings are due to the difficulty in controlling for sampling variations and the differences in SCU care delivery, treatment, and outcome measurement.

STAFFING PATTERNS

Nursing homes have a variety of professionals and paraprofessionals who provide care to their residents. The number of staff in each area depends on the number of beds; those certified by Medicare and Medicaid have to meet certain staffing requirements. Nursing homes generally have departments that are responsible for resident or social services, administrative services, rehabilitation, nursing, supportive services, and dietary services. Social services staff work with residents and their families to assist them in adjusting to the social and emotional aspects of living in the facility. In addition, social service staff offer medically related social and psychological treatment goals for residents. Nursing homes with 120 beds or more must employ a director of social services; smaller homes may employ a social service director on a consultancy basis (Allen, 1987).

For Your Files: Special Care Unit in Lynden, Washington

The Christian Health Care Center (previously known as the Christian Rest Home), a 150-bed nursing home in Lynden, Washington, has had a special care unit since 1988. The 15-bed special care unit was established because of staff concerns about the safety and wellbeing of residents with dementia who wander or have other behavioral symptoms that cannot be handled in the facility's regular units.

The special care unit consists of resident bedrooms, an activity/dining area, and an enclosed outdoor courtyard. Physical changes were made to the building to create the unit: (a) a set of doors was installed in an existing partition off the resident bedrooms and the activity/dining area, (b) a door was made in an exterior wall to give the residents access to the enclosed courtyard, and (c) keypad-operated locks were installed on the exit doors; the doors open when a number code is punched in on the keypad, and the doors open automatically when the alarm goes off. These physical changes cost less than $5,000.

Some residents of the special care unit have been transferred to the unit from other parts of the nursing home; other residents have been admitted directly from home. Although all the special care unit residents have dementia in the opinion of the facility staff, a few have not had a diagnosis of dementia in their medical records.

The objectives of the unit are to ensure the residents' safety, to reduce agitation and behavioral symptoms, to maintain independent functioning, and to improve the residents' quality of life. The staff members perceive resident agitation and behavioral symptoms as significant expressions of feelings and unmet needs. They attempt to understand and respond to those feelings and needs in the belief that, by doing so, they will reduce agitation and behavioral symptoms and improve the residents' quality of life. Although many of the residents exhibited severe behavioral symptoms before coming to the unit, the unit staff report that these symptoms are relatively easily managed in the special care unit.

Formal and informal activity programs are conducted in the unit. Each afternoon, there is a formal activity program, such as a weekly Bible study and music group, a weekly reminiscence group, a weekly "validation" group, and "high tea"—a Monday afternoon event with real china and lace tablecloths. Other activities, such as food preparation and singing, take place informally in the unit. One resident who likes to fold laundry is encouraged to do so. Family members are welcome in the unit at any time. Staff members know the residents' families and involve them in decisions about the residents' care. Staff members report that family members often thank them for the help they give the residents and the emotional support they give the family members. During the day, the staff in the special care unit consists of one registered nurse, who functions as the unit coordinator, and two nurse aides. A licensed practical nurse and two other nurse aides take over for the evening shift. Because staff consistency is considered important for the unit, the unit staff members generally are not rotated to other units. Special care unit residents are discharged from the unit when staff believe that the residents can no longer benefit from the unit. Several spouses of former special care unit residents have created an informal support group that meets almost daily in the facility, presumably to replace the emotional support they previously received from the unit staff.

Source: U.S. Congress, Office of Technology Assessment (1992).

Mental health services may be provided by staff or contracted out with mental health professionals in the community. Facilities are also required to offer residents an activities program that enhances their physical, social, and psychological wellbeing. Staff in the activities department usually have training in recreational or therapeutic programming and are responsible for developing and implementing social and recreational activities for all residents. Activities staff also are responsible for recruiting, training, and using volunteers to assist with activities. Administrative services staff are responsible for processing admissions and financial accounting. Rehabilitation services such as physical, occupational, and speech therapies can be provided by qualified staff or contracted with outside companies. The goal of various therapies is to help the resident achieve the desired level of functioning in ADLs (Allen, 1987).

Support services staff tend to the cleanliness of the facility, laundry, and maintenance of the physical systems in the nursing home. Staff in the dietary department are responsible for the nutritional needs of the residents. Nursing departments are in charge of the delivery of nursing and personal care services to its residents. Nursing homes employ registered nurses and licensed practical nurses to deliver and oversee medical care, whereas certified nurse aides (CNAs) provide much of the personal care of the residents.

Staff retention has been a problem in many nursing homes across the country, in part because of the stressful nature of the work and the low wages (Foner, 1994). Especially problematic are the turnover rates of CNAs. CNAs are responsible for approximately 80% of direct resident care, yet turnover rates in some facilities have been as high as 75% in a given year (Decker et al., 2003; Harrington, 1991). Factors associated with job satisfaction and turnover rates of CNAs include wage levels, job characteristics, interpersonal relationships with nursing staff, lack of involvement in care planning and assessment of residents, lack of advancement opportunities, working in for-profit nursing homes, higher top management turnover, working in larger facilities, and lower facility quality (Banaszak-Holl & Hines, 1994; Castle & Engberg, 2006; Foner, 1994; Wacker, 1996).

Best Practice: Community Certified Nurse Aide Mentoring Training Program

The Foundation for Long Term Care in New York has created a five-part CNA peer mentoring program where veteran CNAs model exemplary care and mentor newly hired CNAs. The idea is that mentors will share their knowledge, compassion, and caring with new CNAs, provide a warm and welcoming environment, and help new CNAs fit in with their peers and develop positive friendships at work. Mentors model correct clinical skills, positive attitudes, and time management. They also reinforce information about formal policies and procedures and explain informal policies. Mentors are compensated for their mentoring through hourly wage increases during the mentoring, permanent salary increases, honorariums for each training session, or/and extra vacation days. The program involves commitment from administrators and nurse supervisors, and training and ongoing support for the mentors. The five-part training program provides information on (1) how to operate the project; (2) a one-hour workshop for supervisors, to ensure their support; (3) six hours of mentor training; (4) three to nine hours of booster training for mentors; and (5) a newsletter for mentors, to help them maintain interest in the project. A 2004 study of the program showed that there was an average 15% increase in the retention of new CNAs in 11 New York nursing homes. In 2005, the Growing Strong Roots program was given the Best Practices in Human Resources and Aging Award from the American Society on Aging, in collaboration with the Brookdale Center on Aging of Hunter College, New York City. See Hegeman (2005) for more program details.

The Foundation for Long Term Care offers a Growing Strong Roots training materials package. For more information, contact the foundation at 150 State Street, Suite 301, Albany, NY, 12207; phone: 518-449-7873; www.nyahsa.org/foundation/n00000025.cfm.

ACTIVITY PROGRAMS

As mentioned above, nursing homes are required to provide activity programs that enhance residents' physical and mental wellbeing. Indeed, researchers have shown that participation in activities is important to residents' quality of life (Lawton, 1989; Riddick & Keller, 1991). Nursing homes frequently offer discussion groups, religious groups and services, music programs, raised garden beds, pet visitation, exercise programs, and of course, bingo. One activity that fosters a helping relationship between nursing home residents and young adults is intergenerational learning programs. The purpose of these programs is to bring young people and older adults together in a way that allows both older and younger adults to assist one another. For example, an intergenerational learning program between one Illinois nursing home and a local elementary school provided both residents and students with positive interactions (Angelis, 1990). Students helped residents with letter writing and other activities, while residents often read to students and engaged in playing games. Students and residents exchanged cards and presents on birthdays and participated in intergenerational group activities. In addition, several residents attended classes at the elementary school, and a school activity newsletter was sent to the residents every month. Intergenerational programs involving students and residents offer students an educational experience and improve resident wellbeing.

Residents' Rights and the Ombudsman Program

As we discussed earlier in the chapter, older adults living in nursing homes suffer from multiple physical or cognitive impairments. By its very nature, institutional living tends to compromise individual choices. Thus long-term care ombudsman programs were created to act as advocates for older adults living in nursing homes and board and care homes. In response to concerns raised about the quality of care provided in nursing homes, the federal government funded seven nursing home ombudsman demonstration projects in the early 1970s to establish a mechanism for receiving and resolving complaints regarding the delivery of nursing home care, to document problems in nursing homes, and to test the effectiveness of using volunteer ombudsmen (U.S. Senate Special Committee on Aging, 1993). By 1975, the Administration on Aging (AoA) funded small residents' rights programs in all 50 states, and in 1978 the ombudsman program was incorporated into the Older Americans Act (OAA). In 1981, ombudsmen were also directed to serve persons living in board and care homes. In 2004, there were 580 local or regional ombudsman programs located in every state in the United States handling some 287,824 complaints (Administration on Aging [AoA], 2004e). The top five complaints made to ombudsmen about nursing home care in 2005 were (1) call lights, requests for assistance; (2) menu-quantity, quality, variation, choice; (3) dignity, respect-staff attitudes; (4) accidents, improper handling; and (5) care plan/resident assessment (AoA, 2005b). These five represent 22% of all complaints. Congress established separate authorization of $20 million for the ombudsman program in 1988; in 1992, Congress appropriated $8.3 million for ombudsman and elder abuse programs. In the reauthorization of the OAA in 2000, ombudsman services are authorized under Title VII and the proposed budget for 2006 is $14.8 million (AoA, 2006g).

Under the OAA as amended, each state must establish and operate a long-term care ombudsman program. Under the direction of a full-time state ombudsman, programs are directed to

- identify, investigate, and resolve complaints made by or on behalf of residents;
- provide information to residents about long-term care services;
- represent the interests of residents before governmental agencies and seek administrative, legal, and other remedies to protect residents;
- analyze, comment on, and recommend changes in laws and regulations pertaining to the health, safety, welfare, and rights of residents;
- educate and inform consumers and the general public regarding issues and concerns related to long-term care and facilitate public comment on laws, regulations, policies, and actions;
- promote the development of citizen organizations to participate in the program; and
- provide technical support for the development of resident and family councils to protect the wellbeing and rights of residents (AoA, 2004e).

Of course, one primary responsibility of ombudsmen is to protect the rights of residents. Resident rights are based on federal and state laws that are designed to protect the basic liberties of nursing home residents (see Exhibit 19.5). For example, resident rights legislation includes the rights to receive information; participate in planning all types of care; make choices and independent personal decisions; enjoy privacy in care and confidentiality regarding medical, personal, and financial matters; be treated with dignity and respect; have personal possessions that are kept safe and secure; and have advance notice of transfer or change of rooms or roommates (Burger, Fraser, Hunt, & Frank, 1996; National Citizens' Coalition for Nursing Home Reform, 2003).

EXHIBIT 19.5 Summary of Nursing Home Residents' Rights

1. The right to be fully informed about
   - all services available and all charges;
   - the facility's rules and regulations;
   - how to contact the state ombudsman, the other advocacy organizations;
   - the state survey reports on the facility.

2. The right to participate in their own care and to
   - receive adequate or appropriate health care;
   - be informed of their medical condition and to participate in treatment planning and be invited to participate in care planning;
   - refuse medication and treatment;
   - participate in discharge planning and review their medical records;
   - have daily communication in their own language;
   - have assistance if there is sensory impairment.

3. The right to make independent choices, including the right to
   - know that choices are available;
   - make independent personal decisions;
   - choose a physician;
   - participate in activities of the community inside and outside the facility, and participate in a Resident Council;
   - vote.

4. The right to privacy and confidentiality, including the right to
   - private and unrestricted communication with any person of their choice, including privacy for telephone calls, unopened mail, privacy for meetings with family and friends and other residents;
   - privacy in treatment and care for personal needs;
   - have reasonable access to any entity or individual that provides health, social, legal, or other services;
   - confidentiality regarding medical, personal or financial affairs.

5. The right to security for possessions, including the right to
   - manage financial affairs;
   - file a complaint with the state agencies for abuse, neglect, or misappropriation of their property;

6. The right to dignity, respect, and freedom, including the right to
   - be treated with consideration, respect, and dignity;
   - be free from mental and physical abuse;
   - be free from physical and chemical restraints;
   - have self-determination.

7. The right to remain in the facility, including the right to
   - be transferred or discharged only for medical reasons, if needs cannot be met in the facility, if the health and safety of other residents is endangered, or for non-payment of stay;

- receive notice of transfer. A 30-day notice for transfer out of the facility is required, and the notice must include (a) reason for transfer, (b) effective date, (c) location to which the resident is discharged, (d) a statement of right to appeal, and (e) the name, address, and telephone number of the state long-term care ombudsman;
- have sufficient preparation to ensure a safe transfer or discharge.

8. The right to raise concerns or complaints including the right to
   - present grievances to the staff of the nursing home, or to any other person, without fear of reprisal;
   - prompt efforts by the facility to resolve grievances.

9. The facility must maintain identical policies and practices regarding transfer, discharge, and provision of services for all residents regardless of payment source.

Source: Adapted from Burger, Fraser, Hunt, & Frank (1996).

For Your Files: National Citizens' Coalition for Nursing Home Reform

The National Citizens' Coalition for Nursing Home Reform, founded in 1975, is a nonprofit consumer advocacy group whose mission is to ensure quality of care for people in the long-term care system. There are more than 300 state and local member groups and approximately 1,000 members in 40 states. The coalition reviews and distributes information on legislative and regulatory issues, develops training and resource materials for those who act as advocates for nursing home residents, and connects local, state, and national organizations with long-term care experts and resources. The coalition also publishes a variety of resource materials and books, including the *Quality Care Advocate*, a bimonthly newsletter on issues relating to nursing home care and the use of restraints, and a recent book titled *Nursing Homes: Getting Good Care There*.

For more information, contact National Citizens' Coalition for Nursing Home Reform, 1424 16th Street N.W., Suite 202, Washington, DC 20036-2211; phone: 202-332-2275; www.nccnhr.org.

Ombudsmen also deal with a wide range of other issues, including resolving problems that residents might have with their public benefits or guardianship procedures. Netting, Paton, and Huber (1992) examined ombudsman program reports sent to the AoA in 1990 to determine the nature of complaints received by long-term care ombudsman programs. They found that the largest number of complaints were related to resident care, and included such things as not being dressed, physical abuse, neglect, and poorly trained staff. The next most frequent category of complaints comprised administrative complaints about understaffing, roommate conflict, and laundry procedures, followed by resident rights. In 1995, the complaints most frequently received by ombudsmen from residents in board and care homes were about menu quality, building disrepair, administration of medication, and staff respect and attitude (AoA, 1995b). Ten years later, the top five complaints made to ombudsmen in 2005 regarding care provided in board and care homes were (1) menu—quantity, quality, variation, and choice; (2) medications— administration, organization; (3) discharge/eviction—planning, notice, procedure; (4) equipment/ building—disrepair, hazards, poor lighting, fire safety; and (5) dignity, respect—staff attitudes. These five represented 22% of all complaints in both nursing homes and board and care homes (AoA, 2005c).

In their study of ombudsman programs, Monk, Kaye, and Litwin (1984) identified two models of ombudsman activities. The *patient rights model* is perceived as a watchdog approach designed to create systemic change in long-term care services. The *quality-of-life model* is based on resolving resident difficulties with staff on a more informal level. Of course, many programs may use both elements in delivering services. Regardless of the model selected by local programs, they all rely on well-trained staff to deliver program services. Some programs use paid staff, volunteers, or a combination of both to deliver their services. In a study of ombudsman programs in 46 states, 26 states reported that they used mostly volunteer staff, and 20 used primarily paid staff (U.S. Senate Special Committee on Aging, 1993). In 2004, there were 8,714 certified ombudsmen volunteers across the country used to investigate nursing home complaints (AoA, 2004e). Although using volunteer ombudsmen has some drawbacks (see Monk et al., 1984), some programs have successfully relied on volunteers to provide services. For example, the East Tennessee Advocates for Elders Program has successfully used volunteer ombudsmen since 1978, and in 1989 had 94 volunteers who were trained or being trained as ombudsmen (Netting & Hinds, 1989). The program covers a 16-county area and serves 60 nursing homes and 160 assisted living care facilities (East Tennessee Human Resource Agency, n.d.). However, the heavy reliance on volunteer ombudsmen requires that trainers must examine personal characteristics and motivations of volunteers in order to better prepare volunteers for the difficult work they do (Keith, 2003).

Best Practice: Tough Enough to Care

The Texas Department of Aging (TDoA) launched the Tough Enough to Care—Be There volunteer ombudsman program. The goal of the program is to increase the number of volunteer ombudsmen to assist the more than 92,000 long-term care residents across the state of Texas. The TDoA developed a statewide media campaign focusing on volunteer recruitment, and a VISTA volunteer dedicated to assist with the campaign was also placed at the TDoA. A theme was selected, a logo was designed, promotional items were developed, and publicity was generated via press conferences, public service announcements, and other activities. All efforts supported participating Area Agency on Aging (AAA) regions. The pilot for the statewide recruitment campaign, "Tough Enough to Care—Be There," was launched in Waco (AAA of the Heart of Texas) on November 1, 1999, via a press conference covered by local newspapers and television stations. The formal campaign kickoff was held in Austin on January 10, 2000, at the Capitol. The 21 press conferences held across Texas generated support and program awareness of local, regional, state, and federal officials. There is also a website: www.toughenoughtocare.org.

For more information, contact the Texas Department on Aging, P.O. Box 12786, Austin, TX 78751; phone: 800-252-9240 or 512-438-3011; www.dads.state.tx.us/index .cfmResident Councils.

In an attempt to give residents input in the quality of care that they receive, resident councils have emerged as a vehicle to voice residents' concerns. Meyer (1991) collected data about the activities of resident councils through participant observations and interviews with residents as well as statewide resident council members and staff. Resident councils usually meet once a month with the activities director facilitating the meetings; meetings are usually attended by 15 to 30 residents. On the basis of her observations, Meyer concluded that resident councils have at least four functions. First, they make modest changes in the care they receive and condition of the home. For example, specific items discussed at council meetings included acquiring shower chairs for frail residents, more frequent adjustment of window blinds by staff, and parking of carts and wheelchairs on only one side of the hallway. Their success in accomplishing these and other goals was mixed. Resident councils were more successful in obtaining products than they were in changing procedures or services. Second, resident councils provide services to residents and the needy living in their communities. Residents make and sell handcrafted items; the funds are used to assist residents who have experienced a financial crisis or are given to charitable organizations. Third, they broaden the scope of social activities available to residents. These activities include feeding birds, planning ethnic and cultural menus and activities, and arranging social outings to nearby restaurants, zoos, and theaters. Finally, resident councils cooperate with resident councils at other nursing homes to lobby for improvements in quality of care.

Although the resident councils studied by Meyer were unsuccessful in changing procedures, participation in resident councils gave residents a sense of having some control over their lives and a chance to participate in beneficial activities. Meyer also identified barriers to participation in resident councils. Many residents have difficulty hearing, are entering nursing homes with more functional limitations, and have shorter average length of stays. Some residents did not participate because they felt that councils were ineffective in creating change, and others feared retaliation for voicing complaints. Overall, resident councils play an important role in improving the lives of nursing home residents. More research is needed, however, to determine ways to improve participation and outcomes.

IMPROVING QUALITY OF LIFE IN NURSING HOMES

The issue of quality of care has been a concern since nursing homes were formally established decades ago. Indeed, substandard resident care and resident abuse have led to nursing homes being one of the most regulated enterprises in the country. Quality of care includes a wide variety of indicators from the small details of accommodating personal preference to the delivery of personal and medical care. The challenge for nursing homes is that they are at once a place where medical care is provided and where people live their lives (Wiener, 2003).

Stop and consider for a moment how you begin a typical day. You get yourself up, shower and dress, and grab a bite to eat before you go on your way. You decide when to get up, what to wear, and what to eat. You also probably have routines built into your morning—perhaps enjoying a cup of coffee and reading the paper before having breakfast. The mere fact of residing in an institution compromises these types of personal freedoms to some extent. Higher-quality homes attempt to accommodate personal differences, employ well-trained staff, and deliver high-quality medical care.

A landmark work, *Improving Quality of Care in Nursing Homes* (Institute of Medicine, 1986), was instrumental in identifying key indicators of quality of care in nursing homes. Specific indicators that measured resident outcome and care process were identified. Negative indicators included excessive use of psychotropic drugs, high incidence of avoidable decubitus ulcers and urinary tract infections, dehydration, and considerable weight loss. Personal care indicators included whether residents' hair was neat and clean, whether they were dressed in their own clothing, whether they received daily oral care, and whether they received prompt responses to resident call lights. Nutritional and dietary indicators included assisting residents who needed help eating, serving food while it was still warm, and giving residents some choice in menu selections. Finally, overall quality-of-care indicators included living in a clean environment in which residents were allowed to have personal possessions and furnishings in their rooms, opportunities for personal choice, participation in social activities, and treatment by staff with dignity.

For Your Files: The Eden Alternative in Nursing Homes

In 1991 Dr. Bill Thomas, his wife Judy and the administrative team at Chase Memorial Nursing Home in New York sought an alternative to caring for the residents of this rural nursing home in order to address what they identified as the three plagues of nursing homes—loneliness, helplessness, and boredom. They incorporated pets (100 birds, to be exact, as well as dogs, cats, and rabbits), plants and gardens, and visiting children, and changed the way in which care was organized and provided. Pets were designed to get people talking, and involved in their environment; helping children care for pets and plants was designed to assist elders to overcome feelings of helplessness; and an environment with all this 'diversity' was expected to provide the unexpected. Residents also bring their own furniture and their favorite pictures, and their rooms are painted in their favorite colors. In addition to introducing the changes in the environment, Eden Alternative homes create nursing care teams where each team is responsible for a small number of residents and the staff (considered to be anyone who comes into contact with the residents) work together to prepare their own schedules and daily assignments. They dubbed this new approach the "Eden Alternative." Persons interested in the Eden Alternative can complete a four-day Associate Training class to learn about the process. One empirical study that compared resident outcomes of an Eden Alternative and a non-Eden Alternative nursing home found no beneficial effects in terms of cognitive function or functional status; however, qualitative data revealed the Eden Alternative nursing home had psychosocial changes that were positive for both staff and residents (Coleman et al., 2002).

For more information, contact Eden Alternative, 11 Blue Oak Lane, Wimberley, TX 78676; phone: 512–847–6061; www.edenalt.com.

Source: Adapted from the National Center on Accessibility (n.d.) and Eden Alternative (n.d.).

The extent to which nursing homes fail to provide good quality of care has been well documented. For example, in a survey of nursing home staff, Pillemer and Moore (1989) found that 36% of nursing home staff had seen at least one resident physically abused in the past year, and 10% admitted to physically abusing residents. Eighty-one percent reported seeing residents psychologically abused—most often in the form of being yelled at. In addition, treatment of residents has been found to be related to personal characteristics. Residents with higher incomes, more personal possessions, had visitors at least once a month, and who were White, received better overall quality of care (Pillemer, 1988). More recent data from the Ombudsman Annual Report for 2005 indicated that, of the 241,684 complaints made to long-term care ombudsmen across the country, some 9,592 complaints were made regarding resident abuse, neglect, or exploitation (AoA, 2005b). Of all the various types of complaints reported (e.g., residents' rights, resident care, quality of life, and administration), physical abuse, verbal/mental abuse, and gross neglect represented 1.8%, 1.3%, and 1.0%, respectively.

Although much of what is reported in the popular press and to some extent in professional publications focuses on poor-quality care provided in some homes, researchers have identified positive outcomes for residents and family members after nursing home placement. For example, Smith and Bengston (1979) found in their two-year study of nursing home residents and their families that 70% reported that the consequences of nursing home placement were positive. Families reported a renewed or continued closeness among family members as well as a reduction in caregiving stress, which in turn resulted in more time to focus on the emotional aspects of the relationship. Families can also see improvements in residents' physical and mental health and see residents developing new relationships with other residents. When the American Association of Retired Persons (1990) conducted interviews of nursing home residents, it found that many residents talked about the positive aspects of residing in a nursing home. For example, one resident stated, "I learned to walk when I got here." Another commented, "I've gained weight. You better believe it. I was going downhill rather rapidly before [moving into the nursing home]" (1990, p. 13). Other researchers found that, after nursing home placement, health and financial stresses were reduced for spouses and that caregivers' quality of life and health improved compared with caregivers who kept their loved one at home (King & Collins, 1991; Pushkar, Gold, & Reis, 1995). Although there is some indication that nursing home placement can reduce some aspects of family stress, other researchers found that the emotional strain of being a caregiver does not decrease (Lieberman & Fisher, 2001).

CHALLENGES FOR NURSING HOMES IN THE FUTURE

For most of the general public, the nursing home stands as a symbol of all that is dreaded about old age—its residents are physically and mentally impaired, they have become dependent on others to accomplish the most basic tasks of daily living, and they appear lonely and discarded by society. Every so often, popular news programs report the abuses that occur within a nursing home's confines. These images are embedded in our collective consciousness. Nursing homes do care for those who are among the most frail and debilitated in our society; some facilities are better than others. But rather than view nursing homes with contempt, we must embrace them as necessary places within the continuum of care and work to enhance the quality of care provided to their residents. Improving quality of care is like putting together the pieces of a puzzle. No one piece will solve the problems that exist in nursing homes because many pieces need to be addressed.

Reforming Reimbursement and Payment of Long-Term Care Facility Services

Having Medicaid as the largest third-party payer of nursing home care causes a number of problems. First, many have observed that Medicaid reimbursement rates are terribly inadequate, especially for those with high care needs (Swan & Benjamin, 1990). For example, the average Medicaid long-term care expenditure on older adults 65 and older varies from $2,270 in New York to $380 in Arizona, and Medicaid reimbursement rates for nursing home care are approximately 70% of private-pay rates (Kane, Kane, Ladd, & Veazie, 1998; Harrington-Meyer, 2001). In turn this has led, according to some scholars, to structural discrimination toward Medicaid residents in the form of long waiting lists and preferential treatment toward private-pay residents (Abend-Wein, 1991; Estes, Swan, & Associates, 1993; Grimaldi, 1982). Second, for middle-class families, the only alternative to paying for nursing home costs has been to impoverish themselves to qualify for nursing home care. About one-third of nursing home residents who are ineligible for Medicaid when they are admitted deplete enough of their assets to meet the eligibility guides for Medicaid (Wiener, Sullivan, & Skaggs, 1996). How many older families—or their children, for that matter—who need to secure extended long-term care services can afford $100 per day—more than $30,000 per year—for nursing home care? Many health scholars have called for developing a more rational system for financing nursing home care—one that combines both public and private financing (Aiken, 1989; Estes et al., 1993). An increase in public support, either directly or through taxation, is needed, along with efforts such as permitting the integration of Medicaid and long-term care insurance mentioned earlier in this chapter to increase the use of private sector insurance to help spread the risk of long-term care across different sectors of society and thus making nursing home care more affordable.

Attracting Qualified Staff and Improving Working Conditions

To increase the number of qualified staff applying for positions and working in nursing homes, we must work to reduce the stigma associated with working in a nursing home among all professional and certified staff. Anecdotal evidence suggests that nursing homes are often the last employment choice of newly graduated nurses. Nursing programs can work to encourage the placement of their students into long-term care. Just as initiatives have been developed to increase the number of nurses placed in rural areas, so too should initiatives be implemented to increase the number of nurses placed in long-term care facilities. Of course, chances of attracting qualified staff are improved if working conditions and benefits are competitive. Salary and benefits must be competitive with both the medical and nonmedical employment sectors, opportunities for professional advancement must exist, and the organizational climate must convey a sense of respect and appreciation for its employees.

Increasing Family and Community Involvement

Researchers have discovered a link between increased volunteer and family visits and improved quality of care. Staff and those in the aging network must work together to improve the amount of community involvement in nursing homes. Something as simple as having the Area Agency on Aging advisory board meet every month in the nursing home's conference room could increase the amount of contact between "outsiders" and the nursing home community. One facility in Boston has started a "Love is Ageless" program that encourages all nursing homes to display a banner proclaiming that love is ageless and inviting visitors from the community. They project that if only three new people visited each nursing home across the country, 15,000 new visitors would result. Kansas Advocates for Better Care documented community-based intergenerational programs in over 100 nursing homes in Kansas. For example, the Generation Bridge program brings the sixth grade class from Goessel Elementary School to Bethesda Nursing Home every Tuesday to play spelling bingo, bake cookies, make crafts, and visit with residents (Kansas Advocates for Better Care, 2002).

Meeting the Care Needs of a Diverse Group of Residents

The changing nature of the health care delivery system means that the type of care provided in nursing homes will have to change as well. As more community-based alternatives emerge for persons who need custodial care, nursing homes will no doubt emerge as primary places for more therapeutic and rehabilitative care. Furthermore, the increased number of persons with AIDS who will need long-term nursing may have a hand in shaping the future of nursing homes (Aiken, 1989). The changing demographics of the older adult population includes an increasing number of ethnically and racially diverse elders who will be in need of long-term care. Cultural competence is a relatively new concept in health care delivery. A culturally competent organization is "committed to serving diverse clients, hiring diverse staff, and establishing programs that address the needs of different client populations" (Management Sciences for Health, n.d., para 1). The Office of Minority Health identifies national standards for culturally and linguistically appropriate care that includes care where patients "receive from all staff members effective understandable, and respectful care that is provided in a manner compatible with their cultural health beliefs and practices and preferred language" (U.S. Department of Health and Human Services, 2001c, p. 7). Culturally competent training must be incorporated in curriculum and ongoing training provided by long-term care facilities.

Supporting the Future of Long-Term Care Facilities

The 2005 White House Conference on Aging delegates passed two resolutions aimed at improving long-term care. They supported policies that

- establish and foster innovations in financing long-term care to increase options available to consumers; and
- develop a coordinated, comprehensive long-term care strategy by supporting public and private sector initiatives that address financing, choice, quality, service delivery, and the paid and unpaid workforce.

As the population ages and becomes more diverse in the coming decades, long-term care facilities will be faced with a myriad of social and organizational challenges.

CASE STUDY

Defending Individual Rights—A Nursing Home's Dilemma

Edna, an 83-year-old with mild dementia, has lived in a nursing home for the past three years. Her only remaining family is an estranged daughter. Although she can walk with assistance, she prefers to use a wheelchair. Edna has formed a strong attachment to George, a 90-year-old with moderate to severe dementia, depending on the day and his stress level. George's chart also documents a diagnosis of transient ischemic attacks. George is quite handsome and is "the catch of the nursing home." Edna feels important when George is pushing her around in her wheelchair. Being with George has become a status symbol for Edna. George's roommate, Bud, has complained that he does not have any privacy. Edna and George neglect to pull the privacy curtain when they are lying in George's bed. Bud's family also has complained about how embarrassing it is, especially for younger family members, to find Edna and George in bed together when they visit. Edna's daughter called the nursing home and told the head nurse that the facility should stop this relationship because Edna and George were too old to have sex. She demanded that something be done immediately and indicated that if some measures were not taken, she would move her mother to another facility.

The staff of the facility have offered Edna and George the opportunity to room together. Some staff members are uncomfortable with this relationship because George is more confused than Edna, and they feel that she dominates the relationship. They suspect that she can be physically abusive to George if he refuses to spend time with her. They have observed such jealous behavior during group activities and in the dining room when other women try to sit next to George. Other staff members believe that to try to separate the couple would be a violation of their rights to choose their own companions. George's two sons are not adamantly opposed to George's being with Edna. They find it amusing and have joked about it in front of the staff.

Edna and George decide to be roommates. After three days together, George has many bruises on his arms and face. Staff members notice that he is attempting to avoid Edna. They ask George if he wants to move back into his old room, and he replies that he does.

Staff members move George back to his room. Within a day, George is seeking Edna out and refuses to leave her. Staff decide to call the local long-term care ombudsman for technical assistance.

Case Study Questions

1. As the long-term care ombudsman, what additional information would you like to know?

2. What resident rights are in question in this case scenario?

3. Whose interests must be considered? Do any of these interests take precedence over any of the others?

4. Do you believe it is a violation of George and Edna's rights to keep them separated? Why or why not?

5. Can you think of a creative compromise that would mostly satisfy all parties in this case? Are there any other community resources or agencies that could be called on to assist staff? Family members? George or Edna? Bud?

Learning Activities

1. Visit a resident council meeting at a local nursing home. What issues were discussed at the meeting? How many residents and staff attended? Interview the chair of the resident council. Have the chair reflect on the council's accomplishments during the past year.

2. Join the Gerinet Listserv discussion group. To subscribe, send mail to LISTSERV@LISTSERV.BUFFALO.EDU with the command: SUBSCRIBE GERINET Monitor the discussion during a two-week period. What issues are discussed by the group?

3. Obtain a map of your city and mark on the map the locations of the nursing homes in your community. On the same map, draw a line around what you believe are low-income or minority neighborhoods. Where are the nursing homes located in relation to these neighborhoods? If you live in a rural area, determine how far away these facilities are from smaller rural towns. What are the implications of the geographic location of these nursing homes?

For More Information

National Resources

1. American Association of Homes and Services for the Aging, 2519 Connecticut Avenue, N.W., Washington, DC 20008–1520; phone: 202-783-2242; www.aahsa.org.
   The American Association of Homes and Services for the Aging is the national association for nonprofit organizations involved in providing health, community, and related services to older adults. It distributes free information on a variety of issues, including long-term care.

2. American Health Care Association, 1201 L Street N.W., Washington, DC 20005; phone: 202-842-4444; www.ahca.org.

   The American Health Care Association provides leadership in dealing with long-term care issues, offers continuing education programs for nursing home professionals, and publishes *Provider*, a monthly magazine for its members.

3. National Citizens' Coalition for Nursing Home Reform, 1828 L Street, N.W., Suite 801 Washington, DC 20036; phone: 202-332-2276; www.nccnhr.org.

   The Coalition works to achieve quality of care in nursing homes by conducting advocacy training, promotes best practices in care delivery, and provides publications on institutional-based long-term care. It also operates the National Long-Term Care Ombudsman Resource Center.

Web Resources

1. http://erc.msh.org/mainpage.cfm?file = 1.0.htm&module = provider&language = English.

   The Provider's Guide to Quality and Culture is a website designed to provide information to health care organizations to assist them in providing culturally competent care to multi-ethnic populations. This website is a joint project of Management Sciences for Health (MSH), U.S. Department of Health and Human Services, Health Resources and Services Administration, and the Bureau of Primary Health Care. The site explains cultural competence and provides information on how to create culturally competent organizations and how to improve the quality of provider/client interaction. It also provides an extensive list of resources.

2. America's Health Insurance Plans: www.hiaa.org.

   The Health Insurance Association of America has a number of consumer guides online, including one on long-term care insurance. The information about long-term care insurance is comprehensive and covers such topics as "Are you likely to need long-term care?" "What kind of insurance is available?" "What do policies cost?" and "What do long-term care insurance policies cover?" It is a good primer on long-term care insurance.

3. The American Health Care Association and the National Center for Assisted Living: www.longtermcareliving.co

   This is a website for consumers interested in information about nursing homes, assisted living/residential care, and other types of long-term care.

4. Office of the Ombudsman: www.ombud.gov.bc.ca/index.html.

   This website does a good job of explaining what an ombudsman is and does and how to use one. The site also has links to other related resources.

5. Nursing Home Compare: www.medicare.gov/NHCompare/home.asp.

   The primary purpose of this site is to provide detailed information about the performance of every Medicare- and Medicaid-certified nursing home in the country. The site also provides links to other resources. A Guide to Choosing a Nursing Home, and a Nursing Home Checklist are also available.

6. Guide to Nursing Homes in Florida: http://ahcaxnet.fdhc.state.fl.us/nhcguide/GuideIntro.aspx.

   Even for nonresidents of Florida, this site is worth a visit. The Agency for Health Care Administration has created a home page with links to information about tips on finding a nursing home. Visitors can search the guide by region or by keyword.

PART III

Preparing for the Future

20

Programs and Services in an Era of Change

In the previous chapters of this book, we described the wide array of programs and services that exist to assist older adults. Yet to end without describing the important issues facing the nation with regard to service delivery of programs would present an incomplete picture. The programs and services we have described throughout this book exist within a social and political context that influences their existence, the nature of what they offer, and those to whom they offer services. In this final chapter, we discuss the social forces that have brought us to a crossroads of aging policy and service delivery. We then discuss some key issues that will need to be addressed with subsequent reauthorizations of the Older Americans Act (OAA). We conclude with some thoughts about the changing nature of U.S. society and its implications for aging professionals.

SOCIAL AND POLITICAL INFLUENCES ON AGING POLICIES AND PROGRAMS

Two key social and political factors that have emerged in the past decade are forcing a re-examination of aging policies and, in turn, the programs and services they fund. First, the number of people 65 and older is steadily increasing and, concomitantly, there has been a steady increase in the percentage of the federal budget spent on older adults. Second, society's current image of older adults commonly portrays them as healthy, wealthy, and self-consumed. Such an image drives the opinion that programs and services for older adults are no longer needed. Thus these social forces have influenced a discussion regarding possible solutions to "fix" Medicare, to stabilize Social Security in the twenty-first century, and to "protect" society from buckling under the weight of its burdensome older population. Many scholars have argued against the assumptions that older adults are a burden to society and that all older adults are financially and socially comfortable and have voiced the need for society to acknowledge the benefits, both direct and indirect, that everyone experiences when society cares for its elders (see Kingston, Hirshorn, & Cornman, 1986; Marmor, Mashaw, & Harvey, 1990).

Because the OAA is the one of the key social policies created to serve older adults, it too has been the focus of much debate. What role should the Older Americans Act play and who should its programs serve? We will examine some of the issues currently being debated that will shape the future of the OAA.

CHALLENGES FOR THE OLDER AMERICANS ACT

Policy makers and advocates of older adults are currently re-examining a number of issues associated with the OAA. The reauthorization of the Act in 2006 has given professionals in the field of aging an opportunity to debate the role of the OAA, to think about new ways of increasing linkages with the private sector, and to re-examine who should be eligible for services.

The Role of the Older Americans Act

The purpose of the OAA is to provide the policy foundation and nationwide infrastructure to advance advocacy, planning, program design, and implementation for older adults (Takamura, 1999). Funding for the OAA direct service programs has not keep pace with the growth of the older adult population for many years, and new amendments expanding the role of the aging network have been added in recent years without an increase in overall funding (Kutza, 1991). It is unlikely that an increase in funding will be forthcoming. Therefore, some have called for a re-examination of the role of the OAA. Kutza has suggested that the OAA be restructured to reflect its strengths: its advocacy role on behalf of older adults, its role in meeting the nutritional needs of older adults, and its role in providing information and referral services. A restructuring of this nature would allow Area Agencies on Aging (AAAs) to concentrate their efforts on fewer services, rather than the multitude that they now cover. Another possible change in the Act could be to allow local AAAs more flexibility in determining what programs their communities need and, consequently, which are funded. More recently, the delegates at the 2005 White House Conference on Aging recommended expanding the role of the OAA and recommended that the Congress establish set authorization levels for all OAA programs throughout the authorization period of the Act by increasing authorization levels for all of the Titles in the OAA by a minimum of 25%, allowing flexibility and capability for local autonomy, ensuring necessary resources to adequately serve the projected growth in the number of older Americans, taking into consideration the growing ethnic and cultural diversity, and particularly the growing ranks of the "old-old"—those age 85 and over—who are the most frail, vulnerable, and in the greatest need of aging support services (2005, p. 31).

Related to how programs are structured and delivered, the WHCOA (2006) recommended that programs serving older adults:

Proactively realign and modernize . . . to be more efficient and effective in their performance, so as to free-up resources for unmet needs . . . such support has greatly served to enhance the quality of their lives. That support should be continued using more modern and integrated approaches. (2006, p. 22)

Reaching Out to the Private Sector

In the era of smaller budgets and greater needs, there has been a call for the aging network to expand its effort to work with the private sector to help meet the needs of older adults. A strong private sector presence currently exists in many areas of service delivery to older adults, including housing, long-term care, case management, transportation services, and recreational opportunities. With the increase in the number of older adults and an increase in the number of older adults who have adequate income, the role of the private sector in service delivery will become even greater. This increase in private sector involvement has several implications. First, the AAAs can increase their role in forging public–private partnerships to create employment opportunities and to create additional housing options (McConnel & Beitler, 1991). AAAs can also occupy leadership positions coordinating the services and programs offered by both the public and private sectors. Second, with the increase in the service options available because of private sector involvement, a central role of AAAs may be to act as a broker of services on behalf of older adults. As the choices for housing, health care, and other services become increasingly more complex, AAAs might become more actively involved in assisting older adults to make lifestyle choices that best fit their needs.

Who Should Be Eligible for Services?

There has been considerable debate about the universality of the OAA programs and services. As we discussed in Chapter 2, until recently OAA eligibility was determined to be adults 60 years of age and older regardless of their income, but specifically targeting low-income older adults and racial and ethnic minority elders. Again, because of the reduction in OAA funding and the need to extend its limited dollars to reach more people, the questions of who should be targeted to receive services and what cost, if any, participants should pay for those services have been posed and have influenced recent amendments to the Act.

Targeting Services

Through the years, the OAA has been amended so that it targets its services to those deemed to be most in need. The idea of redefining who should be targeted to receive services has once again emerged. Should the Act be revised to raise the age of eligibility? Should additional classes of individuals be targeted, such as those living in public-assisted housing, those living alone, or those who are at risk when discharged from the hospital (Administration on Aging [AoA], 1997b)? Ideally, identifying and targeting services to those most in need make programs more effective in assisting the most needy. The outcome of expanding the number of targeted groups of older adults at the exclusion of those who do not occupy those statuses is unclear.

It also has been proposed that the OAA should simply target its services to low-income individuals by developing financial eligibility standards for participation in its programs (see Gelfand & Bechill, 1991). Under the current provisions of the Act, programs and services are meant to serve those who have both economic and social need, but the Act does not yet use means-test cutoffs for programs and services (e.g, 150% poverty level income).

At first glance, establishing specific income-eligibility guidelines seems to be a reasonable solution to shrinking funding levels. There are, however, many issues to consider. Using income as a criterion for eligibility undermines the "social insurance" principle that has provided broad-based support for universal programs from a wide variety of constituencies (Hudson & Kingson, 1991). The inclusion of the middle class along with the lower class broadens the power base that helps protect the program from complete elimination. Moreover, the exclusion of older adults who have more social and financial resources than their less well-off counterparts might have a negative impact on program delivery. Many of these older adults play a key role in volunteering and assisting their less well-off counterparts. In addition, a means-based program might keep older adults from attending to avoid the social stigma attached to "welfare" programs. More important, the development of the definition of need requires a great deal of thought. Clearly, the most convenient definition of need is based on income or asset level. Aside from the concern that collecting financial information from its participants would create an additional level of bureaucracy and a paperwork nightmare, how will programs measure "social need"? How will programs measure the social need of persons for whom attending a congregate meal is their only source of social interaction? If they do not meet the income guidelines developed, are they any less needy?

On the other hand, there are some arguments for implementing income-eligibility criteria. First, insufficient resources force the need to target service to those least able to afford those services. Second, the collective plight of older adults was much worse when the OAA was enacted in 1965 than it is today. Thus, as social and economic conditions of older cohorts change, the OAA must respond in kind. Clearly, any change in the constituency the OAA serves would have to be carefully weighed against the advantages and disadvantages of changing the eligibility criteria.

Cost Sharing

Mandating cost sharing is another option that has been proposed as a way to make program dollars go farther. The 2006 amendments to the OAA included language that permitted the expansion of cost sharing for selected programs (see Chapter 2). Requiring cost sharing also has some advantages and disadvantages. In addition to covering program costs, cost sharing might promote a sense of equity among participants (see Chapter 3) and reduce their feelings of dependency. Evidence shows that cost sharing can be successful. Participants at congregate meal sites are asked to make a suggested donation that helps cover programmatic expenses. As we discussed in Chapter 10, participant contributions play an important role in supporting the congregate meal program. On the other hand, if programs are required to implement cost sharing as a condition of participation, they will spend a great deal of time and money on the task of collecting and managing paperwork, determining the cost-sharing amount, and collecting the fee from participants. A cost-sharing requirement also may keep the most needy from receiving services.

The discussion about creating financial eligibility guidelines or cost-sharing provisions would benefit from research that collects demographic characteristics of all OAA participants, including measures of income and social support, as well as the impact of cost sharing on service use and delivery. If most OAA programs serve primarily older adults with middle to low incomes or those with minimal social support networks, as data suggest the congregate meal programs do, to what extent would eligibility criteria be needed? How much could participants contribute before the contribution became a barrier? The debate about providing services based on need rather than age will no doubt continue.

SERVING A NEW GENERATION OF OLDER ADULTS: PLANNING FOR TWENTY-FIRST CENTURY AGING

We have attempted to illustrate in this text that policy is inextricably linked to the creation of programs which, in turn, directly support the physical, social, and psychological wellbeing of older adults. Thinking first about social policy at the federal, state, or local level, those working with older adults can advocate for positive changes in the way our communities can be "good places to grow up and grow old" (WHCOA, 2006, p. 58). The White House Conference on Aging recommended a new Title within the OAA called "Community Preparedness for an Aging Population" that would fund programs that help communities address the needs of an aging population. Specifically, it recommended that the new Title would create and fund programs that promote "community preparedness" for today and tomorrow's aging population. The new Title would support AAAs to be the liaison to help cities, counties, and tribal councils as well as the private/nonprofit sectors to address the needs of older adults in the areas of housing and transportation, health, human services, public safety, recreation, and workforce development. This is needed since every aspect of a community will be directly and dramatically impacted by an aging population. The goal is to ensure that America's communities are good places to grow up and grow old (2006, p. 58).

Although this suggestion was not included in the 2006 amendments to the OAA, it is reflective of the importance of the connections between policy, programs, and serving the needs of older adults. At the program delivery level, the challenge that aging professionals have always faced, and will continue to face, is how to change the way services are delivered to meet the needs of a new cohort in a new era As we discussed in Chapter 1, the new cohort—the baby boomers—is different in a number of ways. But what about the new era that will emerge in the next century? We will experience societal changes related to the way we interact with one another and the way we do business. Consider the influence technology has had on our lives and will have in the future. Computer technology has made it possible to access information almost immediately (did you notice the number of online resources we accessed in writing this text?), and through chat rooms and discussion lists we now are able to make contact with people previously unknown to us. Assistive technology also holds great promise in helping people of all ages with various functional limitations to live more independently in our communities. The central role that technology now occupies in our lives will challenge professionals to consider ways to use technology in meeting the social, psychological, and physical needs of older adults. How can technology be used to deliver services? To provide information and referral? To reach those who are socially isolated?

A new era will also bring about changes in how we define and redefine what it means to be old. Former president George Bush, at age 73, jumped from an airplane (with a parachute, of course!). A 63-year-old woman gave birth to a child. These are not the activities that come to mind when thinking about the normative behaviors of older adults! Although these activities are not reflective of the behaviors of most older adults, perhaps the importance of these behaviors lies in their symbolism. They make us rethink what we can and cannot do in our old age.

A new era will also give us an opportunity to redefine the timing of our entry into life course transitions (Atchley, 1997). For example, the timing of entering and leaving the workforce, of entering into lifelong partnerships and having children, and of pursuing educational opportunities is changing. How will the aging network respond to these changes? Our challenge will be to make sure that the programs and services we offer to older adults will evolve along with the social changes we encounter in the coming years.

> We should not approach the challenge of aging with fear and apprehension, but rather with creative foresight, optimism, and a sense of determination. (WHCOA, 2005, p. 23)

References

Abend-Wein, M. (1991). Medicaid's effect on the elderly: How reimbursement policy affects priority in the nursing home. *Journal of Applied Gerontology, 10*(1), 71–87.

Abrahams, R., Nonnenkamp, L., Dunn, S., Mehta, S., & Woodard, P. (1988). Case management in the social/health maintenance organization. *Generations, 12*(5), 39–43.

Abramson, T. A., Trejo, L., & Lai, D. W. L. (2002). Culture and mental health: Providing appropriate services for a diverse older population. *Generations, 16*(1), 21–27.

ACTION. (1990a). *Foster Grandparent Program 25th anniversary 1965–1990: Bridging the generations of need.* Washington, DC: ACTION.

ACTION. (1990b). *Senior Companion Program: Serving with compassion, caring as friends.* Washington, DC: ACTION.

ACTION. (1992). *Retired Senior Volunteer Program: A part of ACTION.* Washington, DC: ACTION.

Adams, J. S. (1965). Inequity in social exchange. In L. Berkowitz (Ed.), *Advances in experimental social psychology, Vol. 2* (pp. 267–300). New York: Academic Press.

Adams, P. F., Hendershot, G. E., & Marano, M. A. (1999). *Current estimates from the National Health Interview Survey, 1996. National Center for Health Statistics. Vital Health Statistics 10*(200). Retrieved July 2, 2001 from www.cdc.gov/nchs/data/series/sr_10/sr10_200.pdf.

Aday, R. H. (2003). *Identifying important linkages between successful aging and senior center participation.* Retrieved June 18, 2006 from www.aoa.gov/prof/agingnet/Seniorcenters/NISC.pdf.

Adler, G., Kuskowski, M. A., & Mortimer, J. (1995). Respite use in dementia patients. *Clinical Gerontologist, 15*(3), 17–30.

Administration on Aging (AoA). (n.d.). *FY 2004 profile of United States OAA Program.* Retrieved January 1, 2007 from www.aoa.gov/prof/agingnet/NAPIS/SPR/2004SPR/profiles/US.pdf.

Administration on Aging. (n.d.). *Latest news: President's council on physical fitness and sports 50th anniversary partner invitation to get America moving.* Retrieved January 29, 2007 from www.aoa.gov/youcan/news/news_pf.asp.

Administration on Aging. (1983). *An evaluation of the nutritional services for the elderly: Vol. 3. Descriptive report* (OHDS Pub. No. 83–20917). Washington, DC: Government Printing Office.

Administration on Aging. (1995a, January). *Elder facts: The Administration on Aging.* Washington, DC: AoA.

Administration on Aging. (1995b). *Long-term care ombudsman annual report: Fiscal year 1995.* Washington, DC: AoA.

Administration on Aging. (1995c). *Title III state and community programs.* Retrieved July 30, 2001 from www.aoa.dhhs.gov/aoa/pages/titleiii.html.

Administration on Aging. (1997a). *Resource centers.* Retrieved July 10, 2001 from www.aoa.dhhs.gov.

Administration on Aging. (1997b). *Targeting of Older Americans Act services: Issues for reauthorization.* Washington, DC: AoA.

Administration on Aging. (1998). *The National Elder Abuse Incidence Study; Final report.* Retrieved July 15, 2001 from www.aoa.dhhs.gov/abuse/report.

Administration on Aging. (2000). *AoA awards $1 million to help end health disparities among older racial and ethnic minority populations.* Retrieved September 16, 2001 from www.aoa.dhhs.gov/pr/Pr2000/healthdisparities.html.

Administration on Aging. (2001a). *Achieving cultural competence: A guidebook for providers of services to older Americans and their families.* Retrieved January 22, 2007 from www.aoa.gov/prof/adddiv/cultural/CC-guidebook.pdf.

Administration on Aging. (2001b). *Frequently asked questions about the Older Americans Act Amendments of 2000.* Retrieved August 13, 2001 from www.aoa.dhhs.gov/oaa/status/faq.html.

Administration on Aging. (2001c). *1998 state performance reports.* Retrieved August 1, 2001 from www.aoa.dhhs.gov/napis/98spr/tables/tables1.html.

Administration on Aging. (2001d). *Older adults and mental health: Issues and opportunities.* Retrieved January 25, 2002 from www.aoa.dhhs.gov/mh/report2001/default.htm.

Administration on Aging. (2001e). *Older Americans Act appropriation information.* Retrieved August 13, 2001 from www.aoa.dhhs.gov/Oaa/oaaapp.html.

Administration on Aging. (2001f). *Profile of older Americans: 2000.* Retrieved December 12, 2000, from www.aoa.gov/aoa/stats/profile.

Administration on Aging. (2002a). *Focal points and senior centers: FY 2000.* Retrieved on June 18, 2006 from www.aoa.gov/prof/agingnet/Seniorcenters/Senior%20Center%20Research.pdf.

Administration on Aging. (2002b). *FY 2000 profile of United States OAA programs.* Retrieved November 21, 2006 from www.aoa.gov/prof/agingnet/NAPIS/2000SPR/profiles/US.pdf.

Administration on Aging. (2003a). *Administration on Aging Nutrition Services Incentive Program frequently asked questions.* Retrieved January 1, 2007 from www.aoa.gov/eldfam/Nutrition/NSIP%20FreqAskedQs%20fb%2007%2003rev.pdf.

Administration on Aging. (2003b). *Administration on Aging: Fact sheet, evidenced-based disease prevention program. U.S. Department of Health and Human Services.* Retrieved January 27, 2007 from www.aoa.gov/press/fact/pdf/fs_EvidenceBased.pdf.

Administration on Aging. (2004a). *AoA Grant Programs. Compendium of active grants under Title IV of the Older Americans Act. Fiscal year 2004.* Retrieved February 25, 2007 from www.aoa.gov/doingbus/comp/comp.asp.

Administration on Aging. (2004b). *American Indian, Alaska Native, and Native Hawaiian Program.* Retrieved January 2, 2007 from www.aoa.gov/press/fact/alpha/fact_ain.asp.

Administration on Aging. (2004c). *Guidelines for culturally and/or linguistically competent agencies.* Retrieved January 22, 2007, from www.aoa.gov/prof/adddiv/progmod/addiv_progmod_section_two.asp.

Administration on Aging. (2004d). *The Older Americans Act National Family Caregiver Support Program: Compassion in action.* Retrieved January 2, 2007 from www.aoa.gov/prof/aoaprog/care giver/care-prof/progguidance/resources/FINAL%20NFCSP%20Report%20July22,%202004.pdf.

Administration on Aging. (2004e). *LTC Ombudsman report FY 2004. U.S. Administration on Aging, Department of Health and Human Services,* Washington, DC. Retrieved February 13, 2007 from www.aoa.gov/prof/aoaprog/elder_rights/LTCombudsman/National_and_State_Data/national_and_state_data.asp.

Administration on Aging. (2005a). *A profile of older Americans: 2005.* Retrieved January 5, 2007 from www.aoa.gov/PROF/Statistics/profile/2005/2005profile.pdf.

Administration on Aging. (2005b). *2005 National Ombudsman Reporting System Data Tables, Top 20 complaints by category for nursing facilities (FFY 1996–2005),* Retrieved February 13, 2007 from www.aoa.gov/prof/aoaprog/elder_rights/LTCombudsman/National_and_State_Data/2005nors/200 5%20NF%20top20.xls.

Administration on Aging. (2005c). *2005 National Ombudsman Reporting System Data Tables, Top 20 complaints by category for board and care facilities (FFY 1996–2005).* Retrieved February 13, 2007 from www.aoa.gov/prof/aoaprog/elder_rights/LTCombudsman/National_and_State_Data/2005nors/2005%20BC%20top20.xls.

Administration on Aging. (2006a). *Older Americans Act cost sharing provisions OAA Section 315(a).* Retrieved February 13, 2007 from www.aoa.gov/about/legbudg/oaa/Cost%20Sharing%20statute.doc.

Administration on Aging. (2006b). *Administration on Aging Reauthorization of the Older Americans Act technical clarifying amendments.* Retrieved February 13, 2007 from www.aoa.gov/about/legbudg/oaa/eNews_Technical_Amendments.doc.

Administration on Aging. (2006c). *FY 2006 Appropriation.* Retrieved January 7, 2007 from www.aoa.gov/about/legbudg/current_budg/legbudg_current_budg.asp.

Administration on Aging. (2006d). *FY 2006 Appropriation.* Retrieved January 28, 2007 from www.aoa.gov/about/legbudg/current_budg/legbudg_current_budg.asp.

Administration on Aging. (2006e). *Evidence based disease prevention grants program.* Retrieved January 23, 2007 from www.aoa.gov/prof/evidence/evidence.asp.

Administration on Aging. (2006f). *FY 2004 profile of United States OAA Program.* Retrieved November 17, 2006 from www.aoa.gov/prof/agingnet/NAPIS/SPR/2004SPR/tables/2004tables.asp.

Administration on Aging. (2006g). *Title VII—Allotments for vulnerable elder rights protection activities: FY 2006 annual allocation.* Retrieved January 9, 2007 from www.aoa.gov/about/legbudg/current_budg/docs/AoA%20FY%202008%20CJ%20Final.pdf.

Administration on Aging. (2007). *Justification of estimates for appropriations committees.* Retrieved February 25, 2007 from www.aoa.gov/about/legbudg/current_budg/docs/AoA%20FY%202008%20CJ%20Final.pdf.

Age Discrimination in Employment Act of 1967, 29 U.S.C. § 621 et seq. (1967), as amended 1986.

Aiken, L. H. (1989). An agenda for the year 2000. In M. D. Mezey, J. E. Lynaugh, & M. M. Cartier (Eds.), *Nursing homes and nursing care: Lessons from the teaching nursing homes* (pp. 145–156). New York: Springer.

Akkerman, R. L., & Ostwald, S. K. (2004). Reducing anxiety in Alzheimer's disease family caregivers: The effectiveness of a nine-week cognitive-behavioral intervention. *American Journal of Alzheimer's Disease and Other Dementias, 19,* 117–123.

Alegria, F. (1992). *A guide to state-level policies, practices, and procedures: Enhancing employment opportunities for older workers.* Washington, DC: National Governors' Association.

Alexander, G. J. (1991). Time for a new law on health care advanced directives. *Hastings Law Journal, 42,* 755–778.

Alliance of Information and Referral Systems [AIRS] (2005). *Standards for professional information and referral.* (5th ed.). Retrieved January 15, 2007 from www.airs.org/documents/StandardsFifthEdition.pdf.

Alliance of Information and Referral Systems [AIRS] (2007). *2-1-1 Initiative, I&R/A: the Birthplace of 2-1-1.* Retrieved January 15, 2007 from www.airs.org/lookingfor211.asp.

Allen, J. E. (1987). *Nursing home administration.* New York: Springer.

Amborgi, D. M., & Leonard, F. (1988). The impact of nursing home admission agreements on resident autonomy. *The Gerontologist, 28*(Suppl.), 82–89.

American Association of Homes and Services for the Aging (1988). *Directory of members.* Washington, DC: AAHSA.

American Association of Homes and Services for the Aging (2001a). *Continuing care retirement communities.* Retrieved May 11, 2001 from www.aahsa.org/public/ ccrcbkgd.htm.

American Association of Homes and Services for the Aging (2001b). *Federally subsidized housing for the elderly.* Retrieved May 11, 2001 from www.aahsa.org/public/housebkgd.htm.

American Association of Homes and Services for the Aging (2006). *Aging services in America: The facts.* Retrieved December 31, 2006 from www.aahsa.org/aging_services/default.asp.

American Association of Retired Persons. (n.d.). *Long term care insurance.* Retrieved January 2, 2007 from www.aarp.org/money/financial_planning/sessionfive/longterm_care_insurance.html.

American Association of Retired Persons. (1985). *The right place at the right time: A guide to long-term care choices.* Washington, DC: AARP.

American Association of Retired Persons. (1990). *Nursing home life: A guide for residents and family.* Washington, DC: AARP.

American Association of Retired Persons. (1992). *Understanding senior housing for the 1990s: An American Association of Retired Persons survey on consumer preferences, concerns, and needs.* Washington, DC: AARP.

American Association of Retired Persons. (1994). *Connecting the generations: A guide to intergenerational resources.* Washington, DC: AARP.

American Association of Retired Persons. (1999). *Assisted living in the United States: Public Policy Institute fact sheet.* Washington, DC: AARP.

American Association of Retired Persons. (2001). *In the middle: A report on multicultural boomers coping with family and aging issues.* Washington, DC: AARP.

American Association of Retired Persons. (2003). *Time and money: An in-depth look at 45 + volunteers and donors.* Retrieved December 19, 2006, from http://assets.aarp.org/rgcenter/general/multic_2003.pdf.

American Association of Retired Persons. (2004). *Continuing Care Retirement Communities (CCRC).* Retrieved January 9, 2007 from www.aarp.org/families/housing_choices/other_options/a2004-02-26-retirementcommunity.html.

American Association of Retired Persons. (2005a). *Reimaging America: AARP's blueprint for the future.* Washington, DC: AARP.

America Association of Retired Persons. (2005b). *Beyond 50.05: A report to the nation on livable communities creating environments for successful aging.* Retrieved August 11, 2006 from http://assets.aarp.org/rgcenter/il/beyond_50_communities.pdf.

American Association of Retired Persons. (2006). *We can do better: Lessons learned from protecting older persons in disasters.* Retrieved March 3, 2007 from http://assets.aarp.org/rgcenter/il/better.pdf.

American Association of Retired Persons. (2007). *Medicare prescription drug coverage.* Retrieved February 1, 2007 from www.aarp.org/health/medicare/drug_coverage/how_much_will_medicare_prescription_drug_coverage.html.

American Association of Retired Persons Foundation. (2006). Senior legal hotlines annual report 2005. Available at www.legalhotlines.org/standards/files/senior_hotline_annual_report_2005.doc.

America's Health Insurance Plans. (2004a). *Guide to long term care insurance*. Retrieved January 19, 2007 from www.pueblo.gsa.gov/cic_text/health/ltc/guide.pdf.

America's Health Insurance Plans. (2004b). *Research findings: Long term care insurance in 2002*. Retrieved January 19, 2007 from www.ahipresearch.org/pdfs/18_LTC2002.pdf.

American Psychological Association. (2002). *Guidelines on multi-cultural education, training, research, practice, and organizational change for psychologists*. Washington, DC: APA.

American Public Human Services Association. (1998). *The National Elder Abuse Incidence Study, 1998*. The National Center on Elder Abuse at The American Public Human Services Association, Washington, DC. Available at www.aoa.gov/eldfam/Elder_Rights/Elder_Abuse/AbuseReport_Full.pdf.

American Public Transportation Association. (2003). *Mobility for the aging population*. Retrieved October 15, 2006 from www.apta.com/research/info/online/aging.cfm.

American Public Transportation Association. (2005). *Safe, accountable, flexible, efficient transportation equity act—a legacy for users*. Retrieved October 9, 2006 from www.apta.com/government_affairs/safetea_lu/documents/brochure/pdf.

America's Second Harvest. (2001). *Hunger in America, 2001*. Retrieved January 10, 2007 from www.hungerinamerica.org.

Americans With Disabilities Act, 42 U.S.C. § 12101 et seq. (1990).

Anderson, R. (1995). Revisiting the behavioral model and access to medical care: Does it matter? *Journal of Health and Social Behavior, 36*, 1–10.

Anderson, R., & Newman, J. (1973). Societal and individual determinants of medical care utilization in the United States. *Milbank Memorial Fund Quarterly, 51*, 95–124.

Anderson, S. A. (1990). Core indicators of nutritional state for difficult-to-sample populations. *Journal of Nutrition, 120*, 11S, 1557–1600.

Angelis, J. (1990). *Intergenerational service learning: Strategies for the future*. Carbondale, IL: Author.

Applebaum, R., & Wilson, N. (1988). Training needs for providing case management for the long-term care client: Lessons learned from the National Channeling Demonstration. *The Gerontologist, 28*, 172–176.

Area Agency on Aging of Northwest Arkansas. (2006). *Transportation services*. Retrieved November 15, 2006 from www.aaanwar.org/resource_directory/sub_directory/transportation_services.htm.

Armstrong, F. (2005, November). *Measuring volatility and the cost of retirement. The CPA Journal Online*. Retrieved January 23, 2007 from www.nysscpa.org/cpajournal/2005/1105/perspectives/p10.htm.

Armstrong G. K. & Morgan K. (1998). Stability and change in levels of habitual physical activity in later life. *Age & Ageing, 27*(3), 17–23.

Arneson, B. (1994). State and federal legislation: Nonmedical homecare services. In J. Handy & C. Schuerman (Eds.), *Challenges and innovations in homecare* (pp. 53–55). San Francisco: American Society on Aging.

Arnsberger, P. (2005). Best practices in care management for Asian American elders: The care of Alzheimer's disease. *Care Management Journals, 6*, 171–177.

Arterburn, D. E., Crane, P. K., & Sullivan, S. D. (2004). The coming epidemic of obesity in elderly Americans. *Journal of the American Geriatric Society, 52*, 11, 1907–1912.

Arora, N. S., & Rochester, D. V. (1982). Respiratory muscle strength and maximal voluntary ventilation in undernourished patients. *American Review of Respiratory Diseases, 126*, 5–8.

Ashford, N., Bell, W. G., & Rich, T. A. (1982). *Mobility and transport for elderly and handicapped persons: Proceedings of a conference held at Churchill College, Cambridge, UK, July 1981.* New York: Gordon & Breach Science.

Atchley, R. (1971). Retirement and leisure participation: Continuity or crisis? *The Gerontologist, 11,* 13–17.

Atchley, R. (1989). A continuity theory of normal aging. *The Gerontologist, 29,* 183–190.

Atchley, R. (1997). *Social forces and aging: An introduction to social gerontology* (8th ed.). Belmont, CA: Wadsworth.

Austin, C. (1996). Aging and long-term care. In C. Austin & R. McClelland (Eds.), *Perspectives on case management practice* (pp. 73–98). Milwaukee, WI: Families International.

Baer, D. (1998). *Awareness and Popularity of Property Tax Relief Programs. Research Report. AARP Public Policy Institute.* Retrieved January 1, 2007 from http://assets.aarp.org/rgcenter/econ/9803_tax.pdf.

Bailey, L. (2004). *Aging Americans: Stranded without transportation. Surface Transportation Policy Project.* Retrieved October 23, 2006 from www.apta.com/research/info/online/documents/aging_stranded.pdf.

Balsam, A., & Osteraas, G. (1987). Instituting a continuum of community nutrition services: Massachusetts elderly nutrition programs. *Journal of Nutrition for the Elderly, 6*(4), 51–67.

Balsam, A. L., & Rogers, B. L. (1988). *Service innovations in the elderly nutrition program: Strategies for meeting unmet needs.* Medford, MA: Tufts University School of Nutrition.

Balsam, A. L., & Rogers, B. L. (1991). Serving elders in greatest social and economic need: The challenge to the elderly nutrition program. *Journal of Aging and Social Policy, 3*(1/2), 41–55.

Banaszak-Holl, J., & Hines, M. A. (1994, November). Organizational antecedents of nursing home staff turnover. Paper presented at the annual meeting of the Gerontological Society of America, Atlanta, GA.

Bane, S. (1992). Rural caregiving. *Rural Elderly Networker, 3,* 1–6.

Bane, S. D., Rathbone-McCuan, E., & Galliher, J. (1994). Mental health services for the elderly in rural America. In J. Krout (Ed.), *Providing community-based services to the rural elderly* (pp. 243–266). Thousand Oaks, CA: Sage.

Barocas, V. (1994). *Rethinking retirement income.* New York: Conference Board.

Barrett, A. (2006). *Characteristics of Food Stamp household: Fiscal year 2005. Report submitted to the U.S. Department of Agriculture, Food and Nutrition Service.* Washington, DC: Mathematica Policy Research, September 2006. Retrieved January 7, 2007 from www.fns.usda.gov/oane.

Bartels, S. J., Forester, B., Miles, K. M., & Joyce, T. (2000). Mental health service use by elderly patients with bipolar disorder and unipolar major depression. *American Journal of Geriatric Psychiatry, 8*(2), 160–166.

Bass, S. (1992). Gerontology program succeeds in Boston. *Adult Learning, 3,* 22–23.

Bazelon Center. (2000). *Older mental health consumers create new advocacy group.* Retrieved January 25, 2002 from www.webcom.com/bazelon/ourownvoice.html.

Bechill, W. (1992). At age 27, the Older Americans Act needs spirited advocacy, understanding. *Perspective on Aging, 21,* 9–11.

Bedford, V. H. (1989). Understanding the value of siblings in old age: A proposed model. *American Behavioral Scientist, 33,* 33–44.

Bedient, D., Snyder, V., & Simon, M. (1992). Retirees mentoring at-risk college students. *Phi Delta Kappan, 73,* 462–463, 466.

Belloc, N., & Breslow, L. (1972). Relationship of physical health status and health practices. *Preventive Medicine, 1*, 409–421.

Belza, B., Shumway-Cook, A., Phelan, E., Williams, B., Snyder, S., & LoGerfo, J. P. (2006). The effects of a community-based exercise program on function and health in older adults: the EnhanceFitness Program. *Journal of Applied Gerontology, 25*(4): 291–306.

Benitez-Silva, H., & Heiland, F. (2006). *The Social Security earnings test and work incentives*. Retrieved January 24, 2007 from http://ms.cc.sunysb.edu/ ~ hbenitezsilv/policy.pdf.

Berry, G., Zarit, S., & Rabatin, V. (1991). Caregiver activity on respite and nonrespite days: A comparison of two service approaches. *The Gerontologist, 31*, 830–835.

Biegel, D., Sales, E., & Schultz, R. (1991). *Family caregiving in chronic illness*. Newbury Park, CA: Sage.

Bild, B. R., & Havingurst, R. J. (1976). Senior citizens in great cities: The case of Chicago. *The Gerontologist, 16*(1, Pt. 2), 3–88.

Binney, E., Estes, C., & Ingman, S. (1990). Medicalization, public policy and the elderly: Social services in jeopardy? *Social Science and Medicine, 30*, 761–771.

Black, B. S., Rabins, P. V., German, P., McGuire, M., & Roca, R. (1997). Need and unmet need for mental health care among elderly public housing residents. *The Gerontologist, 37*, 717–728.

Blazer, D. (1994). Epidemiology of late-life depression. In L. S. Schneider, C. F. Reynolds, B. D. Lebowitz, & A. J. Friedhoff (Eds.), *Diagnosis and treatment of depression in late life* (pp. 9–20). Washington, DC: American Psychiatric Press.

Blazer, D. G. (2003). Depression in late life: Review and commentary. *Journal of Gerontology: Medical Sciences, 58*, M249–M265.

Blieszner, R., Roberto, K. A., Wilcox, K. L., Barham, E. J., & Winston, B. L. (2007). Dimensions of ambiguous loss in couples coping with mild cognitive impairment. *Family Relations, 56*, 196–209.

B'nai B'rith (1997). *B'nai B'rith senior housing: An overview*. Retrieved January 25, 2002 from www.bnaibrith.org/sch/over.html.

Bond, J. T., Thompson, C., Galinsky, E., & Prottas, D. (2002). *The national study of the changing workforce: Families and Work Institute*. Retrieved January 25, 2007 from www.familiesandwork.org/announce/2002NSCW.html.

Boondas, J. (1991). Nursing home resident assessment classification and focused care. *Nursing and Health Care, 12*, 308–312.

Borrayo, E. A., Salmon, J. R., Polivka, L., & Dunlap, B. D. (2002). Utilization across the continuum of long-term care services. *The Gerontologist, 42*, 603–612.

Bourgeois, M. S., Schulz, R., & Burgio, L. (1996). Interventions for caregivers of patients with Alzheimer's disease: A review and analysis of content, process, and outcomes. *International Journal of Aging and Human Development, 43*, 35–92.

Bowen, D. J., Andersen, M. R., & Urban, N. (2000). Volunteerism in a community-based sample of women aged 50 to 80 years. *Journal of Applied Social Psychology, 30*, 1829–1842.

Bowers, B. J. (1988). Family perceptions of care in a nursing home. *The Gerontologist, 27*, 4–8.

Bowman, K. W., & Singer, P. A. (2001). Chinese seniors' perspectives on end-of-life decisions. *Social Sciences & Medicine, 53*, 455–464.

Brabazon, K., & Disch, R. (Eds.). (1997). *Intergenerational approaches in aging: Implications for education, policy and practice*. New York: Haworth.

Bratter, B., & Freeman, E. (1990). The maturing of peer counseling. *Generations, 14*(1), 49–52.

Brawley, L. R., Rejeski, W. J. & King, A. C. (2003). Promoting physical activity for older adults: The challenges for changing behavior. *American Journal of Preventive Medicine, 25*(3Sii), 172–183.

Brehm, J. W. (1966). *A theory of psychological reactance.* New York: Academic Press.

Brehm, S. S., & Brehm, J.W. (1981). *Psychological reactance: A theory of freedom and control.* New York: Academic Press.

Briggs, E. (1992). *Nutrition and the black elderly.* San Diego, CA: San Diego State University, National Resource Center on Minority Aging Populations.

Bright, K. (2005). *Section 202 supportive housing for the elderly. AAAP Public Policy Institute.* Retrieved December 28, 2006, from http://assets.aarp.org/rgcenter/il/fs65r_housing.pdf.

Brigl, B. (2001). *Testimony to the Commission on Affordable Housing and Health Facility Needs for Seniors in the 21st Century.* Retrieved January 11, 2007 from http://govinfo.library.unt.edu/seniorscommission/pages/hearings/011107/brignl.html.

Brody, E. M. (1981).Women in the middle and family help to older people. *The Gerontologist, 21,* 471–480.

Brody, E. M. (1985). Parent care as a normative family stress. *The Gerontologist, 25,* 19–29.

Brotman, S., Ryan, B., & Cormier, R. (2003). The health and service needs of gay and lesbian elders and their families in Canada. *The Gerontologist, 43,* 192–202.

Brown, J., Hassett, K., & Smetters, K. (2005). *Top ten myths of social security reform.* Retrieved January 26, 2007 from www.bc.edu/centers/crr/papers/wp_2005–11.pdf.

Brown, R. (1989). *The rights of older persons* (2nd ed.). Carbondale: Southern Illinois University Press.

Brubaker, T., & Roberto, K. A. (1993). Family life education for the later years. *Family Relations, 42,* 212–221.

Bryant, L. J. (2001). *The coming of age. Research and creative activity.* Retrieved January 7, 2007, from www.indiana.edu/ ~ rcapub/v24n2/p20.html.

Bryant, L. L, Altpeter, M., & Whitelaw, N. A. (2006). Evaluation of health promotion programs for older adults: An introduction. *The Journal of Applied Gerontology, 25*(3), 197–213.

Buchanan, R. J., Choi, M., Wang, S., Hysunsu, J., and Graber, D. (2005). Nursing home residents with Alzheimer's disease in special care units compare to other residents with Alzheimer's disease. *Dementia, 4*(2), 249–267.

Buchner, D. M., & Pearson, D. C. (1989). Factors associated with participation in a community senior health promotion program: A pilot study. *American Journal of Public Health, 79,* 775–777.

Buchner, D. M., Cress, M. E., de Lateur, B. J. et al. (1997). The effect of strength and endurance training on gait, balance, fall risk, and health services use in community-living older adults. *Journal of Gerontology: Medical Sciences, 52A,* M218–224.

Buelow, J., & Conrad, K. (1992). Assessing the influence of adult day care on client satisfaction. *Journal of Health and Aging, 4,* 303–321.

Burger, S. G., Fraser, V., Hunt, S., & Frank, B. (1996). *Nursing homes: Getting good care there.* San Luis Obispo, CA: Impact.

Burkhardt, J. (2005). *Seniors benefit from transportation coordination partnerships—a toolbox: Promising practices from the aging network. Report submitted to the Administration on Aging,* Washington, DC: WESTAT, September 2005. Retrieved October 23, 2006 from www.aoa.gov/prof/transportation/transportation.asp.

Burman, L. E. (2004). *Distributional effects of defined contribution plans and individual retirement arrangements. National Tax Journal.* Retrieved January 26, 2007 from http://goliath.ecnext.com/coms2/summary_0199-894088_ITM.

Burnette, D. (1999). Custodial grandparents in Latino families: Patterns of service use and predictors of unmet needs. *Social Work, 44*(1), 22–34.

Cahill, S., South, K., & Spade, J. (2000). *Outing age: Public policy issues affecting gay, lesbian, bisexual and transgender elders. National Gay and Lesbian Task Force.* Retrieved November 1, 2006 from www.thetaskforce.org/downloads/reports/reports/OutingAge.pdf.

Cain, M. (1996). Health maintenance organizations. In L. A. Vitt, J. K. Siegenthaler, N. E. Culter, & S. Golant (Eds.), *Encyclopedia of financial gerontology* (pp. 243–248). Westport, CT: Greenwood.

Calsyn, R. J., Burger, G. K., and Roades, L. A. (1996). Cross-validation of differences between users and non-users of senior centers. *Journal of Social Service Research, 21,* 3, 39–56.

Calsyn, R. J., & Winter, J. P. (1999). Who attends senior centers? *Journal of Social Service Research, 26*(2), 53–69.

Calsyn, R. J., & Winter, J. P. (2001). Predicting four types of service needs in older adults. *Evaluation and Program Planning, 24,* 157–166.

Cantor, M. H. (1979). Neighbors and friends: An overlooked resource in the informal support system. *Research on Aging, 1,* 434–463.

Cantor, M. H. (1983). Strain among caregivers: A study of experience in the United States. *The Gerontologist, 23,* 597–604.

Cantor, M. H. (1991). Family and community: Changing roles in an aging society. *The Gerontologist, 31,* 337–346.

Capretta, J. (2007). *Long-term care insurance partnerships: New choices for consumers—potential savings for federal and state government. AHIP Center for Policy and Research, January 2007.* Retrieved February 2, 2007 from www.ahipresearch.org/PDFs/IssueBriefSavingsfromExpandedLTC Partnerships1–24–2007.pdf.

Carder, P., Morgan, L. A., & Eckert, K. J. (2006). Small board-and-care homes in the age of assisted living. *Generations, 29*(4), 24–31.

Carlton-LaNey, I. (1991). Some considerations of the rural elderly blacks' underuse of social services. *Journal of Gerontological Social Work, 16,* 3–16.

Caro, F., & Bass, S. (1995). Increasing volunteering among older people. In S. Bass (Ed.), *Older and active: How Americans over 55 are contributing to society* (pp. 71–96). New Haven, CT: Yale University Press.

Carter, W. B., Elward, E., Malmgren, J., Martin, M., & Larson, E. (1991). Participation in health promotion programs and research: A critical review of the literature. *The Gerontologist, 31,* 584–592.

Castle, N. G., & Engberg, J. (2006). Organizational Characteristics Associated With Staff Turnover in Nursing Homes. *The Gerontologist, 46,* 62–73.

Castner, L. (2000). *Trends in Food Stamp participation rates: Focus on 1994 to 1998. Report submitted to the U.S. Department of Agriculture, Food and Nutrition Service.* Washington, DC: Mathematica Policy Research, November 2000

Catalano, S. M. (2006). Criminal victimization, 2005. *Bureau of Justice Statistics Bulletin.* U.S. Department of Justice. Washington, DC. Available at www.ojp.usdoj.gov/bjs/pub/pdf/cv05.pdf.

Centaur Associates. (1986). *Report on the 502(e) experimental projects funded under Title V of the Older Americans Act.* Washington, DC: Author.

Center for Mental Health Services. (2004). *Community integration for older adults with mental illnesses: Overcoming barriers and seizing opportunities.* DHHS Pub. No. (SMA) 05–4018. Retrieved March 1, 2007 from www.mentalhealth.samhsa.gov/media/ken/pdf/SMA05–4018/OlderAdults.pdf.

Center for Mental Health Services. (2007). *2005 CMHS Uniform Reporting System (URS) Tables: Mental Health National Outcome Measures*. Retrieved January 23, 2007 from http://download.ncadi .samhsa.gov/ken/pdf/URS_Data05/VA.pdf.

Center on an Aging Society. (2004). *Cultural competence in health care*. Retrieved January 19, 2007 from http://hpi.georgetown.edu/agingsociety/pdfs/cultural.pdf.

Center on an Aging Society. (2005a). *Adult children: The likelihood of providing care for an older parent*. Retrieved June 9, 2006 from http://ihcrp.georgetown.edu/agingsociety/pdfs/CAREGIVERS2.pdf.

Center on an Aging Society. (2005b). *Caregiving and paid work: Are there trade-offs?* Retrieved August 8, 2006 from http://ihcrp.georgetown.edu/agingsociety/pdfs/CAREGIVERS4.pdf.

Centers for Disease Control. (2001). *Basic statistics: Cumulative AIDS cases*. Retrieved August 30, 2001 from www.cdc.gov/hiv/stats.

Centers for Medicare and Medicaid Services [CMS]. (n.d.). *Medicare enrollment: National trends 1966–2005*. Retrieved February 21, 2007 from www.cms.hhs.gov/MedicareEnRpts/Downloads/ HISMI05.pdf.

Centers for Medicare and Medicaid Services. (2003). *Home health quality initiative*. Retrieved January 2, 2007 from www.cms.hhs.gov/HomeHealthQualityInits/downloads/HHQIOverview.pdf.

Centers for Medicare and Medicaid Services. (2004). *Program information on Medicaid and State Children's Health Insurance Program (SCHIP)*. Retrieved January 23, 2007 from www.cms.hhs.gov/ TheChartSeries/downloads/Medicaid_prog_info_pdf.

Centers for Medicare and Medicaid Services. (2005a). *Medicaid at-a-glance 2005: A Medicaid information source. Department of Health and Human Services*. Retrieved January 22, 2007 from www.cms.hhs.gov/MedicaidGenInfo/Downloads/MedicaidAtAGlance.pdf.

Centers for Medicare and Medicaid Services. (2005b). *2005 Medicare managed care enrollment report: Summary statistics as of June 30, 2005*. Retrieved January 22, 2007 from www.cms.hss.gov/ MedicaidDataSourcesGenInfo/Downloads/mmcer05.pdf.

Centers for Medicare and Medicaid Services. (2006). *Nursing home data compendium*. Retrieved February 7, 2007 from www.cms.hhs.gov/CertificationandComplianc/12_NHs.asp.

Centers for Medicare and Medicaid Services. (2007). *Medicare and you*. Retrieved January 22, 2007 from www.medicare.gov/publications/pubs/pdf/10050.pdf.

Chandra, R. K. (1992). Effect of vitamin and trace-element supplementation on immune responses and infection in elderly subjects. *Lancet, 340*, 1124–1127.

Chapman, N. J., & Howe, D. A. (2001). Accessory apartments: Are they a realistic alternative for ageing in place. *Housing Studies, 16*, 637–650.

Chappell, N. L., & Blandford, A. A. (1987). Health service utilization by elderly persons. *Canadian Journal of Sociology, 12*(3), 195–215.

Chappell, N. L., and Reid, R. C. (2000). Dimensions of care of dementia sufferers in long-term care institutions: Are they related to outcomes? *Journal of Gerontology: Social Sciences, 55B*(4), S234–S244.

Chelimsky, E. (1991). *Older Americans Act: Promising practice in information and referral services*. Washington, DC: Government Printing Office.

Chernoff, R. (2001). Nutrition and health promotion in older adults. *Journals of Gerontology, 56A*, 47–53.

Cherry, R., Prebis, J., & Pick, V. (1995). Service directories: Reinvigorating community resource for self-care. *The Gerontologist, 35*, 560–563.

Chicago Department on Aging, National Council on the Aging, and Washington Business Group on Health. (1992). *Public/private partnerships: Examples from the aging network.* Washington, DC: National Eldercare Institute on Business and Aging.

Choi, N. G. (1999). Determinants of frail elders' length of stay in Meals on Wheels. *The Gerontologist, 39,* 4, 397–404.

Christianson, J. B., Warrick, L. H., Netting, F. E., Williams, F. G., Read, W., & Murphy, J. (1991). Hospital case management: Bridging acute and long-term care. *Health Affairs, 10*(2), 173–184.

Chumbler, N. R., Cody, M., Booth, B. M., & Beck, C. K. (2001). Rural–urban differences in service use for memory-related problems in older adults. *Journal of Behavioral Health Services & Research, 28,* 212–221.

Chumbler, N. R., Dobbs-Kepper, D., Beverly, C., & Beck, C. (2000). Eligibility for in-home respite care: Ethnic status and rural residence. *Journal of Applied Gerontology, 19*(2), 151–169.

Civic Ventures. (2006). *Fact sheet on older Americans.* Retrieved January 3, 2007, from www.civicventures.org/publications/articles/fact_sheet_on older_americans.cfm.

Civil Rights Act of 1964, Pub. L. No. 88–352, 78 Stat. 241.

Civil Service Retirement Act of 1920, 5 U.S.C. § 8331 et seq. (1990).

Clark, R. L., & Quinn, J. F. (2002). Patterns of work and retirement for a new century. *Generations, 16,* 17–24.

Cobb, R. L., & Dvorak, S. (2000). *Accessory dwelling units: Model state acts and local ordinances.* Retrieved January 14, 2007 from http://assets.aarp.org/rgcenter/consume/d17158_dwell.pdf.

Cohen, E., & Cesta, T. (1994). Case management in the acute care setting: A model for health care reform. *Journal of Case Management, 3,* 110–116.

Coleman, B. (1989). *Primer on Employee Retirement Income Security Act* (3rd ed.). Washington, DC: Bureau of National Affairs.

Coleman, B. (2000). *Helping the helpers: State-supported services for family caregivers* (AARP Public Policy Institute Issue Paper #2000–07). Washington, DC: American Association of Retired Persons.

Coleman, D., & Iso-Ahola, S. (1993). The role of social support and self-determination. *Journal of Leisure Research, 25,* 111–128.

Coleman, M. T., Looney, S., O'Brien, J., Ziegler, C., Pastorino, C. A., & Turner, C. (2002). The Eden Alternative: Findings after 1 year of implementation. *Journals of Gerontology, Series A: Biological Sciences and Medical Sciences, 57,* M422–M427.

Coleman, N., Wood, E. F., Sabatino, C. P., Nelson, B., & Baker, C. D. (1986). *Assisting the aging network with private Bar involvement and selected legal issues: Final report on a model project.* Washington, DC: American Bar Association.

Colenda, C. C., Bartels, S. J., & Gottlieb, G. L. (2002). The United States system of care. In J. R. M. Copeland, J. T. Abou-Saleh, & D. G. Blazer (Eds.), *Principles and practices of geriatric psychiatry* (2nd ed.) (pp. 689–696). New York: Wiley.

Colorado Department of Health Care Policy and Financing. (2006). *Care management client satisfaction survey project: Final report and recommendations.* Retrieved December 22, 2006, from www.hcbs.org/moreInfo.php/nb/doc/1761/Care_Management_Client_Satisfaction_Survey

Colston, L., Harper, S., & Mitchener-Colston, W. (1995). Volunteering to promote fitness and caring: A motive for linking college students with mature adults. *Activities, Adaptation, and Aging, 20,* 79–90.

Commission on Accreditation of Rehabilitation Facilities. (2007). *Earning CARF-CCAC accreditation.* Retrieved January 14, 2007 from www.carf.org/Providers.aspx?content = content/Accreditation/Opportunities/AS/CCACAccreditation.htm.

Committee for the Study on Improving Mobility and Safety for Older Persons. (1988). *Transportation in an aging society: Improving mobility and safety for older persons (Vol. 1).* Washington, DC: National Research Council, Transportation Research Board.

Commonwealth Fund. (1993). *The untapped resource: The final report of the Americans Over 55 at Work Program.* New York: Author.

Community Mental Health Act of 1963, 42 U.S.C. § 2689 et seq., as amended.

Community service is key. (1994). *Community Transportation Reporter, 13*(4), 5.

Community Transportation Association of America. (1995). Transportation access technologies developed under project ACTION. *Community Transportation Reporter, 13*, 2–4.

Community Transportation Association of America. (2001). *Status of rural public transportation—2000. Report submitted to the U.S. Department of Transportation, Federal Transit Administration, April 2001.* Retrieved October 28, 2006 from www.ctaa.org/ntrc/rtap/pubs/status2000.

Comprehensive Health Planning and Public Health Service Amendments of 1966, 42 U.S.C. §§ 243, 246.

Congressional Budget Office. (2004). *Financing long term care for the elderly.* Washington, DC: Congressional Budget Office. Retrieved February 2, 2007 from www.cbo.gov/showdoc.cfm?index = 5400&sequence = 0.

Conlin, M., Caranasos, G., & Davidson, R. (1992). Reduction of caregiver stress by respite care: A pilot study. *Southern Medical Journal, 85*, 1096–1100.

Connecticut Continuing Care. (1994). *Guidelines for long-term care case management practices.* Bristol, CT: Author.

Connor, S. R., Tecca, M., LundPerson, J, & Teno, J. (2004). Measuring hospice care: The National Hospice and Palliative Care Organization National Hospice Data Set. *Journal of Pain and Symptom Management, 28*, 316–328.

Cooke, D. D., McNally, L., Mulligan, K.T., Harrison, M. J. G., & Newman, S. P. (2001). Psychosocial interventions for caregivers of people with dementia: A systematic review. *Aging and Mental Health, 5*, 120–135.

Cooperative Extension System. (2006). *Aging issues: Resources, contacts, and collaborations.* Retrieved January 12, 2007 from www.csrees.usda.gov/nea/family/pdfs/aging_resources.pdf.

Corder, R. (1991). Getting volunteers involved: San Clemente PD's retired senior volunteers. *Western City, 67*, 21–23.

Corporation for National and Community Service. (2006). *Volunteer growth in America: A review of trends since 1974.* Retrieved January 18, 2007 from www.nationalservice.org/about/role_impact/performance_research.asp#VOLGROWTH

Costo, S. L. (2006). Trends in retirement plan coverage over the last decade. *Monthly Labor Review, 129*, 58–64

Corrigan, P. W., Swantek, S., Watson, A. C., & Kleinlein, P. (2003). When do older adults seek primary care services for depression? *Journal of Nervous and Mental Disease, 191*, 619–622.

Coulton, C., & Frost, A. K. (1982). Use of social and health services by the elderly. *Journal of Health and Social Behavior, 23*, 330–339.

Courtenay, B. (1990). Community education for older adults. In M. Galbraith (Ed.), *Education through community organizations* (pp. 37–44). San Francisco: Jossey-Bass.

Covey, H. C., & Menard, S. (1988). Trends in elderly criminal victimization from 1973 to 1984. *Research on Aging, 10*, 329–341.

Cox, C. (1997). Findings from a statewide program of respite care: A comparison of service users, stoppers, and nonusers. *The Gerontologist, 37*, 511–517.

Cox, C., & Monk, A. (1990). Integrating the frail and well elderly: The experience of senior centers. *Journal of Gerontological Social Work, 15*, 131–147.

Coyne, A. C. (1991). Information and referral service usage among caregivers for dementia patients. *The Gerontologist, 31*, 384–388.

Crandall, R. C. (1991). *Gerontology: A behavioral science approach*. New York: McGraw-Hill.

Craver, R. (2007). *Winston-Salem company hires mostly older workers. The Mercury News.* Retrieved January 17, 2007 from www.mercurynews.com/mld/mercurynews/news/breaking_news/15122580.htm.

Cruzan v. Harmon, 760 S.W.2d 408 (1988).

Crystal, S., & Beck, P. (1992). A room of one's own: The SRO and the single elderly. *The Gerontologist, 32*, 684–692.

Cudney, A. (2002). Case management: A serious solution for serious issues. *Journal of Healthcare Management, 47*(3), 149–152.

Cuellar, J. (1990). Hispanic American aging: Geriatric education curriculum development for selected health professions. In M. S. Harper (Ed.), *Minority aging* (DHHS Pub. No. HRS P-DV-90-4). Washington, DC: Government Printing Office.

Cushing, M., & Long, N. (1974). *Information and referral services: Reaching out* (DHEW Pub. No. OHD 75–110). Washington, DC: Government Printing Office.

Daily, N. (1998). *When baby boom women retire*. Westport, CT: Praeger.

Dansky, K. H., Brannon, D., Shea, D. G., Vasey, J., & Dirani, R. (1998). Profiles of hospital, physician, and home health service use by older persons in rural areas. *The Gerontologist, 38*, 320–330.

Davis, M. A., Murphy, S. P., Neuhaus, J. M., & Lein, D. (1990). Living arrangements and dietary quality of older U.S. adults. *Journal of the American Dietetic Association, 90*, 1667–1672.

Davis, M. A., Randall, E., Forthofer, R. N., Lee, E. S., & Margen, S. (1985). Living arrangements and dietary patterns of older adults in the United States. *Journal of Gerontology, 40*, 434–442.

de Vries, B. (2006). Home at the end of the rainbow. *Generations, 39*(4), 64–69.

Decker, F., & Dollard, K. J. (2001). *Staffing of nursing services in long term care: Present issues and prospects for the future*. Washington, DC: American Health Care Association.

Decker, F. H. (2005). *Nursing homes, 1977–1999: What has changed, what has not? Hyattsville, Maryland, National Center for Health Statistics.* Retrieved February 4, 2007 from www.cdc.gov/nchs/about/major/nnhsd/Trendsnurse.htm.

Decker, F. H., Gruhn, P., Matthews-Martin, L., Dollard, K. J., Tucker, A. M., & Bizette, L. (2003). *Results of the 2002 AHCA survey of nursing staff vacancy and turnover in nursing homes. Health Services Research and Evaluation, American Health Care Association*, Washington, DC, Retrieved February 12, 2007 from www.ahca.org/research/rpt_vts2002_final.pdf.

Degenholtz, H., Kane, R. A., & Kivnick, H. Q. (1997). Care-related preferences and values of elderly community-based LTC consumers: Can case managers learn what's important to clients? *The Gerontologist, 37*, 767–776.

Dellasega, C., & Stricklin, M. L. (1993). Cognitive impairment in elderly home health clients. *Home Health Care Services Quarterly, 14*, 81–92.

DeLong, D. & Associates. (2006). *Living longer, working longer: The changing landscape of the aging work-force*. New York: MetLife Mature Market Institute. Retrieved January 16, 2007 from www.metlife.com/WPSAssets/11931727601144937501V1FLivingLonger.pdf.

Demmer, C. (2003). A national survey of hospice bereavement services. *OMEGA: The Journal of Death and Dying, 47,* 4, 327–341

DePaulo, B. M. (1978). Help seeking from the recipient's point of view. *JSAS Catalogue of Selected Documents in Psychology, 8,* 62 (Ms. No. 1721b).

DePaulo, B. M., & Fisher, J. D. (1980). The cost of asking for help. *Basic and Applied Social Psychology, 1,* 23–35.

Di, J., & Berman, J. (2000, October). Older New Yorkers' use of senior center services: Effect of family support networks. *The Gerontologist, 40,* 390.

Dickerson, B., Myers, D., Seelbach, W., & Johnson-Dietz, S. (1990). A 21st century challenge to higher education: Integrating the older person into academia. In R. Sherron & D. B. Lumsden (Eds.), *Introduction to educational gerontology* (3rd ed., pp. 297–331). New York: Hemisphere.

Diebert, L. (1996). *Options for funding rural transit programs: A community transit funding primer*. Boulder, CO: Boulder County Colorado Transit.

Dilworth-Anderson, P., Williams, I. C., & Gibson, B. E. (2002). Issues of race, ethnicity, and culture in caregiving research: A 20-year review (1980–2000). *The Gerontologist, 42,* 237–272.

DiPietro, L. (2001). Physical activity in aging: Changes in patterns and their relationship to health and function. *Journal of Gerontology, 56A* (Special Issue II), 13–22.

Dispute Resolution Center. (2000). *Dispute Resolution Center. Saint Paul, MN: Author*. Retrieved May 26, 2001 from www.disputeresolutioncenter.org.

Diwan, S. (1999). Allocation of case management resources in long-term care: Predicting high use of case management of time. *The Gerontologist, 39,* 580–590.

Doolin, J. (1985). America's untouchables: The elderly homeless. *Perspective on Aging, 9*(2), 8–12.

Doty, P. (1986). Family care of the elderly: The role of public policy. *Milbank Memorial Fund Quarterly, 64,* 34–75.

Downing, R. (1985). The elderly and their families. In M. Weil, J. Karls, & Associates (Eds.), *Case management in human service practice: A systematic approach to mobilizing resources for clients* (pp. 145–169). San Francisco: Jossey-Bass.

Drenning, S., & Getz, L. (1992). Computer ease. *Phi Delta Kappan, 74,* 471–472.

Dumazadier, J. (1967). *Towards a society of leisure*. New York: Free Press.

Duquin, M., McCrea, J., Fetterman, D., & Nash, S. (2004). A faith-based intergenerational health and wellness program. *Journal of Intergenerational Relationships: Programs, Policy, and Research, 2,* 105–118.

Dwyer, J. (1991). *Screening older Americans' nutritional health: Current practices and future possibilities*. Washington, DC: Nutrition Screening Initiative.

Dwyer, J. (1994). Nutritional problems of elderly minorities. *Nutrition Reviews, 52*(8), S24–S27.

Dychtwald, K. (2000). *Age power: How the 21st century will be ruled by the new old*. New York: Tarcher/Putnam.

East Tennessee Human Resource Agency. (n.d.). *Long term care ombudsman*. Retrieved February 13, 2007 from www.ethra.org/HTML.Pgms/Ombuds.htm.

Eaton J., & Salari, S. (2005). Environments for lifelong learning in senior centers. *Educational Gerontology, 31,* 461–480.

Edelstein, S. (1996). Legal issues and resources: An introduction for professionals in aging. Unpublished manuscript.

Eden Alternative. (n.d.). *Welcome to the Eden Alternative*. Retrieved February 18, 2007 from www.edenalt.com.

Eldeman, T. S. (1990). The nursing home reform law: Issues for litigation. *Clearinghouse Review, 24*, 545–550.

Elderhostel. (2006a). *What is Elderhostel?* Retrieved December 18, 2006 from www.elderhostel .org/about/what_is.asp.

Elderhostel. (2006b). *Frequently asked questions for the media*. Retrieved December 18, 2006 from www.elderhostel.org/about/media_faq.asp.

Emlet, C., & Hall, A. M. (1991). Integrating the community into geriatric case management: Public health interventions. *The Gerontologist, 31*, 556–560.

Employee Benefit Research Institute. (2003). Private Pension Plans, Participation, and Assets: Update. Facts from EBRI. Available at www.ebri.org/publications/facts/index.cfm?fa = 0103fact

Employment Benefit Research Institute. (2005). Employment-base retirement plan participation: Geographic differences and trends, 2004. EBRI Issue Brief #286, October. Available at www.ebri.org/publications/ob/index.cfm?fa + ibPrint&content_id + 3590.

Employee Retirement Income Security Act of 1974, 29 U.S.C. §§ 1001–1461 (1974), as amended.

Enguidanos, S. M., Gibbs, N. E., Simmons, W. J., Savoni, K. J., Jamison, P. M., Hackstaff, L. et al. (2003). Kaiser Permanente Community Partners Project: Improving geriatric care management practices. *Journal of the American Geriatrics Society, 51*, 710–714.

Erickson, R., & Eckert, J. K. (1977). The elderly poor in downtown San Diego hotels. *The Gerontologist, 17*, 440–446.

Eschtruth, A. (2006). *Myths and realties about retirement preparedness*. Retrieved January 12, 2007 from www.bc.edu/centers/crr/facts/NRRI%20Myths_Realities.pdf.

Estes, C. (1979). *The aging enterprise*. San Francisco: Jossey-Bass.

Estes, C. L., Swan, J. H., & Associates (1993). *The long term care crisis: Elders trapped in the no-care zone*. Newbury Park, CA: Sage.

Ettinger, W., Burns, R. et al. (1997). A randomized trial comparing aerobic exercise and resistance exercise with a health education program in older adults with knee osteoarthritis: The Fitness Arthritis and Senior Trial (FAST). *Journal of the American Medical Association, 277*, 25–31.

Experience Works. (2006). *2005 Annual report*. Retrieved January 16, 2007 from www.experienceworks .org/site/DocServer/web-2005_AReport.pdf?docID = 601.

The extra mile: Overnight and weekend care. (1996, Fall/Winter). *Respite Report, 1–2*, 6.

Factor, A. (1993). Translating policy into practice. In E. Sutton, A. Factor, B. Hawkins, T. Heller, & G. Seltzer (Eds.), *Older adults with developmental disabilities: Optimizing choices and change* (pp. 257–275). Baltimore: P. H. Brookes.

FallCreek, S. J., Allen, B. P., & Halls, D. M. (1986). *Health promotion and aging: A national directory of selected programs* (DHHS Pub. No. OHDS 86–950). Washington, DC: U.S. Department of Health and Human Services, Office of Human Development Services, Administration on Aging.

FallCreek, S. J., & Franks, P. (1984). *Health promotion and aging: Strategies for action* (DHHS Pub. No. OHDS 84–818). Washington, DC: U.S. Department of Health and Human Services, Office of Human Development Services, Administration on Aging.

FallCreek, S. J., & Mettler, M. (1982). *A healthy old age: A sourcebook for health promotion with older adults* (DHHS Pub. No. 447-a-1). Washington, DC: U.S. Department of Health and Human Services, Office of Human Development Services, Administration on Aging.

Family Caregiver Alliance. (2002). *Caregiver depression.* Retrieved January 12, 2007 from www.caregiver.org/caregiver/jsp/content_node.jsp?nodeid = 393.

Family and Medical Leave Act of 1993, 5 U.S.C. § 6381 et seq., 29 U.S.C. §§ 2601 et seq., 2631 et seq. (1993).

Federal Bureau of Investigation. (2005). *Financial Crimes Report to the Public.* U.S. Department of Justice, Washington, DC. Available at www.fbi.gov/publications/financial/fcs_report052005/fcs_report052005.htm.

Federal Funding Resources. (1995, January). *Community Transportation Reporter, 13,* 21–30.

Federal Interagency Forum on Aging-Related Statistics. (2000). *Older Americans 2000: Key indicators of well-being.* Hyattsville, MD: Author.

Federal Interagency Forum on Aging-Related Statistics. (2004). *Older Americans 2004: Key indicators of well-being.* Washington, DC: U.S. Government Printing Office.

Federal Interagency Forum on Aging-Related Statistics. (2006). *Older Americans update 2006: Key indicators of well-being.* Washington, DC: U.S. Government Printing Office.

Federal Transit Act of 1988, 49 U.S.C. § 1601 et seq. (1988).

Feldman, N. S. (1991). Lifelong education: The challenge of change. In *Resourceful aging: Today and tomorrow: Vol. 5. Lifelong education* (pp. 17–31). Washington, DC: American Association of Retired Persons.

Fellin, P., & Powell, T. (1988). Mental health services and older adult minorities: An assessment. *The Gerontologist, 28,* 442–447.

Ficke, S. C. (1985). *Older Americans Act 1965–1985: 20th anniversary: An orientation to the Older Americans Act.* Washington, DC: National Association of State Units on Aging.

Finkel, S. (1993). Mental health and aging: A decade of progress. *Generations, 17*(1), 25–30.

Fischer, C. A., Crockett, S. J., Heller, K. E., & Skauge, L. H. (1991). Nutrition knowledge, attitudes and practices of older and younger elderly in rural areas. *Journal of the American Dietetic Association, 91,* 1398–1401.

Fischer, D. L. (1978). *Growing old in America.* New York: Oxford University Press.

Fischer, L., Mueller, D., & Cooper, P. (1991). Older volunteers: A discussion of the Minnesota Senior Study. *The Gerontologist, 31,* 183–194.

Fischer, L. R., & Schaffer, K. B. (1993). *Older volunteers: A guide to research and practice.* Newbury Park, CA: Sage.

Fischer, R. (1992). Post-retirement learning. In R. Fischer, M. Blazey, & H. Lipman (Eds.), *Students of the third age* (pp. 13–21). New York: Macmillan.

Fisher, J. D., & Nadler, A. (1976). The effect of donor resources on recipient self-esteem and self-help. *Journal of Experimental Social Psychology, 12,* 139–150.

Fisher, J. D., Nadler, A., & Whitcher-Alagna, S. (1983). Four conceptualizations of reactions to aid. In J. D. Fisher, A. Nadler, & B. M. DePaulo (Eds.), *New directions in helping, Vol. 1* (pp. 51–84). New York: Academic Press.

Fiske, S. T., & Taylor, S. E. (1991). *Social cognition* (2nd ed.). New York: McGraw-Hill.

Folkemer, D. (2006). *Home care quality: Emerging state strategies to deliver person-centered services.* Retrieved January 2, 2007 from www.cms.hhs.gov/HomeHealthQualityInits/downloads/HHQIOverview.pdf.

Foner, N. (1994). *The caregiving dilemma.* Los Angeles: University of California Press.

Food Stamp Act of 1964, 7 U.S.C. § 2011 et seq. (1995).

Fox, P. J., Breuer, W., & Wright, J. A. (1997). Effects of a health promotion program on sustaining health behaviors in older adults. *American Journal of Preventive Medicine, 13*(4), 257–264.

Franco, S. J. (2004). *Medicare home health care in rural America. NORC Walsh Center for Rural Health Analysis.* Retrieved December 18, 2006 from www.norc.org/issues/NseriesJan04v1.pdf.

Freedman, M. (1994). *Seniors in national and community service: A report prepared for the Commonwealth Fund's Americans Over 55 at Work Program.* Philadelphia: Public/Private Ventures.

Freiman, M., & Brown, E. (1999). *Special care units in nursing homes: Selected characteristics, 1996.* Retrieved December 1, 2000 from www.meps.ahrq.gov/mepsweb/data_files/publications/ rf6/rf6.pdf.

Freiman, M., Cunningham, P., & Cornelius, L. (1993). The demand for health care for the treatment of mental problems among the elderly. *Advances in Health Economics and Health Services Research, 14,* 17–36.

Friedan, B. (1995). *The fountain of age.* New York: Simon & Schuster.

Fuller-Thompson, E., Minkler, M., & Driver, D. (1997). A profile of grandparents raising grandchildren in the United States. *The Gerontologist, 37,* 406–411.

Gabrel, C. S. (2000a). *Characteristics of elderly nursing home current residents and discharges: Data from the 1997 National Nursing Home Survey (Advance Data From Vital and Health Statistics No. 312).* Hyattsville, MD: National Center for Health Statistics.

Gabrel, C. S. (2000b). *An overview of nursing home facilities: Data from the 1997 National Nursing Home Survey (Advance Data From Vital and Health Statistics No. 312).* Hyattsville, MD: National Center for Health Statistics.

Gage, B., Pilkauskas, N., Dalton, K., Constantine, R., Leung, M., Hoover, S., & Green, J. (2007). *Long-Term Care Hospital (LTCH) payment system monitoring and evaluation PHASE II REPORT: January 2007.* RTI International Health, Social, and Economics Research, Waltham, MA. Available at www.cms.hhs.gov/LongTermCareHospitalPPS/Downloads/RTI_LTCHPPS_Final_Rpt.pdf.

Galambos, C. M. (1997). Resolving ethical conflicts in providing case management services to the elderly. *Journal of Gerontological Social Work, 27*(4), 57–67.

Gallagher-Thompson, D., Arean, P., Coon, D., Menéndez, A., Tagaki, K., Haley, W. E. et al., (2000). Development and implementation of intervention strategies for culturally diverse caregiving populations. In R. Schulz (Ed.), *Handbook on dementia caregiving* (pp. 151–186). New York: Springer.

Gallagher-Thompson, D., Arean, P., Rivera, P., & Thompson, L. W. (2001). Reducing distress in Hispanic caregivers using a psychoeducational intervention. *Clinical Gerontologist, 23,* 17–32.

Gambone, J. V. (2001). *Retirement: A boomer's guide to life after 50.* Minneapolis, MN: Kirkhouse.

Garson, A. (1994, September). RSVP International: Putting seniors to work as volunteers. *Transitions Abroad, 18,* 53.

Gaugler, J. E., Jarrott, S. E., Zarit, S. H., Stephens, M. A. P., Townsend, A., & Greene, R. (2003). Respite for dementia caregivers: the effects of adult day service use on caregiving hours and care demands. *International Psychogeriatrics, 15,* 37–58.

Gelfand, D. E., & Bechill, W. (1991). The evolution of the Older Americans Act: A 25-year review of the legislative changes. *Generations, 15*(3), 19–22.

George, L. (1987). Respite care. In G. Maddox (Ed.), *The encyclopedia of aging* (pp. 576–577). New York: Springer.

Gerber, I. (1969). Bereavement and the acceptance of professional service. *Community Mental Health Journal, 5,* 487–495.

Gergen, K. J., Morse, S. J., & Kristeller, J. L. (1973). The manner of giving: Crossnational continuities in reactions to aid. *Psychologia, 16,* 121–131.

Geron, S., & Chassler, D. (1995). Advancing the state of the art: Establishing guidelines for long-term care case management. *Journal of Case Management, 4,* 9–13.

Gigliotti, C. M., Jarrott, S. E., & Yorgason, J. (2004). Harvesting health: Effects of three types of horticultural therapy for persons with dementia. *Dementia, 3,* 161–180.

Given, B. A., & Given, C. W. (2001). Health promotion for older adults in a managed care environment. In E. A. Swason, T. Tripp-Reimer, & K. Buckwalter (Eds.), *Health promotion and disease prevention in the older Adult: Interventions and recommendations.* New York: Springer.

Glass, T. A. (2006). Disasters and older adults: Bringing a policy blindspot into the light. *Public Policy and Aging Report, 16,* 2, 1–7.

Goggin, J., & Ronan, B. (2004). *Our next chapter: Community colleges and the aging baby boomers. Leadership Abstracts, 17,* 11–15. Retrieved December 18, 2006 from www.civicventures.org/articles.cfm.

Goins, R. T., Mitchell, J., & Wu, B. (2006). Service issues among rural racial and ethnic minority elders. In R. T. Goins & J.A. Krout (Eds.), *Service delivery to rural older adults: Research, policy, and practice* (pp. 55–78). New York: Springer.

Golant, S. M., & LaGreca, A. J. (1994). Housing quality of U.S. elderly households: Does aging or place matter? *The Gerontologist, 34,* 803–814.

Gold, M., Hudson M. C., & Davis, S. (2006). *Medicare Advantage benefits and premiums. Mathematica Policy Research, Inc.* Retrieved January 17, 2007 from http://assets.aarp.org/rgcenter/health/2006_23_medicare.pdf.

Gonyea, J. (1988). Acceptance of hospital-based respite care by families and elders. *Health and Social Work, 3,* 201–208.

Goodwin, J. S. (1989). Social, psychological and physical factors affecting the nutritional status of elderly subjects: Separating cause and effect. *American Journal of Clinical Nutrition, 50,* 1201–1209.

Goyer, A. (1998–99). Intergenerational shared-site programs. *Generations, 22*(4), 79–80.

Grabbe, L., Demi, A., Whittington, F., Jones, J., Branch, L., & Lambert, R. (1995). Functional status and the use of formal home care in the year before death. *Journal of Aging and Health, 7,* 339–364.

Grabowski, D. C. (2006). The cost-effectiveness of noninstitutional long-term care services: Review and Synthesis of the most recent evidence. *Medical Care Research and Review, 63,* 3–28

Gräsell, E. (1997). Temporary institutional respite in dementia cases: Who utilizes this form of respite care and what effect does it have? *International Psychogeriatrics, 9,* 437–448.

Greater Boston Food Bank. (2001). *Let's bag it brown bag program.* Retrieved August 1, 2001 from www.gbfb.org.

Green, L., Fitzhugh, E., Wang, M. Q., Perko, J., Eddy, J., & Westerfield, C. (1993). Influence of living arrangements on dietary adequacy for U.S. elderly: 1987–1988 nationwide food consumption survey. *Wellness Perspectives: Research, Theory and Practice, 10*(1), 32–40.

Green Thumb, Inc. (2001). *Green Thumb, Inc.* Retrieved May 9, 2001 from www.experience works.org.

Greenberg, M. S., & Shapiro, S. P. (1971). Indebtedness: An adverse aspect of asking for and receiving help. *Sociometry, 34*, 290–301.

Greenberg, M. S., & Westcott, D. R. (1983). Indebtedness as a mediator of reactions to aid. In J. D. Fisher, A. Nadler, & B. M. DePaulo (Eds.), *New directions in helping, Vol. 1* (pp. 85–112). New York: Academic Press.

Grimaldi, P. L. (1982). *Medicaid reimbursement of nursing home care.* Washington, DC: American Enterprise Institute.

Grinstead, L., Leder, S., Jensen, S., & Bond, L. (2003). Review of the research on the health of caregiving grandparents. *Journal of Advanced Nursing, 44*, 318–326.

Gross, D. (1998). *Different needs, different strategies: A manual for training low-income, older workers.* Retrieved May 9, 2001 from http://wdsc.doleta.gov/seniors/ html_docs/dnds.html.

Grove, N. C., & Spier, B. E. (1999). Motivating the well elderly to exercise. *Journal of Community Health Nursing, 16*(3), 179–189.

Guttman, D. (1980). *Perspective on equitable shares in public benefits by minority elderly: Executive summary.* Washington, DC: Catholic University of America.

Hale, N. (1990). *The older worker.* San Francisco: Jossey-Bass.

Halpain, M. C., Harris, M. J., McClure, F. S., & Jeste, D. V. (1999). Training in geriatric mental health: Needs and strategies. *Psychiatric Services, 50*, 1205–1208.

Halpren, D. (2005). *Social capital.* Polity Press: Malden, MA.

Hamburg, D., Elliot, G., & Parron, D. (1982). *Health behavior: Frontiers of research in the biobehavioral sciences.* Washington, DC: National Academy Press.

Hampton, N. (2006, June). *Aging network supports caregivers.* Retrieved January 12, 2007 from www.ncsu.edu/project/calscommblogs/archives/2006/06/aging_network_s.html.

Hanssen, A., Meima, N., Buckspan, L., Henderson, B., Helbig, T., & Zarit, S. (1978). Correlates of senior center participation. *The Gerontologist, 18*, 193–199.

Hardin, J., Tucker, L., & Callejas, L. (2001). *Assessment of operational barriers and impediments to transit use: Transit information and scheduling for major activity centers. Report submitted to the U.S. Department of Transportation, Federal Transit Administration. December 2001 by the National Center For Transit Research (NCTR).* Retrieved October 28, 2006 from http://ntl.bts.gov/lib/12000/12000/12049/392–11.pdf.

Hare, P. (1990). The echo housing/granny flat experience in the US. *Journal of Housing for the Elderly, 7*(2), 57–70.

Harper, B. (1995). Report from the national task force on access to hospice care by minority groups. *Hospice Journal, 10*, 1–9.

Harper, M. S. (1991). Delivery of mental health services in the home, and other community-based health services. In M. S. Harper (Ed.), *Management and care of the elderly* (pp. 320–331). Newbury Park, CA: Sage.

Harper, N., McDowell, D., Turner, J., & Sharma, A. (1988). Planned short-stay admissions to a geriatric unit: One aspect of respite care. *Age and Ageing, 3*, 199–203.

Harrington, C. (1991). The nursing home industry: A structural analysis. In M. Minkler & C. L. Estes (Eds.), *Critical perspectives on aging: The political and moral economy of growing old.* Amityville, MD: Baywood.

Harrington, C., Carrillo, H., Wellin, V., Miller, N., & LeBlanc, A. (2000). Predicting state Medicaid home and community expenditures, 1992–1997. *The Gerontologist, 40,* 673–686.

Harrington-Meyer, M. (2001). Medicaid reimbursement rates and access to nursing homes: Implications for gender, race, and marital status. *Research on Aging, 23,* 532–539.

Harris-Kojetin, L., Lipson, D., Fielding, J., Kiefer, K., & Stone, R. (2004). *Recent findings on frontline long-term care workers: A research synthesis 1999–2003.* Washington, DC: U.S. Department of Health and Human Services.

Harris & Associates. (1975). *The myth and reality of aging in America.* Washington, DC: National Council on the Aging.

Harvard School of Public Health. (2004). *Reinventing aging: Baby boomers and civic engagement. Harvard School of Public Health–MetLife Foundation Initiative on Retirement and Civic Engagement Report.* Boston, MA: Harvard School of Public Health.

Hasler, B. S. (1990). *Reporting of minority participation under Title III of the Older Americans Act.* Washington, DC: Public Policy Institute/American Association of Retired Persons.

Hatfield, E., & Sprecher, S. (1983). Equity theory and recipient reactions to aid. In J. D. Fisher, A. Nadler, & B. M. DePaulo (Eds.), *New directions in helping, Vol. 1* (pp. 113–141). New York: Academic Press.

Haupt, B. (1997). *Characteristics of patients receiving hospice care services: United States, 1994 (Advance Data From Vital and Health Statistics, No. 282).* Hyattsville, MD: National Center for Health Statistics.

Hawes, C., Wildfire, J. B., & Lux, L. J. (1993). *The regulation of board and care homes: Results of a survey in the 50 states and the District of Columbia: National summary.* Washington, DC: American Association of Retired Persons.

Hawranik, P. (2002). In home service use by caregivers and their elders: Does cognitive status make a difference? *Canadian Journal on Aging, 21,* 257–271.

He, W., Sengupta, M., Velkoff, V. A., & DeBarros, K. A. (2005). *65 + in the United States.* Retrieved on January 9, 2007, from www.census.gov/prod/2006pubs/p23-209.pdf.

Health Care Financing Administration. (1996a). *Medicaid eligibility.* Retrieved January 27, 2002 from www.hcfa.gov/medicaid/meligib.htm.

Health Care Financing Administration. (1996b). *Medicare and Medicaid: Brief summaries of Title XVIII and Title XIX of the Social Security Act.* Retrieved January 27, 2002 from www.hcfa.gov/pubforms/actuary/ormedmed/default.htm.

Health Care Financing Administration. (1997). *National Health Expenditures Projections: 1998–2008, freestanding home health agencies.* Retrieved January 25, 2002 from www.hcfa.gov/stats.

Health Care Financing Administration. (2000a). *Medicare enrollment trends.* Retrieved August 1, 2001 from www.hcfa.gov/stats/enrltrnd.htm.

Health Care Financing Administration. (2000b). *Medicare 2000: 35 years of improving American's health and security.* Retrieved August 1, 2001 from www.hcfa.gov/stats/35chartbk.pdf.

Health Care Financing Administration. (2000c). *A profile of Medicaid chart book.* Retrieved August 15, 2001 from www.hcfa.gov/stats/2Tchartbk.pdf.

Health Care Financing Administration. (2001a). *Medicaid eligibility.* Retrieved September 1, 2001 from www.hcfa.gov/medicaid/meligib.htm.

Health Care Financing Administration. (2001b). *The Medicare + Choice program in 2001 and 2002.* Retrieved September 15, 2001 from www.hcfa.gov/facts/fs010829.htm.

Health Care Financing Administration. (2001c). *Your Medicare benefits.* Retrieved September 15, 2001 from www.medicare.gov/Publications/Pubs/pdf/yourmb.pdf.

Heath, A. (1993). *ElderTransit facts: Increasing minority participation in transportation programs* (Brochure). Washington, DC: National Eldercare Institute on Transportation.

Hedge, J. W., Borman, W. C., & Lammlein, S. E. (2006). *The aging workforce: Realities, myths, and implications for organizations.* Washington, DC: American Psychological Association.

Hegeman, C. R. (2005). *Turnover turnaround. Health Progress, 86*(6), n.p. Retrieved February 18, 2007 from www.chausa.org/Pub/MainNav/News/HP/default.htm.

Helpguide (2006). *Board and care homes for seniors.* Retrieved December 28, 2006 from http://helpguide .org/elder/board_care_homes_senior _residential.htm.

Henry, M. E., & Capitman, J. (1995). Finding satisfaction in adult day care: Analysis of a national demonstration of dementia care and respite services. *Journal of Applied Gerontology, 14,* 302–320.

Herdt, G., & de Vries, B. (2004). *Gay and lesbian aging: Research and future directions.* New York: Springer.

Herman, C. J., & Wadsworth, N. (1992). *Action for health: Older women's project.* Cleveland, OH: Case Western Reserve University School of Medicine.

Herz, D. E., Meisenheimer, J. R., & Weinstein, H. G. (2000). *Health and retirement benefits: data from two BLS surveys.* Retrieved January 21, 2002, from www.bls.gov/opub/mlr/2000/03/art1full.pdf.

Hetzel, L., & Smith, A. (2001). *The 65 years and over population: 2000. US Census Bureau.* Retrieved February 4, 2007 from www.census.gov/prod/2001pubs/c2kbr01-10.pdf

Heumann, L. F. (1990). The housing and support costs of elderly with comparable support needs living in long-term care and congregate housing. *Journal of Housing for the Elderly, 6*(1/2), 45–71.

Hibbard, J., Greene, J., & Tusler, M. (2006). *An assessment of beneficiary knowledge of Medicare coverage options and the prescription drug benefit. AARP Public Policy Institute,* Washington, DC. Retrieved January 28, 2007 from http://assets.aarp.org/rgcenter/health/2006_12_ medicare.pdf.

Hickey, T., & Stilwell, D. L. (1991). Health promotion for older people: All is not well. *The Gerontologist, 31,* 822–829.

High, L. (2000). CCRCs: Surviving the evolving landscape. *Assisted Living Today, 7*(8), 61–63.

Higher Education Act, 20 U.S.C. § 1001 et seq. (1965).

Hirshorn, B., & Hoyer, D. (1994). Private sector hiring and use of retirees: The firm's perspective. *The Gerontologist, 34,* 50–58.

Hirshorn, B. A., & Piering, P. (1998–99). Older people at risk: Issues and intergenerational responses. *The Generations, 22*(4), 49–53.

Hodgson, L. G. (1995). Adult grandchildren and their grandparents: The enduring bond. *International Journal of Aging and Human Development, 34,* 209–225.

Home and Community Based Services. (2000). *Board and care homes.* Retrieved January 20, 2002 from www.hcbs.org/resources/four/board_and_care_homes.htm.

Hoffman, E. D., Klees, B. S., & Curtis, C. A. (2006). *Brief summaries of Medicare and Medicaid Title XVIII and Title XIX of The Social Security Act.* Centers for Medicare & Medicaid Services, Department of Health and Human Services. Available at www.cms.hhs.gov/MedicareProgramRatesStats/downloads/ MedicareMedicaidSummaries2006.pdf

Hooper, K., & Hamberg, J. (1986). The making of America's homeless: From skid row to the new poor, 1945–1984. In R. Bratt, C. Hartman, & A. Meyerson (Eds.), *Critical perspectives in housing.* Philadelphia: Temple University Press.

Hooyman, N. R., & Kiyak, H. A. (1996). *Social gerontology: A multidisciplinary perspective* (4th ed.). Needham Heights, MA: Simon & Schuster.

Hooyman, N. R., & Kiyak, H. A. (2002). *Social gerontology: A multidisciplinary perspective* (6th ed.). Needham Heights, MA: Simon & Schuster.

Hopp, F. P. (1999). Patterns and predictors of formal and informal care among elderly persons living in board and care homes. *The Gerontologist, 39*, 167–176.

Hopp, F. P. (2000). Preferences for surrogate decision makers, informal communication, and advance directives among community-dwelling elders: Results from a national study. *The Gerontologist, 40*(4), 449–457.

Horowitz, A. (1985). Family caregiving to the frail elderly. In C. Eisdorfer (Ed.), *Annual review of gerontology and geriatrics, Vol. 5* (pp. 194–246). New York: Springer.

Horvath, B., Silberg, M., Landerman, L. R., Johnson, F. S., & Michener, J. L. (2006). Dynamics of patient targeting for care management in Medicaid: A case study of the Durham Community Health Network. *Care Management Journals, 7*, 107–114.

Hospice Association of America. (2006). *Hospice facts and statistics*. Retrieved December 18, 2006 from www.nahc.org/hospicefs06.pdf.

Houser, A. (2005). *Community mobility options: The older person's interest*. Washington, DC: *The American Association of Retired Persons, AARP Public Policy Institute, August 2005*. Retrieved October 20, 2006 from www.aarp.org/ppi.

Howe, R. (1994). A framework for case management. In R. Howe (Ed.), *Case management for health care professionals* (pp. 3–12). Chicago: Precept.

Hoyert, D. L., Heron, M. P., Murphy, S. L., & Kung, H. (2006). Deaths: Final Data for 2003. *National Vital Statistics Reports, 54, 13, 27*. Retrieved January 27, 2007 from http://wonder.cdc.gov/wonder/sci_data/natal/linked/type_txt/lbd03/Mortality.pdf.

Hudson, R. B., & Kingson, E. R. (1991). Inclusive and fair: The case for universality in social programs. *Generations, 15*(3), 51–56.

Hunt, M. (1998). Naturally occurring retirement communities. In *Encyclopedia of American Cities and Suburbs* (pp. 517–518). New York: Garland.

Hushbeck, J. (1990). American business, public policy, and the older worker. *Virginia Journal of Science, 41*, 169–181.

Huttman, E. D. (1985). *Social services for the elderly*. New York: Free Press.

Independent Sector Institute of Medicine. (1986). *Improving the quality of care in nursing homes*. Washington, DC: National Academy Press.

Independent Sector Institute of Medicine. (1991). *Disability in America: Toward a national agenda for prevention*. Washington, DC: National Academy Press.

Independent Sector. (2001). *Giving and Volunteering in the United States, 2001*. Washington, DC: Author.

Institute of Medicine. (1991). *Disability in America: Toward a National Agenda for Prevention*. Washington, DC: Institute of Medicine.

Intermodal Surface Transportation Efficiency Act of 1991, Pub. L. No. 102–240, 105 Stat. 1914.

International Longevity Center–Schmieding Center Health and Education Task Force. (2006). *Caregiving in America*. Retrieved October 10, 2006, from www.ilcusa.org/_lib/pdf/Caregiving%20in%20America-%20Final.pdf.

Jaffe, D. J., & Howe, E. (1988). Agency-assisted shared housing: The nature of programs and matches. *The Gerontologist, 28*, 318–324.

Janke, M., Davey, A., & Kleiber, D. (2006). Modeling change in older adults' leisure activities. *Leisure Sciences, 28*, 285–303.

Jarrott, S. E. (2005). Evaluation. In S. Steinig (Ed.), *Under one roof: A guide to starting and strengthening intergenerational shared site programs* (pp. 85–97). Washington, DC: Generations United.

Jarrott, S. E., Gigliotti, C. M., & Smock, S. A. (2006). Where do we stand? Testing the foundation of a shared site intergenerational program. *Journal of Intergenerational Relationships, 4*(2), 73–92.

Jarrott, S. E., Zarit, S. H., Stephens, M. A. P., Townsend, A., & Greene, R. (1999). Caregiver satisfaction with adult day service programs. *American Journal of Alzheimer's Disease, 14*, 233–244.

Jeste, D. V., Alexopoulos, G. S., Bartels, S. J., Cummings, J. L., Gallo, J. J., Gottlieb, G. L. et al., (1999). Consensus statement on the upcoming crisis in geriatric mental health: Research agenda for the next two decades. *Archives of General Psychiatry, 56*, 848–853.

Jette, A., & Branch, L. (1992). A ten-year follow-up of driving patterns among the community-dwelling elderly. *Human Factors, 34*(1), 25–31.

Jirovec, R. L., Erich, J. A., & Sanders, L. J. (1989). Patterns of senior center participation among low income urban elderly. *Journal of Gerontological Social Work, 13*, 115–132.

Job Training Partnership Act of 1982, Pub. L. No. 97–300, 96 Stat. 1322 (1982).

Johnson, R. W., & Favreault, M. M. (2001). *Retiring together or working alone: The impact of spousal employment and disability on retirement decisions.* Washington, DC: Urban Institute.

Johnson, R.W., & Schaner, S. G. (2005). V*alue of unpaid activities by older Americans tops $160 billion per year.* Retrieved January 3, 2007 from www.urban.org/publications/311227.html.

Johnson, R.W., & Uccello, C.E. (2005). *Is private long-term care insurance the answer? An Issue in Brief, March 2005, Number 29. Center for Retirement Research at Boston College.* Retrieved February 4, 2007 from www.urban.org/UploadedPDF/1000795.pdf.

Johnson, R.W., & Weiner, J. M. (2006). A profile of frail older Americans and their caregivers. *The Urban Institute.* Retrieved March 9, 2006 from www.urban.org/UploadedPDF/311284_older_americans.pdf.

Jones, D. C., & Vaughan, K. (1990). Close friendships among senior adults. *Psychology and Aging, 3*, 451–457.

Justice, D. (1993). *Case management standards in state community based long-term care programs.* Washington, DC: Congressional Research Service.

Kaiser Commission. (2006). *Medicaid 1915c home and community-based service programs: Data update.* Retrieved December 28, 2006 from www.kff.org/medicaid/upload/7575.pdf.

Kane, R. A. (2000). *Assuring quality in care at home.* New York: Springer.

Kane, R., & Caplan, A. (Eds.). (1993). *Ethical conflict in the management of home care: Case manager's dilemma.* New York: Springer.

Kane, R., & Frytak, J. (1994). *Models for case management in long-term care: Interactions of case managers and home care providers.* Minneapolis, MN: National Long-Term Care Resource Center.

Kane, R., Illston, L., & Miller, N. (1992). Qualitative analysis of the program of all-inclusive care for the elderly (PACE). *The Gerontologist, 32*, 771–780.

Kane, R., & Kane, R. (1981). *Assessing the elderly: A practical guide for measurement.* Lexington, MA: Lexington.

Kane, R., Kane, R., Kaye, N., Mollica, R., Riley, T., Saucier, P. et al., (1996). *Managed care: Handbook for the aging network.* Minneapolis, MN: National Long-Term Care Resource Center.

Kane, R. L., Kane, R. A., Ladd, R. C., & Veazie, W. (1998). Variations in state spending for long-term care: Factors associated with more balanced systems. *Journal of Health Politics, Policy, and Law, 23*, 363–390.

Kannel, W. B. (1986). Nutritional contributors to cardiovascular disease in the elderly. *Journal of the American Geriatrics Society, 34*, 27–36.

Kansas Advocates for Better Care. (2002). *Intergenerational initiatives in Kansas nursing homes.* Retrieved on February 17, 2007 from www.kabc.org.

Kaplan, J., & Shore, H. (1993). The Jewish nursing home: Innovations in practice and policy. In C. M. Barresi & D. E. Stull (Eds.), *Ethnic elderly and long-term care* (pp. 115–129). New York: Springer.

Kaplan, M. (1997). The benefits of intergenerational community service projects: Implications for promoting intergenerational unity, community activism, and cultural continuity. In K. Brabazon & R. Disch (Eds.), *Intergenerational approaches in aging* (pp. 211–228). New York: Haworth.

Karlin, B. E., & Norris, M. B. (2006). Public mental health care utilization by older adults. *Administration and Policy in Mental Health and Mental Health Services Research, 33,* 730–735.

Karner, T., & Hall, L. C. (2002). Successful strategies for serving diverse populations. *Home Health Care Services Quarterly, 21*(3/4), 107–131.

Karoly, L. A., & Zissimopoulos, J. (2004). *Self-employment among older U.S. workers. Monthly Labor Review.* Retrieved January 26, 2007 from www.bls.gov/opub/mlr/2004/07/art3full.pdf.

Kart, C. S. (1997). *The realities of aging: An introduction to gerontology* (5th ed.). Needham Heights, MA: Allyn & Bacon.

Kassner, E. (2006a). *Consumer-directed home and community-based services. AARP Public Policy Institute.* Retrieved July 17, 2006 from http://assets.aarp.org/rgcenter/il/fs128_cons_dir.pdf.

Kassner, E. (2006b). *Home and community-based long-term services and supports for older people. AARP Public Policy Institute.* Retrieved July 17, 2006 from http://assets.aarp.org/rgcenter/il/fs90r_hcbltc.pdf.

Kaufman, A. V., Scogin, F. R., MaloneBeach, E. E., Baumhover, L. A., & McKendree-Smith, N. (2000). Home-delivered mental health services for aged rural home health care recipients. *Journal of Applied Gerontology, 19,* 460–475.

Keith, P. M. (2003). Interests and skills of volunteers in an ombudsman program: Opportunities for participation. *International Journal of Aging and Human Development, 57*(1), 1–20.

Keith, P. M., & Wacker, R. R. (1994). *Older wards and their guardians.* New York: Praeger.

Kelley, H. H. (1967). Attribution theory in social psychology. In D. Levin (Ed.), *Nebraska Symposium on Motivation* (pp. 151–174). Lincoln: University of Nebraska Press.

Kelly, J. R., Steinkamp, M. W., & Kelly, J. R. (1986). Later life leisure: How they play in Peoria. *The Gerontologist, 26,* 531–537.

Kelly, J. R., Steinkamp, M. W., & Kelly, J. R. (1987). Later life satisfaction: Does leisure contribute? *Leisure Sciences, 9,* 189–200.

Kemper, P. (1988). The evaluation of the National Long Term Care Demonstration: Overview of the findings. *Health Services Research, 23,* 161–174.

Kennet, J., Burgio, L., & Schulz, R. (2000). Interventions for in-home caregivers: A review of research 1990 to present. In R. Schulz (Ed.), *Handbook of dementia caregiving* (pp. 61–125). New York: Springer.

Kenney, G. M. (1993). Is access to home health care a problem in rural areas? *American Journal of Public Health, 83*(3), 412–414.

Kent, D. (1978). The how and why of senior centers. *Aging,* May–June, 2–6.

Kessler, R. C., Berglund, P. A., Glantz, M. D., Koretz, D. S., Merikangas, K. R., Walters, E. E. et al., (2002). *Estimating the prevalence and correlates of serious mental illness in community epidemiological surveys. In R.W. Manderscheid & M. J. Henderson (Eds.), Mental Health, United States, 2002.* Retrieved January 25, 2007 from http://mentalhealth.samhsa.gov/publications/allpubs/SMA04-3938/Chapter12.asp.

Kim, E., Kleiber, D. A., & Kropf, N. (2001). Leisure activity, ethnic preservation, and cultural integration of older Korean Americans. *Journal of Gerontological Social Work, 36*(1/2), 107–129.

Kimball, B., & O'Neill, E. (2002). *Health care's human crisis: The American nursing shortage.* Princeton, NJ: The Robert Wood Johnson Foundation.

King, A. C., Haskell, W. L., Taylor, C. B., Kraemer, H. C., & DeBusk, R. F. (1991). Group versus home-based exercise training in healthy older men and women: A community-based clinical trial. *Journal of the American Medical Association, 266,* 1535–1542.

King, A. C., Rejeski, J., & Buchner, D. M. (1998). Physical activity interventions targeting older adults: A critical review and recommendations. *American Journal of Preventive Medicine, 15*(4), 316–333.

King, S., & Collins, C. (1991). Institutionalization of an elderly family member: Reactions of spouse and nonspouse caregivers. *Archives of Psychiatric Nursing, 5,* 323–330.

Kingston, E. R., Hirshorn, B. A., & Cornman, J. M. (1986). *Ties that bind: The interdependence of generations.* Cabin John, MD: Seven Locks.

Kirschner Associates, Inc. (1983). A*n evaluation of the nutritional services for the elderly* (Vols. 1–5). Washington, DC: U.S. Department of Health and Human Services, Administration on Aging.

Kochera, A., Straight, A., & Guterbock, T. (2005). *A report to the nation on livable communities: Creating environments for successful aging.* Retrieved December 28, 2006 from http://assets.aarp.org/rgcenter/il/beyond_50_communities.pdf.

Koffman, D., Raphael, D., & Weiner, R. (2004). *The impact of federal programs on transportation for older adults. Report submitted to the American Association of Retired Persons, San Francisco, CA: Nelson/Nygaard Consulting Associates.* Retrieved January 15, 2006 from http://assets.aarp.org/rgcenter/post-import/2004_17_transport.pdf.

Korim, A. (1974). *Older Americans and community colleges: A guide for program implementation.* Washington, DC: American Association of Community and Junior Colleges.

Kosloski, K., & Montgomery, R. (1993). The effects of respite on caregivers of Alzheimer's patients: One-year evaluation of the Michigan model of respite programs. *Journal of Applied Gerontology, 12,* 4–17.

Kosloski, K., & Montgomery, R. (1995). The impact of respite use on nursing home placement. *The Gerontologist, 35,* 67–74.

Kosloski, K., Montgomery, R. J. V., & Youngbauer, J. G. (2001). Utilization of respite services: A comparison of users, seekers, and nonseekers. *Journal of Applied Gerontology, 20*(1), 111–132.

Kramarow E., Lentzner, H., Rooks, R., Weeks, J., & Saydah, S. (1999). *Health and Aging Chartbook. Health, United States, 1999.* Hyattsville, Maryland: National Center for Health Statistics.

Kramer, A. (2006). *Uniform patient assessment for post-acute care: Final report. Division of Health Care Policy and Research, University of Colorado at Denver and Health Sciences Center, Aurora, CO.* Retrieved February 5, 2007 from www.cms.hhs.gov/QulaityInitiativesGenInfo/downloads/QualityPACFullReport.pdf.

Krout, J. (1981). *Service utilization patterns of the rural elderly: Final report to the Administration on Aging.* Fredonia, NY: Author.

Krout, J. (1982). *Determinants of service use by the aged: Final report to the AARP Andrus Foundation.* Fredonia, NY: Author.

Krout, J. (1983a). Correlates of senior center utilization. *Research on Aging, 5,* 339–352.

Krout, J. (1983b). Knowledge and use of services by the elderly: A critical review of the literature. *International Journal of Aging and Human Development, 17,* 153–167.

Krout, J. (1984). Knowledge of senior center activities among the elderly. *Journal of Applied Gerontology, 3,* 71–81.

Krout, J. (1985a). Senior center activities and services. *Research on Aging, 7*, 455–471.

Krout, J. (1985b). Service awareness among the elderly. *Journal of Gerontological Social Work, 9*, 7–19.

Krout, J. (1987a). Rural versus urban differences in senior center activities and services. *The Gerontologist, 27*, 92–97.

Krout, J. (1987b). *Senior center linkages and the provision of services to the elderly: Final report to the AARP Andrus Foundation*. Fredonia, NY: Author.

Krout, J. (1988). *The frequency, duration, stability, and discontinuation of senior center participation: Causes and consequences: Final report to the AARP Andrus Foundation*. Fredonia, NY: Author.

Krout, J. (1989a). *Area Agencies on Aging: Service planning and provision for the rural elderly: Final report to the Retirement Research Foundation*. Fredonia, NY: Author.

Krout, J. (1989b). *Senior centers in America*. Westport, CT: Greenwood.

Krout, J. (1990). *The organization, operation, and programming of senior centers in America: A seven-year follow-up: Final report to the AARP. Andrus Foundation*. Fredonia, NY: Author.

Krout, J. (1993a). Case management activities for the rural elderly: Findings from a national study. *Journal of Case Management, 2*, 137–146.

Krout, J. (1993b). *Senior centers and at-risk older persons: A national agenda*. Washington, DC: National Institute on the Aging.

Krout, J. (1995). Senior centers and services for the frail elderly. *Journal of Aging and Social Policy, 7*(2), 59–76.

Krout, J., Cutler, S. J., & Coward, R. T. (1990). Correlates of senior center participation: A national analysis. *The Gerontologist, 30*, 72–79.

Krout, J. A., Moen, P., Holmes, H. H., Oggins, J., & Bowen, N. (2002). Reasons for relocation to a continuing care retirement community. *The Journal of Applied Gerontology, 21*, 236–256.

Kuehne, V. S. (2000). *Intergenerational programs: Understanding what we have created*. New York: Haworth.

Kuhn, B. A., Dunn, P. A., Smallwood, D., Hanson, K., Blaylock, J., & Vogel, S. (1996). Policy watch: The food stamp program and welfare reform. *Journal of Economic Perspectives, 10*(2), 189–198.

Kuiken, D. (2004). *A systems integration of mental health services for older adults in community based long term care. White House Conference on Aging: Listening session*. Retrieved January 23, 2007 from www.whcoa.gov/about/policy/meetings/summary/ILkuikentestimony.pdf.

Kutner, M., Greenberg, E., & Baer, J. (2005). *A first look at the literacy of America's adults in the 21st century. National Center for Education Statistics*. Retrieved January 22, 2007 from http://nces.ed .gov/NAAL/PDF/2006470.PDF.

Kutner, G., & Love, J. (2003). *Time and money: An in-depth look at 45+ volunteers and donors*. Washington, DC: AARP.

Kutza, E. A. (1991). The Older Americans Act of 2000: What should it be? *Generations, 15*(3), 65–68.

LA4Seniors. (2006). *Single room occupancy housing corporation: Project Hotel Alert*. Retrieved December 28, 2006 from www.la4seniors.com/single_room_corp.htm.

Lachs, M. S., & Pillemer, K. (2004). Elder abuse. *The Lancet, 364*, 1192–1263.

Lalonde, B., Hooyman, N., & Blumhagen, J. (1988). Long-term outcome effectiveness of a health promotion program for the elderly: The Wallingford Wellness Project. *Journal of Gerontological Social Work, 13*, 95–112.

Larkin, E. (1998–99). The intergenerational response to childcare and after-school care. *Generations, 22*(4), 33–36.

Larkin, J. P., & Hopcroft, B. M. (1993). In-hospital respite as a moderator of caregiver stress. *Health and Social Work, 18*, 132–138.

Lawton, M. P. (1980). Housing elderly: Residential quality and residential satisfaction. *Research on Aging, 2*, 309–328.

Lawton, M. P. (1982). Competence, environmental press, and the adaptation of older people. In M. P. Lawton, P. G. Windley, & T. O. Byerts (Eds.), *Aging and the environment: Theoretical approaches* (pp. 33–59). New York: Springer.

Lawton, M. P. (1989). Three functions of the residential environment. In L. A. Pastalan & M. E. Cowart (Eds.), *Lifestyles and housing of older adults* (pp. 35–50). New York: Haworth.

Lawton, M. P., Brody, E., & Saperstein, A. (1991). *Respite for caregivers of Alzheimer's patients: Research and practice*. New York: Springer.

Lawton, M. P., Moss, M., & Fulcomer, M. (1982). *Determinants of the leisure activities of older people*. Philadelphia: Philadelphia Geriatrics Center.

Lawton, M. P., & Nahemow, L. (1973). Ecology and the aging process. In C. Eisdorfer & M. P. Lawton (Eds.), *Psychology of adult development and aging* (pp. 619–674). Washington, DC: American Psychological Association.

Leanse, J., Tiven, M., & Robb, T. B. (1977). *Senior center operation*. Washington, DC: National Council on the Aging.

Leanse, J., & Wagner, L. (1975). *Senior centers: A report of senior group programs in America*. Washington, DC: National Council on the Aging.

Leavitt, M. O. (2006). *Report to Congress: Patient classification under Medicare's Prospective Payment System for Skilled Nursing Facilities*. Washington, DC: Department of Health and Human Services. Retrieved February 8, 2007 from www.cms.hhs.gov/SNFPPS/Downloads/RC_2006_PC-PPSSNF.pdf.

Lebowitz, B., & Niederehe, G. (1992). Concepts and issues in mental health and aging. In J. Birren, R. B. Sloane, & G. Cohen (Eds.), *Handbook of mental health and aging* (2nd ed., pp. 3–26). New York: Academic Press.

Lee, G. R. (1983). Social integration and fear of crime among older persons. *Journal of Gerontology, 38*, 745–750.

Lee, J. (1991). *Development, delivery, and utilization of services under the Older Americans Act: A perspective of Asian American elderly*. New York: Garland.

Lee, J. (1993). *ElderTransit facts: Analysis of area agency on aging transportation survey* (Brochure). Washington, DC: National Eldercare Institute on Transportation.

Lee, R. E., & King, A. C. (2003). Discretionary time among older adults: How do physical activity promotion interventions affect sedentary and active behaviors? *Annals of Behavioral Medicine, 25*(2), 112–119.

Lefebvre, R. C., Harden, E. A., Rawkowski, W., Lasater, T. M., & Careton, R. A. (1987). Characteristics of participants in community health programs: Four-year results. *American Journal of Public Health, 77*, 1342–1344.

Legal Services Corporation Act, 42 U.S.C. § 2996 et seq. (1974).

Legal Services Corporation. (1997). *LSC Acts/Regulations*. Retrieved February 2, 1997, from www.lsc.gov.presser/pr_act.html.

Legal Services Corporation. (2006). *Legal Services Corporation fact book 2005*. Washington, DC. Available at www.rin.lsc.gov/Rinboard/2005FactBook.pdf.

Legal Services of Northern California. (2001). *About the senior legal hotline*. Retrieved August 15, 2001 from www.seniorlegalhotline.org.

Levinson, R. W. (1988). *Information and referral networks*. New York: Springer.

Lewin Group (2006a). *Nursing home use by "oldest old" sharply declines*. Retrieved January 8, 2007 from www.lewin.com/NR/rdonlyres/9A0A92A2-4D76-4397-A0A2-04EB20700795/0/NursingHomeUseTrendsPaper.pdf.

Lewin Group. (2006b). *The Aging and Disability Resource Center (ADRC) Demonstration grant initiative: Interim outcomes report*. Retrieved November 30, 2006 from www.adrc-tae.org/documents/InterimReport.pdf?PHPSESSID = 67420645e557c26c56f4b9c7a957a77b.

Lichtenberg, P. (1994). *A guide to psychological practice in geriatric long-term care*. New York: Haworth.

Lichtenstein, J. H. & Verma, S. (2003). Older workers' pension plan and IRA coverage. Washington, DC: Public Policy Institute, American Association of Retired Persons. Available at http://assets.aarp.org/rgcenter/econ/dd91_retire.pdf.

Lieberman, M. A., & Fisher, L. (2001). The effects of nursing home placement on family caregivers of patients with Alzheimer's disease. *The Gerontologist, 41*, 819–826.

Liebig, P. S., Koenig, T., & Pynoos, J. (2006). Zoning, accessory dwelling units, and family caregiving: Issues, trends, and recommendations. *Journal of Aging and Social Policy, 18*(3/4), 155–172.

Lifelong Learning Act, Pub. L. No. 94–482 (1976).

Lifelong Learning Institutes. (2006a). *Facts about the Elderhostel Institute network*. Retrieved December 18, 2006 from www.elderhostel.org/ein/factsheet.asp.

Lifelong Learning Institutes. (2006b). *The LLI movement across college and university campuses*. Retrieved December 18, 2006 from www.elderhostel.org/ein/ilrmovement.asp.

Lifelong Learning Institutes. (2006c). *A brief overview of the LLI movement*. Retrieved December 18, 2006 from www.elderhostel.org/ein/overview.asp.

LIHEAP Clearinghouse. (2006). *Low-income energy program funding history: 1977–2006*. Retrieved December 28, 2006 from http://liheap.ncat.org/Funding/lhhist.htm.

Lincoln Area Agency on Aging. (2006). *ActivAge Centers*. Retrieved June 19, 2006 from www.lincoln.ne.gov/city/mayor/aging/centers.htm.

Lindquist, J. H., & Duke, J. M. (1982). The elderly victim at risk: Explaining the fear victimization paradox. *Criminology, 20*(1), 115–126.

Lipman, A., & Longino, C. F., Jr. (1982). Formal and informal support: A conceptual clarification. *Journal of Applied Gerontology, 1*, 141–146.

Lipman, A., & Sterne, R. (1962). Aging in the United States: Ascription of a terminal sick role. *Sociology and Social Research, 53*, 194–203.

Lipsky, M., & Thibodeau, M. A. (1990). Domestic food policy in the United States. *Journal of Health Politics, Policy and Law, 15*(2), 319–339.

Litwak, E. (1985). *Helping the elderly: The complementary roles of informal networks and formal systems*. New York: Guilford.

Litwak, E., & Misseri, P. (1989). Organizational theory, social supports, and mortality rates: A theoretical convergence. *American Sociological Review, 54*, 49–66.

Long, N. (1975). *Information and referral services: Research findings* (DHEW Pub. No. OHDS 77–410). Washington, DC: Government Printing Office.

Long, N., Anderson, J., Burd, R., Mathis, M. E., & Todd, S. P. (1971). Information and referral centers: A functional analysis (DHEW Pub. No. OHDS 75–235). Washington, DC: Government Printing Office.

Lowenthal, B., & Egan, R. (1991). Senior citizen volunteers in a university day-care center. *Educational Gerontology, 17*, 363–378.

Lowy, L. (1980). *Social policies and programs on aging.* Lexington, MA: Lexington.

Lowy, L., & Doolin, J. (1985). Multipurpose and senior centers. In A. Monk (Ed.), *Handbook of gerontological services* (pp. 342–376). New York: Van Nostrand Reinhold.

Lucas, J. A., Scotto R. N., Andrew, L. J., & Howell-White, S. (2002). *Review of adult day health services: A review of the literature. Rutgers Center for Health Policy.* Retrieved September 28, 2006, from www.cshp.rutgers.edu/PDF/AdultDaycareLitRev.pdf.

Lund, D. A., Hill, R. D., Caserta, M. S., & Wright, S. D. (1995). Video Respite™: An innovated resource for family, professional caregivers, and person with dementia. *The Gerontologist, 35*, 683–687.

Lutzky, S., Alecxih, L. M. B., Duffy, J., & Neill, C. (2000). *Review of the Medicaid 1915(c) Home and Community Based Services waiver program literature and program data.* Washington, DC: U.S. Department of Health and Human Services.

Maas, M. (1988). Management of patients with Alzheimer's disease in long-term care facilities. *Nursing Clinics of North America, 23*, 57–68.

MacAdam, M., Capitman, J., Yee, D., Prottas, J., Leutz, W., & Westwater, D. (1989). Case management for frail elders: The Robert Wood Johnson Foundation's program for hospital initiatives in long-term care. *The Gerontologist, 29*, 737–744.

MacDonald, D. (1992). Hospice patients without primary caregivers: A critique of prevailing intervention strategies. *Home Healthcare Nurse, 10*, 24–26.

MacNeil, R. D. (2001). Bob Dylan and the baby boom generation: The times they are a-changin'—again. *Activities, Adaptation & Aging, 25*(3/4), 45–58

MaloneBeach, E., Zarit, S., & Shore, D. (1992). Caregivers' perceptions of case management and community-based services: Barriers to service use. *Journal of Applied Gerontology, 11*, 145–159.

Management Sciences for Health. (n.d). *Provider's guide to quality and culture.* Retrieved February 2, 2007 from http://erc.msh.org/mainpage.cfm?file = 9.0.htm&module = provider&language = English&ggroup = &mgroup = .

Manheimer, R. (1992). Creative retirement in an aging society. In R. Fischer, M. Blazey, & H. Lipman (Eds.), *Students of the third age* (pp. 122–131). New York: Macmillan.

Manheimer, R. J. (2002). *Older adult education in the United States: Trends and predictions. North Carolina Center for Creative Retirement.* Retrieved on January 13, 2007 from www.unca.edu/ncccr/Reports/older_adult_education_in_the_US.htm

Manheimer, R., Snodgrass, D., & Moskow-McKenzie, D. (1995). *Older adult education: A guide to research, programs, and policies.* Westport, CT: Greenwood.

Mantell, J., & Gildea, M. (1989). Elderly shared housing in the United States. In D. J. Jaffe (Ed.), *Shared housing for the elderly* (pp. 13–23). New York: Greenwood.

Manton, K. I. (1987). Patterns and psychological correlates of material support within a religious setting: The bidirectional support hypothesis. *American Journal of Community Psychology, 15*, 185–207.

Mark Battle Associates. (1977). *Evaluation of information and referral services for the elderly: Final report* (DHEW Pub. No. OHDS 77-20109). Washington, DC: Government Printing Office.

Marken, D. M. (2005). One step ahead: Preparing the senior center for 2030. *Activities, Adaptation & Aging, 29*, 4, 69–84.

Marks, N. F. (1998). Does it hurt to care? Caregiving, work–family conflict, and midlife well-being. *Journal of Marriage and the Family, 60*, 951–966.

Marmor, T. R., Mashaw, J. L., & Harvey, P. L. (1990). *America's misunderstood welfare state: Persistent myths, enduring realities*. New York: Basic Books.

Matthews, D. H., & Sprey, J. (1984). The impact of divorce on grandparenthood: An exploratory study. *The Gerontologist, 24*, 41–47.

Matthews, J. (1992). *Social Security, Medicare, and pensions: A sourcebook for Older Americans* (5th ed.). Berkeley, CA: Nolo.

Matthews, J., & Berman, D. M. (1990). *Social Security, Medicare and pensions* (3rd ed.). Berkeley, CA: Nolo.

Matthews, J., & Berman, D. M. (1996). *Social Security, Medicare, and pensions* (6th ed.). Berkeley, CA: Nolo.

Matthews, S. H., & Rosner, T. T. (1988). Shared filial responsibility: The family as the primary caregiver. *Journal of Marriage and the Family, 50*, 185–195.

Mauser, T. (1994). *Colorado transit overview*. Denver: Colorado Department of Transportation.

Maxwell, J. (1962). *Centers for older people: Guide for programs and facilities*. Washington, DC: National Council on the Aging.

McCaslin, R. (1981). Next steps in information and referral for the elderly. *The Gerontologist, 21*, 184–193.

McCaslin, R. (1989). Service utilization by the elderly: The importance of orientation to the formal system. *Journal of Gerontological Social Work, 14*, 153–174.

McClusky, H. (1974). Education for aging: The scope of the field and perspectives for the future. In S. M. Grabowski & W. D. Mason (Eds.), *Learning for aging* (pp. 324–355). Washington, DC: Adult Education Association of the USA.

McConnel, S., & Beitler, D. (1991). The Older Americans Act after 25 years: An overview. *Generations, 15*(3), 5–10.

McConnell, S., & Ponza, M. (1999). *The reaching the working poor and poor elderly study: What we learned and recommendations for future research*. Report submitted to the U.S. Department of Agriculture, Food and Nutrition Service. Washington, DC: Mathematica Policy Research, June.

McCrea, J. M., Nichols, A., & Newman, S. (Eds.). (1998). *Intergenerational service learning in gerontology: A compendium, Vol. 1*. Washington, DC: Association for Gerontology in Higher Education.

McCrea, J. M., Nichols, A., & Newman, S. (Eds.). (1999). *Intergenerational service learning in gerontology: A compendium, Vol. 2*. Washington, DC: Association for Gerontology in Higher Education.

McCrea, J. M., Nichols, A., & Newman, S. (Eds.). (2000). *Intergenerational service learning in gerontology: A compendium, Vol. 3*. Washington, DC: Association for Gerontology in Higher Education.

McGinnis, J. (1988). *Year 2000 health objectives for the nation: Proceedings of the Surgeon General's Workshop: Health Promotion and Aging*. Washington, DC: Government Printing Office.

McGuire, M. (2002). *Food donation initiatives assessment and food recovery infrastructure evaluation: Revised final report*. Portland, OR: Metro Regional Environmental Management. Retrieved on January 7, 2007 from http://www.metro-region.org/library_doc/recycling/food_assess_rpt_0402_revised.pdf.

McKee, P. (1995). Gardening: An equal opportunity joy. *Activities, Adaptation, and Aging, 20*, 71–78.

McNeil, J. (2001). *Americans with disabilities: 1997*. Current Population Reports, P70–73, U.S. Census Bureau. Washington, DC: Government Printing Office.

Meals on Wheels America: A history of success, (1996, Spring). Alexandria, VA: Meals on Wheels America, pp. 1–2.

Medicare Rights Center. (2006). *Eligibility for home health care and hospice*. Retrieved January 19, 2007, from www.medicarerights.org/maincontenteligibility.html.

Menec, V. H. (2003). The Relation Between Everyday Activities and Successful Aging: A 6-Year Longitudinal Study. *Journal of Gerontology, 58B*(2), S74–S82.

MetLife. (2005a). *Demographic profile of American babyboomers*. Retrieved December 19, 2006, from www.metlife.com/WPSAssets/34442486101113318029V1FBoomer%20Profile%202005.pdf.

MetLife. (2005b). *The MetLife market survey of nursing home and home health care costs*. Westport, CT: MetLife Mature Market Institute. Retrieved on February 13, 2007 from www.magaltc.com/mature-marketsurveycharts.pdf.

MetLife. (2006a). *The MetLife market survey of assisted living costs: October 2006*. Retrieved December 17, 2006, from www.metlife.com/WPSAssets/13288174261105724366V1FMetLife%20Market%20Survey.pdf.

MetLife. (2006b). The MetLife study of Alzheimer's disease: *The caregiving experience*. Retrieved August 25, 2006, from www.metlife.com/WPSAssets/14050063731156260663V1FAlzheimerCaregiving Experience.pdf.

Mettler, M., & Kemper, D. W. (1995). Healthwise study shows rural self-care training pays off. *Aging Today*, January/February, 5.

Meyer, M. D. (1991). Assuring quality of care: Nursing home resident councils. *Journal of Applied Gerontology, 10*(1), 103–116.

Middlecamp, M., & Gross, D. (2002). Intergenerational daycare and preschoolers' attitudes about aging. *Educational Gerontology, 28*, 271–288.

Milbank Memorial Fund. (2006). *Public housing and supportive services for the frail elderly: A guide for housing authorities and their collaborators*. Retrieved January 2, 2007 from www.milbank.org/reports/0609publichousing/0609publichousing.pdf.

Miller, D., & Goldman, L. (1989). Perceptions of caregivers about special respite services for the elderly. *The Gerontologist, 29*, 408–410.

Mills, E. (1993). *The story of Elderhostel*. Hanover, NH: University Press of New England.

Milne, K. (1994). The evolution of case management to care management. In R. Howe (Ed.), *Case management for health care professionals* (pp. 179–190). Chicago: Precept.

Miner, S., Logan, J. R., & Spitz, G. (1993). Predicting the frequency of senior center attendance. *The Gerontologist, 33*, 650–657.

Minkler, M., & Pasick, R. J. (1985). Health promotion and the elderly: A critical perspective on the past and future. In K. Dychtwald (Ed.), *Wellness and health promotion for the elderly* (pp. 39–51). Rockville, MD: Aspen.

Minkler, M., & Roe, K. M. (1996). Grandparents as surrogate parents. *Generations, 20*(1), 34–37.

Minnesota Board on Aging. (n.d.). *MinnesotaHelp.info*. Retrieved on February 12, 2007 from www.minnesotahelp.info/en/mn/cgi-bin/location.asp.

Mitchell, J. (1995). Service awareness and use among older North Carolinians. *Journal of Applied Gerontology, 14*(2), 193–209.

Moen, E. (1978). The reluctance of the elderly to accept help. *Social Problems, 25*, 293–303.

Mollica, R. (2003). Coordinating services across the continuum of health, housing, and supportive services. *Journal of Aging and Health, 15*, 165–188.

Monk, A., & Kaye, L. W. (1991). Congregate housing for the elderly: Its need, function, and perspective. *Journal of Housing for the Elderly, 9*(1/2), 5–20.

Monk, A., Kaye, L.W., & Litwin, H. (1984). *Resolving grievances in the nursing home: A study of the ombudsman program.* New York: Columbia University Press.

Montgomery, R. (1992). Examining respite: Its promise and limits. In M. Ory & A. Dunker (Eds.), *In-home care for older people: Health and supportive services* (pp. 75–96). Newbury Park, CA: Sage.

Montgomery, R. J., & Kamo, Y. (1989). Parent care by sons and daughters. In J. A. Mancini (Ed.), *Aging parents and adult children* (pp. 213–228). Lexington, MA: Lexington.

Montgomery, R. V., Marquis, J., Schaefer, J. P., & Kosloski, K. (2002). Profile of respite users. *Home Health Care Services Quarterly, 21*(3/4), 33–63.

Moody, H. R. (1976). Philosophical presuppositions of education for older adults. *Educational Gerontology, 2,* 1–16.

Moody, H. R. (1988). *Abundance of life: Human development policies for an aging society.* New York: Columbia University Press.

Moon, M., & Ruggles, P. (1994). The needy or the greedy? Assessing the income support of an aging population. In T. Marmor, T. Smeeding, & V. Greene (Eds.), *Economic security and intergenerational justice: A look at North America* (pp. 207–226). Washington, DC: Urban Institute.

Moore, M., & Piland, W. (1994). Impact of campus physical environment on older adult learners. *Community College Journal of Research and Practice, 18,* 307–317.

Moore, W. (1989). Assessing the unmet legal needs of older persons: What will it cost to meet that need? *Elder Law Forum, 1*(2), 4.

Moore, W. (1992). Improving the delivery of legal services for the elderly: A comprehensive approach. *Emory Law Journal, 41,* 805–861.

Mor, V., & Allen, S. (1995). Hospice. In G. Maddox (Ed.), *The encyclopedia of aging* (2nd ed., pp. 475–477). New York: Springer.

Morgan, L. A., Gurber-Baldini, A. L., & Magaziner, J. (2001). Resident characteristics. In S. I. Zimmerman, P. D. Sloane, & J. K. Eckert (Eds.), *Assisted living: Residential care in transition* (pp. 144–172) Baltimore, MD: Johns Hopkins University Press.

Mosher-Ashley, P., & Allard, J. (1993). Problems facing chronically mentally ill elders receiving community-based psychiatric services: Need for residential services. *Adult Residential Care Journal, 7,* 23–30.

Moulton, P., McDonald, L., Muus, K., Knudson, A., Wakefield, M., & Ludtke, R. (2005). *Prevalence of Chronic Disease Among American Indian and Alaska Native Elders. Center for Rural Health, University of North Dakota, School of Medicine & Health Sciences.* Retrieved January 27, 2007 from www.med.und.nodak.edu/depts/rural/nrcnaa/pdf/chronic_disease1005.pdf.

Mullins, L. C., Cook, C., Mushel, M., Machin, G., & Georgas, J. (1993). A comparative examination of the characteristics of participants of a senior citizens nutrition and activities program. *Activities, Adaptation, and Aging, 17*(3), 15–37.

Munnell, A. H., Webb, A., & Delorme, L. (2006). *A new national retirement risk index.* Retrieved January 12, 2007 from www.bc.edu/centers/crr/issues/ib_48.pdf.

Murakami, E. (1994). *Elder transit facts: Improving travel for the elderly* (Brochure). Washington, DC: National Eldercare Institute on Transportation.

Murtaugh, C., Kemper, P., & Spillman, B. (1990). The risk of nursing home use in later life. *Medical Care, 28,* 952–962.

Musick, M. A., & Wilson, J. (2003). Volunteering and depression: the role of psychological and social resources in different age groups. *Social Science and Medicine, 56*(2), 259–69.

Nadler, A., Fisher, J. D., & Streufest, S. (1976). The donor's dilemma: Recipients' reactions to aid from friend or foe. *Journal of Personality, 44*, 392–409.

Nadler, A., & Mayseless, O. (1983). Recipient self-esteem and reactions to help. In J. D. Fisher, A. Nadler, & B. M. DePaulo (Eds.), *New directions in helping, Vol. 1* (pp. 167–188). New York: Academic Press.

Nadler, A., Sheinberg, L., & Jaffe, Y. (1981). Coping with stress by help seeking: Help seeking and receiving behavior in male paraplegics. In C. Spielberger, I. Sarason, & N. Milgram (Eds.), *Stress and anxiety, Vol. 8* (pp. 375–386). Washington, DC: Hemisphere.

Narrow, W. E., Rae, D. S., Robins, L. N., & Regier, D. A. (2002). Revised prevalence estimates of mental disorders in the United States: Using a clinical significance criterion to reconcile 2 surveys' estimates. *Archives of General Psychiatry, 59*(2), 115–123.

National Adult Day Services Association. (2006). *Trends in ADS*. Retrieved December 28, 2006 from www.nadsa.org/adsfacts/default.asp.

National Aging I&R/A Support Center. (2001). *Aging Specialty Information and Referral Certification Program. Competencies*. Retrieved on January 15, 2007 from www.nasua.org/informationand referral/pdf/AgingCertificationcompetencies.pdf.

National Alliance for Caregiving/AARP. (2004). *Caregiving in the U.S.* Retrieved January 25, 2007 from http://assets.aarp.org/rgcenter/il/us_caregiving.pdf.

National and Community Service Trust Act of 1993, 42 U.S.C. § 12571 et seq. (1996).

National Association for Home Care & Hospice. (2004). *Basic statistics about home care*. Retrieved December 18, 2006 from www.nahc.org/04HC_Stats.pdf.

National Association for Home Care & Hospice. (2007). *Welcome to NAHC*. Retrieved January 10, 2007 from www.nahc.org.

National Association of Area Agencies on Aging. (1996). *Legislative briefing: Advocate's guide to 1996 national policy priorities*. Washington, DC: NAAoA.

National Association of Home Builders Research Center. (2002). *National older adult housing survey report 2002: Summary of findings*. Retrieved January 9, 2007 from www.nahbrc.org/docs/MainNav/Seniors/3743_noahssummary.pdf.

National Association of State Units on Aging. (n.d.). *Eldercare locator*. Retrieved January 16, 2007 from www.nasua.org/informationandreferral/locator.cfm.

National Association of State Units on Aging. (2000). *Vision 2010: Toward a comprehensive aging information resource system for the 21st century*. Retrieved January 23, 2007 from www.nasua.org/vision_2010.pdf.

National Association of State Units on Aging. (2006). *Medicare Empowerment Program. Part I: Overview of N4A and NASUA Role*. Retrieved January 23, 2007 from www.nasua.org/informationandreferral/pdf/medicareempowerment.pdf.

National Center on Accessibility. (n.d.). *The Eden Alternative—Renewing Life in Nursing Homes*. Retrieved February 18, 2007 from www.ncaonline.org/ncpad/eden.shtml.

National Chronic Care Consortium. (1997). *Care management for the frail elderly: A literature review on selected topics*. Retrieved December 22, 2006 from www.nccconline.org/products/M10097.pdf.

National Center for Assisted Living. (2006a). *Assisted living facility profile*. Retrieved January 9, 2007, from www.ncal.org/about/facility.htm.

National Center for Assisted Living. (2006b). *Assisted living resident profile*. Retrieved January 9, 2007 from www.ncal.org/about/resident.htm.

National Center for Assisted Living. (2006c). *Assisted living state regulatory review 2006.* Retrieved January 9, 2007 from www.ncal.org/about/2006_reg_review.pdf.

National Center for Health Statistics. (1990). *Current estimates from the National Health Interview Survey: 1989* (Vital and Health Statistics, Series 10, No. 176). Washington, DC: Government Printing Office.

National Center for Health Statistics. (1993). *Health: United States.* Hyattsville, MD: Public Health Service.

National Center for Health Statistics. (2000). *Nursing home residents 65 years old and over by selected characteristics: 1997.* (Advance Data From Vital and Health Statistics, No. 312). Hyattsville, MD: NCHS.

National Center for Health Statistics. (2002). *2000 National Home and Hospice Care Survey: Data tables.* Retrieved January 2, 2007, from www.cdc.gov/nchs/data/nhhcsd/curhomecare00.pdf.

National Center for Health Statistics. (2004a). Respondent-assessed health by age, sex, and race/ethnicity: United States, 1997–2004. *National Health Interview Survey, Trends in Health and Aging.* Retrieved January 22, 2007 from www.cdc.gov/nchs/agingact.htm.

National Center for Health Statistics. (2004b). Prevalence of selected chronic conditions by age, sex, and race/ethnicity: United States, 1997–2004. *National Health Interview Survey, Trends in Health and Aging.* Retrieved January 22, 2007 from www.cdc.gov/nchs/agingact.htm.

National Center for Health Statistics. (2004c). *Difficulty performing activities of daily living by age, residence, sex, race and ethnicity: Medicare beneficiaries from the Medicare current beneficiaries survey, 1992–2004. National Health Interview Survey, Trends in Health and Aging.* Retrieved January 22, 2007 from www.cdc.gov/nchs/agingact.htm.

National Center for Health Statistics. (2004d). *Difficulty performing instrumental activities of daily living by age, residence, sex, race and ethnicity: Medicare beneficiaries from the Medicare current beneficiaries survey, 1992–2004. National Health Interview Survey, Trends in Health and Aging.* Retrieved on January 22, 2007 from www.cdc.gov/nchs/agingact.htm.

National Center for Health Statistics. (2004e). *Needing help with routine needs by age, sex, and race/ethnicity: United States, 1997–2005. National Health Interview Survey, Trends in Health and Aging.* Retrieved January 27, 2007 from www.cdc.gov/nchs/agingact.htm.

National Center for Health Statistics. (2004f). *Needing help with personal care needs by age, sex, and race/ethnicity: United States, 1997–2005. National Health Interview Survey, Trends in Health and Aging.* Retrieved January 27, 2007 from www.cdc.gov/nchs/agingact.htm.

National Center for Health Statistics. (2005). *Health, United States, 2005. Nursing homes, beds, occupancy, and residents, according to geographic division and state: United States, 1995–2003, Table 116.* Retrieved February 4, 2007 from www.cdc.gov/nchs/data/hus/hus05.pdf#116.

National Citizens' Coalition for *Nursing Home Reform. (2003). Residents' rights: An overview. Consumer Fact Sheet No. 2 August 2003,* Retrieved February 13, 2007 from www.nccnhr.org/uploads/ResRights03.pdf.

National Cooperative Highway Research Program. (2006). *Estimating the impacts of the aging population on transit ridership. Report submitted to the Transportation Research Board of the National Academies.* Fairfax, VA: ICF Consulting.

National Council on Aging. (1998). *National quality standards for nation's 16,000 senior centers get boost from new accreditation process.* Retrieved August 25, 2001 from www.ncoa.org/news/archives/national_quality.htm.

National Council on Aging. (2005). *Fact Sheets—Senior Centers: Background/History.* Retrieved on June 18, 2006 from www.ncoa.org/content.cfm?sectionID = 103&detail = 1177.

National Council on Aging. (2006a). *Special report—Accredited senior centers: A snapshot, January 12, 2006.* Retrieved on June 18, 2006 from www.ncoa.org/content.cfm?sectionID = 134& detail = 1307.

National Council on Aging. (2006b). *Special report—tomorrow's senior center: Dynamic, accessible, and perhaps not even called senior.* Retrieved June 19, 2006 from www.ncoa.org/content.cfm?sectionID = 134&detail = 1308.

National Council on Aging. (2007). *Congress passes Older Americans Act reauthorization.* Retrieved February 24, 2007 from www.ncoa.org/content.cfm?sectionID = 2&detail = 1712.

National Eldercare Institute on Health Promotion. (1995). Telephone links reduce isolation. *Perspectives in Health Promotion and Aging, 10*(1), 2.

National Eldercare Institute on Transportation. (1992). *Focus group report.* Washington, DC: NEIT.

National Eldercare Institute on Transportation. (1994). *Meeting the challenge: Mobility for elders* (prepared for the Administration on Aging). Washington, DC: NEIT.

National Fraud Information Center. (2004). *Telemarketing Fraud Report.* Washington, DC: National Consumer League.

National Governors' Association. (2004). *State support for family caregivers and paid home-care workers.* Retrieved January 2, 2007 from www.subnet.nga.org/ci/assets/4-caregivers.pdf.

National Highway Transportation Safety Administration. (2001). *Traffic Safety Facts 2000: Older Population.* Retrieved November 13, 2006 from www.nhtsa.dot.gov.

National Household Transportation Survey. (2001). Cited in L. Bailey, L. (2004). *Aging Americans: Stranded without transportation. Surface Transportation Policy Project.* Retrieved October 23, 2006 from www.apta.com/research/info/online/documents/aging_stranded.pdf.

National Hospice and Palliative Care Organization. (2001). *Facts and figures on hospice care in America.* Retrieved January 25, 2002 from www.nhpco.org.

National Hospice and Palliative Care Organization. (2006). *2006 in review.* Retrieved December 18, 2006 from www.nhpco.org/files/public/2006review.pdf.

National Institute of Senior Centers. (1978). *Senior center standards: Guidelines for practice.* Washington, DC: National Council on the Aging.

National Institute on Aging and Administration on Aging. (1996). *Resource directory for older people* (NIH Pub. No. 95–738). Washington, DC: Government Printing Office.

National Long-Term Care Ombudsman Resource Center. (n.d.). *What does an ombudsman do?* Retrieved February 2, 2007 from www.ltcombudsman.org/ombpublic/49_151_855.cfm.

National Low Income Housing Coalition. (2006). *Section 202 Supportive Housing for the Elderly.* Retrieved January 9, 2007 from www.nlihc.org/detail/article.cfm?article_id = 2803&id = 46.

National PACE Association. (2006). *National PACE Association applauds $7.5 million in grants to expand pace to rural areas.* Retrieved January 14, 2007 from www.npaonline.org/website/article.asp?id = 4.

National Policy and Resource Center on Nutrition and Aging. (1996). *Use of medical food and food for special dietary uses in elderly nutrition programs.* Miami: Florida International University.

National Senior Service Corps. (1997a). *Foster Grandparent Program: Fact sheet.* Retrieved May 4, 2001 from www.cns.gov/news/factsheets/fgp.pdf.

National Senior Service Corps. (1997b). *Senior Companion Program: Fact sheet.* Retrieved May 4, 2001 from www.cns.gov/news/factsheets/scp.pdf.

Neese, J. B., Abraham, I. L., & Buckwalter, K. C. (1999). Utilization of mental health services among rural elderly. *Archives of Psychiatric Nursing, 13*(1), 30–40.

Netting, F. E., & Hinds, H. (1989). Rural volunteer ombudsman programs. *Journal of Applied Gerontology, 8*, 419–427.

Netting, F. E., Paton, R. N., & Huber, R. (1992). The long-term care ombudsman program: What does the complaint reporting system tell us? *The Gerontologist, 32*, 843–848.

Newman, S., & Riess, J. (1992). Older workers in intergenerational child care settings. *Journal of Gerontological Social Work, 19*, 45–66.

Newman, S., Ward, C., Smith, T., Wilson, J., & McCrea, J. (Eds.). (1997). *Intergenerational programs: Past, present, and future*. Bristol, PA: Taylor & Francis.

Nijssen, J. (2004, November). *This is not your father's retirement. AARP Opinion*. Retrieved January 12, 2007 from www.aarp.org/research/work/retirement/a2004–11–11-gra-fathersretirement.html.

Noggle, B. (1995). Identifying and meeting needs of ethnic minority patients. *Hospice Journal, 10*, 85–93.

Nord, M. (2002). Food security rates are high for elderly households. *Food Review, 25*(2), 19–24.

Nord, M., Andrews, M., & Carlson, S. (2002). *Household food security in the United States, 2001. ERS Food Assistance and Nutrition Research Report No. 29*. Washington, DC: *U.S. Department of Agriculture*. Retrieved January 5, 2007 from www.ers.usda.gov/publications/fanrr29.

North Carolina Division of Aging. (2001). *Model senior centers*. Retrieved August 25, 2001 www.dhhs.state.nc.us/aging/srcen.pdf.

Novak, M. (2001). New older learner. *Continuing Higher Education Review, 65*, 98–105.

Office of the Assistant Secretary for Planning and Evaluation. (1995). *Subacute care: Policy synthesis and market area analysis*. Retrieved January 27, 2002 from http://aspe.hhs.gov/search/daltcp/Reports/XSUBACUT.HTM.

O'Keeffe, J., & Siebenaler, K. (2006). *Adult day services: A key community service for older adults*. Retrieved September 28, 2006 from http://aspe.hhs.gov/daltcp/reports/2006/keyADS.htm.

Older Adult Service and Information System. (2006). *Welcome to OASIS*. Retrieved January 10, 2007 from www.oasisnet.org.

Older Americans Act of 1965, Pub. L. No. 89–73, 42 U.S.C. § 3001 et seq., as amended or reauthorized 1967, 1968, 1972, 1973, 1974, 1975, 1977, 1978, 1984, 1987, 1992, 1997, 2000, 2006.

Older Workers Benefit Protection Act of 1990, 29 U.S.C. §§ 623, 626, 630 (1990).

Olson, L. K. (Ed.). (2001). *Age through ethnic lenses: Caring for the elderly in a multicultural society*. Laham, MD: Rowman & Littlefield.

Omnibus Budget Reconciliation Act of 1980, 5 U.S.C. § 8340 et seq., as amended.

Omnibus Budget Reconciliation Act of 1981, Pub. L. No. 97–35, 95 Stat. 357, 5 U.S.C. § 8340 et seq., as amended.

Omnibus Budget Reconciliation Act of 1987, 5 U.S.C. § 8340 et seq., as amended.

Omnibus Budget Reconciliation Act of 1989, 5 U.S.C. § 8340 et seq., as amended.

Omnibus Budget Reconciliation Act of 1990, 5 U.S.C. § 8340 et seq., as amended.

Ong, P. M., & Haselhoff, K. (2005). *Barriers to transit use. SCS Fact Sheet, 1(11)*. Retrieved October 29, 2006 from http://respositories.cdlib.org/lewis/scs/V011_N011.

Ormond, B. A., Black, K. J., Tilly, J., & Thomas, S. (2004). *Supportive services programs in naturally occurring retirement communities*. Retrieved January 2, 2007 from http://aspe.hhs.gov/daltcp/reports/NORCssp.pdf.

Ovrebo, B., Minkler, M., & Liljestrand, P. (1991). No room in the inn: The disappearance of SRO housing in the United States. *Journal of Housing for the Elderly, 8*(1), 77–92.

Palley, H. A., & Oktay, J. S. (1983). *The chronically limited elderly: The case for a national policy for in-home and supportive community based services.* New York: Haworth.

Pandya, S. M. (2005). *Caregiving in the United States.* Washington, DC: *AARP Public Policy Institute.* Retrieved January 25, 2007 from http://assets.aarp.org/rgcenter/il/fs111_caregiving.pdf.

Pardasani, M. P. (n.d). Senior centers: Patterns of programs and services. Retrieved December 1, 2006 from www.ncoa.org/attachments/Senior_Center_Services.pdf.

Pardasani, M. P. (2004). Senior centers: Increasing minority participation through diversification. *Journal of Gerontological Social Work, 43*(2/3), 41–56.

Parmalee, P. A., Katz, I. R., & Lawton, M. P. (1992). Incidence of depression in long-term care settings. *Journal of Gerontology, 47*, M189–M196.

Parmelee, P. A., & Lawton, M. P. (1990). The design of special environments for the aged. In J. E. Birren & K. W. Schaie (Eds.), *Handbook of the psychology of aging* (3rd ed., pp. 464–487). San Diego, CA: Academic Press.

Pascucci, M. (1992). Measuring incentives to health promotion in older adults: Understanding neglected health promotion in older adults. *Journal of Gerontological Nursing, 18*, 16–23.

Patterson, A. H. (1985). Fear of crime and other barriers to use of public transportation by the elderly. *Journal of Architectural Planning and Research, 2*, 277–288.

Payette, H. (2005). Nutrition as a determinant of functional autonomy and quality of life in aging: A research program. *Canadian Journal of Physiology & Pharmacology, 83*, 1061–1070.

Peng, T. R., Navaie-Waliser, M., & Feldman, P. H. (2003). Social support, home health service use, and outcomes among four racial-ethnic groups. *The Gerontologist, 43*, 503–513.

Pension Benefit Guaranty Corporation. (2006). *Pension insurance data book 2005.* Retrieved January 12, 2007 from www.pbgc.gov/docs/2005databook.pdf.

Personal Responsibility and Work Opportunity Reconciliation Act of 1996, Pub. L. No. 104–193, H.R. 3734, 104th Cong., 1st Sess., Cong. Rec. H8831 (1996).

Perspective on Aging. (1993). The first half-century of senior centers charts the way for decades to come. *Perspective on Aging, 22*(3), 16–25.

Peterson, D. (1985). A history of education for older learners. In D. Lumsden (Ed.), *The older adult as learner* (pp. 1–23). New York: Hemisphere.

Peterson, D. (1990). A history of the education of older learners. In R. Sherron & D. Lumsden (Eds.), *Introduction to educational gerontology* (3rd ed., pp. 1–21). New York: Hemisphere.

Peterson, J. (1995). The faces of community transportation. *Community Transportation Reporter, 13*(3), 10–12.

Peterson, S. A. (1989). Elderly women and program encounters: A rural study. *Journal of Women and Aging, 1*(4), 41–56.

Peterson, S. A., & Maiden, R. (1991). Older Americans' use of nutrition programs. *Journal of Nutrition for the Elderly, 11*(1/2), 49–67.

Petty, D. (1990). Respite care: A flexible response to service fragmentation. In N. Mace (Ed.), *Dementia care: Patient, family, and community* (pp. 243–269). Baltimore: Johns Hopkins University Press.

Pettey, S. M. (2003). Report recommends standards for assisted living. *Caring for the Aged, 4*(7), 6–10.

Pierce, D. (1993). Edu-tourism. *Winds of Change, 8*, 62–65.

Pillemer, K. (1988). Maltreatment of patients in nursing homes: Overview and research agenda. *Journal of Health and Social Behavior, 29*, 227–238.

Pillemer, K., & Finkelhor, D. (1989). The prevalence of elder abuse: A random sample survey. *The Gerontologist, 28*, 51–57.

Pillemer, K., & Moore, D. W. (1989). Abuse of patients in nursing homes: Findings from a survey of staff. *The Gerontologist, 29*, 132–135.

Pirie, P. L., Elias, W. S., Wackman, D. B., Jacobs, D. R., Murray, D. M., Mittelmark, M. B. et al., (1986). Characteristics of participants and non-participants in a community cardiovascular disease risk factor screening: The Minnesota Heart Health Program. *American Journal of Preventive Medicine, 2*, 20–25.

Ponza, M., Ohls, J. C., & Millen, B. E. (1996). *Serving elders at risk: The Older Americans Act Nutrition Program's national evaluation of the Elderly Nutrition Program, 1993–1995.* Washington, DC: U.S. Department of Health and Human Services.

Ponza, M., Ohls, J. C., Millen, B. E., McCool, A. M., Needels, K. E., Rosenberg, K. et al., (1996). *Serving elders at risk: The Older Americans Act Nutrition Program: National evaluation of the Elderly Nutrition Program 1993–1995. Report submitted to the U.S. Department of Health and Human Services.* Washington, DC: *Mathematica Policy Research.* Retrieved January 5, 2007 from www.aoa.gov/ prof/aoaprog/nutrition/program_eval/eval_report.asp.

Porell, F. W., & Miltiades, H.B. (2001). Disability outcomes of older Medicare HMO enrollees and fee-for-service Medicare beneficiaries. *Journal of the American Geriatrics Society, 49*, 615–631.

Posner, B. M. (1979). *Nutrition and the elderly.* Lexington, MA: Lexington.

Powers, E., & Bultena, G. (1974). Correspondence between anticipated and actual uses of public services by the aged. *Social Service Review, 48*, 245–254.

Prohaska, T., Belansky, E., Belza, B., Buchner, D., Marshall, V., McTigue, K. et al. (2006). Physical activity, public health, and aging: Critical issues and research priorities. *Journals of Gerontology, 61B*(5), S267–S273.

Purcell, P. J. (2000). Older workers: Employment and retirement trends. *Monthly Labor Review*, 19–30.

Pushkar, S., Gold, D., & Reis, M. (1995). When home caregiving ends: A longitudinal study of outcomes for caregivers of relatives with dementia. *Journal of the American Geriatrics Society, 43*, 10–16.

Putnam, R. (1993). *Making democracy work: Civic traditions in modern Italy.* Princeton, NJ: Princeton University Press.

Putnam, R. (2000). *Bowling alone: The collapse and revival of American community.* New York: Simon and Schuster.

Qualls, S. H., & Roberto, K. A. (2006). Diversity and caregiving support interventions: Lessons from elder care research. In B. Hayslip & J. Hicks Patrick (Eds.), *Custodial grandparents: Individual, cultural, and ethnic diversity* (pp. 37–54). New York: Springer.

Quandt, S. A., & Rao, P. (1999). Hunger and food security among older adults in a rural community. *Human Organization, 58*(1), 28–35.

Quinn, J. (1993). *Successful case management in long-term care.* New York: Springer.

Quinn, M. E., Hohnson, M. A., Andress, E. L., McGinnis, P., & Ramesh, M. (1999). Health characteristics of elderly personal care home residents. *Journal of Advanced Nursing, 30*, 410–417.

Quirk, D. A., Whaley, J. S., & Hutchinson, A. B. (1994). *Enhancing the capacity of state aging information and referral systems to meet the future needs of an aging society.* Washington, DC: National Association of State Units on Aging.

Rabins, P. V. (1986). Establishing Alzheimer's units in nursing homes: Pros and cons. *Hospital and Community Psychiatry, 37*, 120–121.

Railroad Retirement Act of 1937, 45 U.S.C. § 201 et seq. (1995).

Ralston, P. (1982). Perceptions of senior centers by the black elderly: A comparative study. *Journal of Gerontological Social Work, 4*, 127–137.

Ralston, P. (1985). Determinants of senior center attendance. Paper presented at the Annual Scientific Meeting of the Gerontological Society of America, New Orleans, LA.

Ralston, P. (1991). Senior centers and minority elderly: A critical review. *The Gerontologist, 31*, 325–331.

Ralston, P. (1993). Health promotion for rural black elderly: A comprehensive review. *Journal of Gerontological Social Work, 20*, 53–78.

Ralston, P., & Cohen, N. L. (1994). Nutrition and the rural elderly. In J. Krout (Ed.), *Providing community-based services to the rural elderly* (pp. 202–220). Thousand Oaks, CA: Sage.

Raphael, D. (2001). *Medicaid transportation: Assuring access to health care. A primer for states, health plans, providers and advocates.* Washington, DC: *Community Transportation Association of America.* Retrieved October 23, 2006 from www.ctaa.org/ntrc/medical.

Rapp, S. R., & Chao, D. (2000). Appraisals of strain and gain. Effects on psychological well-being of caregivers of dementia patients. *Aging & Mental Health, 4*, 142–147.

Rasmussen, W. (1989). *Taking the university to the people: Seventy-five years of cooperative extension.* Ames: Iowa State University Press.

Region VIII Office, Administration on Aging. (n.d.). *Title IV research and development: History of making a difference.* Denver, CO: Author.

Regnier, V. (1988). Sensitive environments that overcome barriers. *Architecture California, 10*, 18–26.

Regnier, V., & Culver, J. (1994). Single room occupancy: SRO-type housing for older people. *Supportive Housing Connection: A Technical Assistance Quarterly From the National Eldercare Institute on Housing and Supportive Services*, February, 1–3.

Rejecki, W., & Brawley, L. R. (1997). Shaping active lifestyles in older adults: A group-facilitated behavior change intervention. *Annals of Behavioral Medicine, 19*(Suppl), S106

Reschovsky, J. D., & Newman, S. J. (1991). Home upkeep and housing quality of older homeowners. *Journal of Gerontology, 46*, S288–S297.

Rethinking an old notion. (1996). *Hospital Care Management, 4*, 29–30.

Revenue Act of 1921, Pub. L. No. 136, 42 Stat. 227 (1921).

Retired Senior and Volunteer Program International. (2001). *RSVPI.* Retrieved January 13, 2007 from www.hhp.umd.edu/AGING/RSVPI/index.html.

Rhoades, J. A. (2005). *Overweight and obese elderly and near elderly in the United States, 2002: Estimates for the noninstitutionalized population age 55 and older. Medical Expenditures Panel Survey, Statistical Brief No. 68. Agency for Healthcare Research and Quality.* Retrieved February 2, 2007 from www.meps.ahrq.gov/mepsweb/data_files/publications/st68/ stat68.pdf.

Rich, B. M., & Baum, M. (1984). *The aging: A guide to public policy.* Pittsburgh, PA: University of Pittsburgh Press.

Riddick, C., & Keller, J. (1991). The benefits of therapeutic recreation in gerontology. In C. P. Coyle, W. B. Kinney, B. Riley, & J. Shank (Eds.), *Benefits of therapeutic recreation: A consensus view* (pp. 151–204). Philadelphia: Temple University Press.

Riddick, C. C., & Stewart, D. G. (1994). An examination of the life satisfaction and importance of leisure in the lives of older female retirees: A comparison of blacks to whites. *Journal of Leisure Research, 26*(1), 75–87.

Rife, J. (1992). Case managers' perceptions of case management practice: Implications for educational preparation. *Journal of Applied Social Sciences, 16*, 161–176.

Rix, S. (1994). *Older workers: How do they measure up? An overview of age differences in employee cost and performance*. Washington, DC: American Association of Retired Persons.

Rizzuto, T. E., & Mohammed, S. (2005). Workplace technology and the myth about older workers. Paper presented at the Society for Industrial and Organizational Psychology conference, Los Angeles, CA, April.

Roadscholar. (2006). *Roadscholar*. Retrieved December 18, 2006 from www.roadscholar.org.

Roberto, K. A., & Scott, J. (1986). Equity considerations in the friendships of older adults. *Journal of Gerontology, 41*, 241–247.

Roberto, K. A., & Stroes, J. (1992). Grandchildren and grandparents: Roles, influences, and relationships. *International Journal of Aging and Human Development, 34*, 227–239.

Roff, L. L., Burgio, L. D., Gitlin, L., Nichols, L., Chaplin, W., & Hardin, J. M. (2004). Positive aspects of caregiving: The role of race. *Journal of Gerontology: Psychological Sciences, 59*, P185–P190.

Rogers, C. R. (1991). Health and social characteristics of the nonmetro elderly. *Agriculture Outlook, 92*(4), 21–29.

Rollinson, P. A. (1990). The story of Edward: The everyday geography of elderly single room occupancy (SRO) hotel tenants. *Journal of Contemporary Ethnography, 19*(2), 188–206.

Rollinson, P. A. (1991a). Elderly single room occupancy (SRO) hotel tenants: Still alone. *Social Work, 36*, 303–308.

Rollinson, P. A. (1991b). The spatial isolation of elderly single-room-occupancy hotel tenants. *Professional Geographer, 43*, 457–464.

Ronch, J. (1987). Specialized Alzheimer's units in nursing homes: Pros and cons. *American Journal of Alzheimer's Care and Research, 2*, 10–19.

Rook, K. S. (1987). Reciprocity of social exchange and social satisfaction among older women. *Journal of Personality and Social Psychology, 52*, 145–154.

Roots&Branches Theatre. (2001). *Roots&Branches: New York's intergenerational theater*. Retrieved May 5, 2001 from www.rootsandbranches.org.

Rosenbloom, S. (1993a). *ElderTransit facts: What you should know about the Americans With Disabilities Act* (Brochure). Washington, DC: National Eldercare Institute on Transportation.

Rosenbloom, S. (1993b). *Will older persons lose mobility?* Washington, DC: American Association of Retired Persons.

Rosenbloom, S., & Waldorf, B. (1999). *Older travelers: Does place or race make a difference?* U.S. Department of Transportation, Conference Proceedings, Personal travel: The long and short of it. Retrieved August 1, 2001 from http://trb.org/trb/publications/ec026/01_rosenbloom.pdf.

Rosenheimer, L., & Francis, E. (1992). Feasible with subsidy: Overnight respite for Alzheimer's. *Journal of Gerontological Nursing, 18*, 21–29.

Rosenzwieg, E. (1995). Trends in home care entitlements and benefits. *Journal of Gerontological Social Work, 24*, 9–29.

Rucker, G. (1995a). *ElderTransit facts: Legislation of interest to community transportation: Intermodal Surface Transportation Efficiency Act (ISTEA)* (Brochure). Washington, DC: National Eldercare Institute on Transportation.

Rucker, G. (1995b). *Rural transit: Stretching to meet the needs of the neediest* (National Transit Resource Center Fact Sheet 9). Washington, DC: National Transit Resource Center.

Ryan, V. C., & Bower, M. E. (1989). Relationship of socioeconomic status and living arrangements to nutritional intake of the older persons. *Journal of the American Dietetic Association, 89,* 1805–1807.

Sahyoun, N. R., Pratt, L. A., Lentzner, H., Dey, A., & Robinson, K. N. (2001). *The changing profile of nursing home residents: 1985–1997* (Aging Trends, No. 4). *Hyattsville, MD: National Center for Health Statistics.* Retrieved August 15, 2001 from www.cdc.gov/nchs/data/agingtrends/ 04nursin.pdf.

Samuelson, R. J. (2005). *The debate we're not having. Newsweek, April 9.* Retrieved January 10, 2007, from www.msnbc.msn.com/id/7409313/site/newsweek.

Sangl, J. (1985). The family support system of the elderly. In R. J. Vogel & H. C. Palmer (Eds.), *Long-term care: Perspectives from research and demonstration* (pp. 307–336). Rockville, MD: Aspen.

Saunders, J. (1997). *Continuing care retirement communities: A background and summary of current issues.* Retrieved January 14, 2007 from http://aspe.hhs.gov/daltcp/reports/ccrcrpt.htm.

Saxon-Harrold, S. K. E., & Weitzman, M. (2000). *Giving and volunteering in the United States: 1999 edition.* Washington, DC: Independent Sector.

Saxton, S. V., & Etten, M. J. (1994). *Physical change and aging: A guide for the helping professions* (3rd ed.). New York: Tiresias.

Schafer, R. B., & Keith, P. M. (1982). Social-psychological factors in the dietary quality of married and single elderly. *Journal of the American Dietetic Association, 81,* 30–34.

Schaie, K. W. (1994). The course of adult intellectual development. *American Psychologist, 49,* 304–313.

Scharlach, A., & Boyd, S. C. (1989). Caregiving and employment: Results of an employee survey. *The Gerontologist, 29,* 382–387.

Scharlach, A., & Frenzel, C. (1986). An evaluation of institutional-based respite care. *The Gerontologist, 26,* 77–82.

Schlenker, R. E., Shaughnessy, P. W., & Crisler, K. S. (1995). Outcome-based continuous quality of improvement as a financial strategy for home health care agencies. *Journal of Home Health Care, 7*(4), 1–15.

Schmall, V., & Webb, L. (1994). Respite and adult day care for rural elders. In J. Krout (Ed.), *Providing community-based services to the rural elderly* (pp. 156–178). Thousand Oaks, CA: Sage.

Schneider, F., Landon, B., Tobias, C., & Epstein, A. (2004). Quality oversight in Medicaid primary care case management programs. *Health Affairs, 23,* 235–242.

Schoeffler, R. W. (1995). Senior centers as brokers of home and community-based long term care. In D. Shollenberger (Ed.), *Senior centers in America: A blueprint for the future: Outcomes of a national meeting convened to develop recommendations for programs, policies, and funding of senior center programs of the future.* Washington, DC: National Council on the Aging.

Schraeder, C., Fraser, C., Bruno, C., & Dworak, D. (1990). *Case management in primary care: A manual.* Englewood, CO: Center for Research in Ambulatory Health Care Administration.

Schultz, J. (2001). *The economics of aging* (7th ed.). Westport, CT: Auburn House.

Schulz, J. H., & Binstock, R. H. (2006). *Aging nation: The economics and politics of growing older in America.* Westport, CT: Praeger.

Schulz, R., Belle, S. H., Czaja, S. J., Gitlin, L. N., Wisniewski, S. T., & Ory, M. G. (2003). Introduction to the special section on Resources for Enhancing Alzheimer's Caregiver Health (REACH). *Psychology and Aging, 18,* 357–360.

Schulz, R., & Martire, L. (2004). Family caregiving of persons with dementia: Prevalence, health effects, and support strategies. *American Journal of Geriatric Psychiatry, 12,* 240–249.

Schwenk, F. N. (1992). Economic status of rural older adults. *Agriculture Outlook, 92*(4), 3–14.

SCORE. (2006a). *Media fact sheet.* Retrieved December 18, 2006 from www.score.org/media_fact_sheet.html.

SCORE. (2006b). *Live your dream. SCORE can help. FY05 Annual Report.* Retrieved December 18, 2006 from www.score.org/pdf/SCORE_FY05_Annual_Report.pdf.

Second, L. (1987). *Private case management for older persons and their families: Practice, policy, potential.* Excelsior, MN: Interstudy Center for Aging and Long-Term Care.

Senior Citizens' Freedom to Work Act. (2000). Pub. L. No. 106–182.

Senior Corps—Foster Grandparents. (2005). *Accomplishments of Foster Grandparents Program.* Retrieved December 18, 2006 from www.seniorcorps.gov/pdf/06_0327_SC_FGP.pdf.

Senior Corps—RSVP. (2005). *Accomplishments of RSVP.* Retrieved December 18, 2006, from http://www.seniorcorps.gov/pdf/06_0327_SC_RSVP.pdf

Senior Corps—Senior Companions. (2005). *Accomplishments of the Senior Companion Program.* Retrieved December 18, 2006 from www.seniorcorps.gov/pdf/06_0327_SC_SCP.pdf.

SeniorNet. (2006). *Computers and internet education for seniors and older adults.* Retrieved May 6, 2001 from www.seniornet.org.

Shagrin, S. S. (2000). Retirement saving and financial planning: Different from a decade ago. *Generations, 16,* 40–44

Shanas, E. (1979). Older people and their families: The new pioneers. *Journal of Marriage and the Family, 42,* 9–15.

Shapiro, E. (1983). Embarrassment and help-seeking. In J. D. Fisher, A. Nadler, & B. M. DePaulo (Eds.), *New directions in helping* (Vol. 2). New York: Academic Press.

Shapiro, E. (1995). Case management in long-term care: Exploring its status, trends, and issues. *Journal of Case Management, 4,* 43–47.

Sharkey, J. R., & Haines, P. S. (2002). Use of telephone-administered survey for identifying nutritional risk indicators among community-living older adults in rural areas. *Journal of Applied Gerontology, 21*(3), 385–403.

Shelton, P., Schraeder, C., Britt, T., & Kirby, R. (1994). A generalist physician-based model for a rural geriatric collaborative practice. *Journal of Case Management, 3,* 98–104.

Shepherd Centers of America. (2006). *Living a life that matters.* Retrieved January 9, 2007 from www.shepherdcenters.org/index.aspx,

Sherman, S. R., & Newman, E. S. (1988). *Foster families for adults: A community alternative in long-term care.* New York: Columbia University Press.

Silvey, R. (1962). Participation in a senior citizen day center. In J. Kaplan & G. J. Aldridge (Eds.), *Social welfare of the aging.* New York: Columbia University Press.

Sing, M., Cody, S., Sinclair, M., Cohen, R., & Ohls, J. (2005). *The Food Stamp Program's elderly nutrition pilot demonstration: Initial evaluation design.* Princeton, NJ: Mathematica Policy Research. Retrieved January 7, 2007 from www.ers.usda.gov.

Singleton, J. F., Forbes, W. F., & Agwani, N. (1993). Stability of activity across the lifespan. *Activities, Adaptation & Aging, 18*(1), 19–26.

Sinnen, M., & Schifalacqua, M. (1991). Coordinated care in a community hospital. *Nursing Administration, 22,* 38–42.

Sirrocco, A. (1988). *Nursing and related care homes as reported from the 1986 inventory of long-term care places.* Hyattsville, MD: National Center for Health Statistics.

Skilton-Sylvester, E., & Garcia, A. (1998–99). Intergenerational programs to address the challenge of immigration. *Generations, 22*(4), 58–63.

Sloan Work and Family Research Network. (2006). *A Sloan network fact sheet on older workers.* Retrieved January 16, 2007 from http://wfnetwork.bc.edu/pdfs/olderworkers.pdf.

Slone, P. D., Lindeman, D. A., Phillips, C., Moritz, D. J., & Koch, G. (1995). Evaluating Alzheimer's special care units: Reviewing the evidence and identifying potential sources of study bias. *The Gerontologist, 35*, 103–111.

Small, N. R. (1988). Evolution of nursing homes. In N. R. Small & M. B. Walsh (Eds.), *Teaching nursing homes: The nursing perspective* (pp. 31–46). Owings Mills, MD: National Health Publishing.

Smallegan, M. (1985). There was nothing else to do: Needs for care before nursing home admission. *The Gerontologist, 25*, 364–369.

Smith, G., Smith, M., & Toseland, R. (1991). Problems identified by family caregivers in counseling. *The Gerontologist, 31*, 15–22.

Smith, K. F., & Bengston, V. L. (1979). The positive consequences of institutionalization: Solidarity between elderly parents and their middle-aged children. *The Gerontologist, 19*, 438–447.

Smith, K. (2003). *How will recent patterns of earnings inequality affect future retirement incomes? Working Paper No. 2003–06, AARP.* Retrieved January 10, 2007 from www.urban.org/Uploaded PDF/411164_future_retire_incomes.pdf.

Smith, T., & Newman, S. (1992). Older adults in Head Start. *National Head Start Association Journal, 10*, 33–35.

Smith, T., & Newman, S. (1993). Older adults in early childhood programs: Why and how. *Young Children, 48*, 32–35.

Smyer, M. A., Shea, D. G., & Streit, A. (1994). The provision and use of mental health services in nursing homes: Results from the National Medical Expenditure Survey. *American Journal of Public Health, 84*, 284–287.

Social Security Act of 1935, 42 U.S.C. § 301 et seq. (1935), as amended 1939, 1950, 1956, 1961, 1965, 1972, 1974.

Social Security Administration. (1996). *Social Security: You may be able to get benefits.* Washington, DC: Social Security Administration.

Social Security Administration. (1997). *History of Social Security.* Retrieved March 26, 1997 from www.ssa.gov/history/history6.html.

Social Security Administration. (2000c). *Income of the aged chartbook, 1998.* Retrieved January 21, 2002 from www.ssa.gov/statistics/income_aged/1998/iac98.pdf.

Social Security Administration. (2000e). *Social Security News Release: Kenneth S. Apfel, Commissioner of Social Security, Praises Senate action and announces implementation plan for the repeal of the retirement earnings test, March 24, 2000.* Retrieved September 21, 2001 from www.ssa.gov/pressoffice/retiretest.htm.

Social Security Administration. (2001/02). Modeling SSI financial eligibility and simulating the effect of policy options. *Social Security Bulletin, 64*, 16–45.

Social Security Administration. (2001). *SSI in California* (SSA Pub. No. 05–11125), January. Retrieved July 15, 2001 from www.ssa.gov/pubs/11125.html.

Social Security Administration. (2002). *Income of the population 55 or older, 2002.* Retrieved January 23, 2007 from www.ssa.gov/policy/docs/statcomps/income_pop55/2002/incpop02.pdf.

Social Security Administration. (2004). *Importance of income sources relative to total income. Income of the Population 55 or Older, 2004.* Washington, DC: *Social Security Administration.* Retrieved January 23, 2007 from www.ssa.gov/policy/docs/statcomps/income_pop55/2004/sect06a.html.

Social Security Administration. (2005). *Trends in the Social Security and Supplemental Security Income Disability Programs: Changes in incentives influencing program size.* Retrieved January 26, 2007 from www.ssa.gov/policy/docs/chartbooks/disability_trends/sect05.html.

Social Security Administration. (2006a). *Annual statistical supplement, 2006.* Retrieved January 12, 2007 from www.socialsecurity.gov/policy/docs/statcomps/supplement/2006/index.html.

Social Security Administration. (2006b). *2007 legislation fact sheet.* Retrieved January 22, 2007 from www.ssa.gov/legislation/2007FactSheet.pdf.

Social Security Administration. (2007). *Social Security/SSI information.* Retrieved February 20, 2007 from www.ssa.gov/legislation/2007FactSheet.pdf.

Society for Human Resource Management. (1998). *Many older worker myths are challenged by SHRM/AARP Survey.* Retrieved May 9, 2001 from www.shrm.org/press/releases/default.asp?page = 980515-3.htm.

Song, J. G. (2003-2004). Evaluating the initial impact of eliminating the retirement earnings test. *Social Security Bulletin, 65*, 1-15.

Sörenson, S., Pinquart, M., & Duberstein, P. (2002). How effective are interventions with caregivers? An updated meta-analysis. *The Gerontologist, 42*, 356-372.

Special Committee on Aging. (1963). *A compilation of materials relevant to the message of the president of the United States on our nation's senior citizens.* Washington, DC: Government Printing Office.

Spense, S. A. (1992). Use of community-based social services by older rural and urban blacks: An exploratory study. *Human Services in the Rural Environment, 15*(4), 16-19.

Spillman, B. C., & Lubitz, J. (2002). New estimates of lifetime nursing home use: Have patterns of use changed? *Medical Care, 40*, 10, 965-975.

Spitz, B., & Abramson, J. (1987). Competition, capitation, and case management: Barriers to strategic reform. *Millbank Quarterly, 65*, 348-370.

Stanford, P., & Bois, B. (1992). Gender and ethnicity patterns. In J. Birren, R. B. Sloane, & C. Cohen (Eds.), *Handbook of mental health and aging* (2nd ed., pp. 99-117). New York: Academic Press.

Stanley, D., & Freysinger, V. J. (1995). The impact of age, health, and sex on the frequency of older adults' leisure activity participation: A longitudinal study. *Activities, Adaptation, and Aging, 19*, 31-42.

Starret, R. A., Wright, R., Mindle, C. H., & Van Tran, T. (1989). The use of social services by Hispanic elderly: A comparison of Mexican American, Puerto Rican and Cuban elderly. *Journal of Social Service Research, 13*(1), 1-25.

Steele, M. F., & Bryan, J. D. (1986). Dietary intake of homebound elderly recipients and nonrecipients of home-delivered meals. *Journal of Nutrition and the Elderly, 5*, 23-35.

Stein, S., & Bonuck, K. (2001). Attitudes on end-of-life care and advance care planning in the lesbian and gay community. *Journal of Palliative Medicine, 4*, 173-190.

Steinig, S., & Simon, J. (Eds.). (2005). *Under one roof: A guide to starting and strengthening intergenerational shared site programs.* Washington, DC: Generations United.

Stephens, B. W., McCarthy, D. P., Marsiske, M., Shechtman, O., Classen, S., Justiss, M. et al., (2005). International older driver consensus conference on assessment, remediation and counseling for transportation alternatives: Summary and recommendations. *Physical and Occupational Therapy in Geriatrics, 23*(2/3), 103-121.

Sterns, H., & McDaniel, M. (1994). Job performance and the older worker. In S. Rix (Ed.), *Older workers: How do they measure up?* Washington, DC: American Association of Retired Persons.

Stevens, D. A., Grivetti, L. E., & McDonald, R. B. (1992). Nutrient intake of urban and rural elderly receiving home-delivered meals. *Journal of the American Dietetic Association, 92,* 714–718.

Stevens, E. (1991). Toward satisfaction and retention of senior volunteers. *Journal of Gerontological Social Work, 16*(3/4), 33–41.

Stoller, E. P. (1989). Formal services and informal helping: The myth of service substitution. *Journal of Applied Gerontology, 8,* 37–52.

Stoller, E. P., & Pugliesi, K. (1988). Informal networks of community based elderly: Changes in composition over time. *Research on Aging, 10,* 499–516.

Stone, D. (2000). *Reframing home health care policy.* Retrieved January 2, 2007 from www.radcliffe.edu/research/pubpol/Reframing_Home_Health_Care.pdf.

Stone, R. (2006). Linking services to housing: Who will provide the care? A competent, stable, and committed workforce is in short supply. *Generations, 29*(4), 44–51.

Stone, R., Cafferata, G., & Sangl, J. (1987). Caregivers of the frail elderly: A national profile. *The Gerontologist, 27,* 616–626.

Stone, R., Reinhard, S. C., Machemer, J., & Rudin, D. (2002). *Geriatric care managers: A profile of an emerging profession.* Retrieved January 23, 2007 from http://assets.aarp.org/rgcenter/il/dd82_care.pdf.

Storey, R. (1962). Who attends a senior activity center? A comparison of Little House members with non-members in the same community. *The Gerontologist, 2,* 216–222.

Strain, L. A. (2001). Senior centres: Who participates? *Canadian Journal on Aging, 20*(4), 471–491.

Strain, L., & Blanford, A. (2002). Community-based services for the taking but few takers: Reasons for nonuse. *Journal of Applied Gerontology, 21*(2), 220–235.

Strauss, P. J., Wolf, R., & Schilling, D. (1990). *Aging and the law.* Chicago: Commerce Clearing House.

Strawbridge, W., & Wallhagen, M. (1991). Impact of family conflict on adult child caregivers. *The Gerontologist, 31,* 770–777.

Strum, R., Ringel, J. S., & Andreyeva, T. (2004). Increasing obesity rates and disability trends. *Health Affairs, 23*(2), 199–205.

Struntz, K. A., & Reville, S. (1985). *Growing together: An intergenerational sourcebook.* Washington, DC: American Association of Retired Persons.

Substance Abuse and Mental Health Services Administration (SAMHSA). (2004). *A vulnerable population. Community integration for older adults with mental illnesses: Overcoming barriers and seizing opportunities.* Retrieved May 30, 2006, from www.mentalhealth.samhsa.gov/media/ken/pdf/SMA05–4018/OlderAdults.pdf.

Substance Abuse and Mental Health Services Administration. (2005). *Successful strategies for recruiting, training, and utilizing volunteers: A guide for faith- and community-based service providers.* Retrieved December 10, 2006 from www.hhs.gov/fbci/docs/Volhandbook.pdf.

Suitor, J. J., & Pillemer, K. (1990). Transitions to the status of family caregiver: A new framework for studying social support and well-being. In S. M. Stahl (Ed.), *The legacy of longevity* (pp. 310–320). Newbury Park, CA: Sage.

Summer, L. L., & Ihara, E. S. (2004). *State-funded home and community-based service programs for older people.* Retrieved January 2, 2007 from www.pascenter.org/state_funded/State-only_Funded_2006_TEXT.pdf.

Swan, J. H., & Benjamin, A. E. (1990). Nursing costs of skilled nursing care for AIDS. *AIDS and Public Policy Journal, 5*, 64–67.

Taggart, C. (2005, March). *Retired nurses to help fill in gaps at KMC. The Spokane Spokesman Review.* Retrieved January 20, 2007 from http://findarticles.com/p/articles/mi_qn4186/is_20050309/ai_n12945616.

Taietz, P. (1976). Two conceptual models of the senior center. *Journal of Gerontology, 31*, 219–222.

Takamura, J. C. (1991). Dana is joy: A volunteer caregivers' program in the Buddhist tradition. *Generations, 15*(4), 79.

Takamura, J. C. (1999). Getting ready for the 21st Century: The aging of America and the Older Americans Act. *Health and Social Work, 24*(3), 232–238.

Tax Equity and Fiscal Responsibility Act of 1982, Pub. L. No. 97–248, 96 Stat. 324 (1982).

Teague, M. L. (1987). *Health promotion programs: Achieving high-level wellness in the later years.* Indianapolis, IN: Benchmark.

Tessler, R. C., & Schwartz, S. H. (1972). Help seeking, self-esteem, and achievement motivation: An attributional analysis. *Journal of Personality and Social Psychology, 21*, 318–326.

Thomas, N. K. (2006). *Elderly legal assistance program: Report on the legal needs of seniors in Georgia.* Atlanta, GA: Department of Human Resources, Division of Aging Services. Available at www.tcsg.org/GALegalNeedsSurvey.pdf.

Tokarek, J. (1996). Keeping frail seniors independent through money management. *Aging, 367*, 84–86.

Torti, F. M., Jr., Gwyther, L. P., Reed, S. D., Friedman, J. Y., & Schulman, K. A. (2004). Multinational review of recent trends and reports in dementia caregiver burden. *Alzheimer's Disease and Associated Disorders, 18*, 99–109.

Tourigny, L., & Pulich, M. (2006). Improving retention of older employees through training and development. *The Health Care Manager, 25*, 43–52.

Townsend, D., & Kosloski, K. (2002). Factors related to client satisfaction with community-based respite services. *Health Care Services Quarterly, 21*(3/4), 89–106.

Travis, S. S. (1995). Families and formal networks. In R. Blieszner & V. H. Bedford (Eds.), *Handbook of aging and the family* (pp. 459–473). Westport, CT: Greenwood.

Trella, R. (1993). A multidisciplinary approach to care management of frail, hospitalized older adults. *Journal of Nursing Administration, 23*, 20–26.

Trice, L. (2006). PACE: A model for providing comprehensive healthcare for frail elders. *Generations, 30*(3), 90–92.

Trotman, F. K., & Brody, C. M. (2002). *Psychotherapy and counseling with older women: Cross-cultural, family, and end-of-life issues.* New York: Springer Publishing Company.

Turner, K. W. (2004). Senior citizens centers: What they offer, who participates, and what they gain. *Journal of Gerontological Social Work, 43*(1), 37–47.

United Way of Connecticut. (2001). *A national initiative to link people with community services.* Retrieved June 13, 2001 from www.211.org.

University of Miami Ethics Programs. (n.d.). Schiavo case resources. Accessed 13 January 2007 from www6.miami.edu/ethics/terri_schiavo_case.html.

Urban Institute. (1993). *Hunger and food insecurity among the elderly.* Washington, DC: Urban Institute.

Urban Institute. (2004). *Volunteer management capacity in America's charities and congregations: A briefing report.* Washington, DC: Urban Institute.

Urban Mass Transportation Act of 1964, 49 U.S.C. § 1601 et seq. (1964).

Urv-Wong, E., & McDowell, D. (1994). Case management in a rural setting. In J. Krout (Ed.), *Providing community-based services to the rural elderly* (pp. 65–89). Thousand Oaks, CA: Sage.

U.S. Bureau of the Census. (1996a). *65 + in the United States (Current Population Reports, Special Studies, Series P-23, N0.20190)*. Washington, DC: Government Printing Office.

U.S. Bureau of the Census. (1996b). *Statistical abstract of the United States* (116th ed.). Washington, DC: U.S. Bureau of the Census.

U.S. Bureau of the Census. (2000a). *Current Population Survey, Racial and ethnic composition*. Washington, DC: Government Printing Office.

U.S. Bureau of the Census. (2000b). *Population projections of the United States by age, sex, race, Hispanic origin, and nativity: 1999 to 2000*. Retrieved January 25, 2002, from www.census.gov/population/www/projections/natproj.html.

U.S. Bureau of the Census. (2001). *The older population in the United States: March 2000. Detailed Tables (PPL-147)*. Retrieved December 21, 2006, from www.census.gov/population/www/socdemo/age/ppl-147.html.

U.S. Bureau of the Census. (2003). *Current Population Survey, Annual Social and Economic Supplement*. Washington, DC: Government Printing Office.

U.S. Bureau of the Census. (2003). *Grandparents living with grandchildren: 2000* (Publication No. C2KBR-31). Retrieved November 30, 2006 from www.census.gov/prod/2003pubs/c2kbr-31.pdf.

U.S. Bureau of the Census. (2004a). *U.S. Interim projections by age, sex, race, and Hispanic origin*. Washington, DC: Government Printing Office.

U.S. Bureau of the Census. (2004b). *Age and sex of all people, family members and unrelated individuals iterated by income-to-poverty ratio and race, 2004*. Retrieved January 23, 2007 from www.pubds3.census.gov/macro/032004/pov/toc.htm.

U.S. Bureau of the Census. (2005). *Current Population Survey, 2005 Annual Social and Economic Supplement*. Retrieved January 23, 2007 from http://www.census.gov/population/www/socdemo/education/cps2005.html

U.S. Bureau of the Census. (2006a). *Current Population Survey, 2006 Annual Social and Economic Supplement*. Retrieved January 10, 2007 from www.census.gov/hhes/www/cpstc/cps_table_creator.html.

U.S. Bureau of the Census. (2006b). Marital status of people 15 years and over, by age, sex, personal earnings, race, and Hispanic origin: 2005. *Current Population Survey, 2005 Annual Social and Economic Supplement*. Available at www.census.gov/population/socdemo/hh-fam/cps2005/tabA1-all.csv.

U.S. Bureau of Labor Statistics. (2006c). Employed and unemployed full- and part-time workers by age, sex, race, and Hispanic or Latino ethnicity. *Current Population Survey*. Available at www.bls.gov/cps/cpsaat8.pdf.

U.S. Bureau of Labor Statistics (2005). *Economic dependency ratio, 1975–2004 and projected 2014, by age*. Retrieved from www.bls.gov/emp/emplab10.htm.

U.S. Bureau of Labor Statistics. (2006a). *Unemployed persons by age, sex, race, Hispanic or Latino ethnicity, marital status, and duration of unemployment*. Retrieved January 25, 2007 from http://stats.bls.gov/web/cpseea36.pdf.

U.S. Bureau of Labor Statistics. (2006b). Employment status of the civilian noninstitutional population by age, sex, and race. *Current Population Survey*. Available at www.bls.gov/cps/cpsaat3.pdf.

U.S. Bureau of the Census. (2006c). *American housing survey for the United States: 2005*. Current Housing Reports, Series H150/05. Retrieved December 28, 2006 from www.census.gov/prod/2006pubs/h150–05.pdf.

U.S. Conference of Mayors. (2002). *A status report on hunger and homelessness in America's cities, 2002.* Washington DC. Retrieved on January 6, 2007 from www.mayors.org/uscm/hungersurvey/2002/onlinereport/HungerandHomelessReport2002.pdf.

U.S. Commission on Civil Rights. (1982). *Minority elderly services: New programs, old problems: A report of the United States Commission on Civil Rights.* Washington, DC: U.S. Commission on Civil Rights.

U.S. Congress, Office of Technology Assessment. (1987). *Losing a million minds: Confronting the tragedy of Alzheimer's disease and other dementias.* Washington, DC: Government Printing Office.

U.S. Congress, Office of Technology Assessment. (1990). *Health care in rural America* (Pub. No. OTA-H-434). Washington, DC: Government Printing Office.

U.S. Congress, Office of Technology Assessment. (1992). *Special care units for people with Alzheimer's and other dementias: Consumer education, research, regulatory, and reimbursement issues* (Pub. No. OTA-H-543). Washington, DC: Government Printing Office.

U.S. Department of Agriculture. (2001a). *Characteristics of food stamp households: Fiscal year 2000 (advance report).* Retrieved August 1, 2001 from www.fns.usda.gov/oane/MENU/Published/FSP/FILES/Participation/2000advrpt.pdf.

U.S. Department of Agriculture. (2001b). *Commodity Supplemental Food Program: Frequently asked questions.* Retrieved July 2, 2001 from www.fns.usda.gov/fdd/MENU/APPLICANTS/SUPPLEMENTAL/csfpfaq.htm.

U.S. Department of Agriculture. (2006a). *Cooperative state research, education, and extension service: About us.* Retrieved January 10, 2007 from www.csrees.usda.gov/qlinks/partners/state_partners.html.

U.S. Department of Agriculture. (2006b). *The commodity supplemental food program. Food and nutrition service, food distribution fact sheet, August 2006.* Retrieved January 7, 2007 from www.fns.usda.gov/fdd/programs/csfp/pfs-csfp.pdf.

U.S. Department of Agriculture. (2006c). *The emergency food assistance program. Food and nutrition service, food distribution fact sheet, August 2006.* Retrieved January 7, 2007 from www.fns.usda.gov/fdd/programs/tefap/pfs-tefap.pdf.

U.S. Department of Defense. (2001). *Tricare for life.* Retrieved September 16, 2001 from www.tricare.osd.mil.

U.S. Department of Education (1998). *Vocational and adult education.* Retrieved from www.ed.gov/offices/OVAE/98age.html.

U.S. Department of Energy. (2006). *Weatherization Assistance Program 2006.* Retrieved December 28, 2007 from www1.eere.energy.gov/office_eere/pdfs/wap_fs.pdf.

U.S. Department of Health and Human Services. (1990). *Healthy people 2000: National health promotion and disease prevention objectives.* Washington, DC: Government Printing Office.

U.S. Department of Health and Human Services. (1991). *Mental illness in nursing homes: United States, 1985* (DHHS Pub. No. PHS 91–1766). Washington, DC: Government Printing Office.

U.S. Department of Health and Human Services. (1993). *Growing older: Healthy Black lifestyles: The health promotion programs in historically Black colleges and universities* (DHHS Pub. No. MF 0447-A-01). Washington, DC: Government Printing Office.

U.S. Department of Health and Human Services. (2001a). *Mental health: Culture, race, and ethnicity: A report of the Surgeon General.* Retrieved January 22, 2007 from www.surgeongeneral.gov/library/mentalhealth/cre.

U.S. Department of Health and Human Services/Administration on Aging. (2001b). *Older adults and mental health: Issues and opportunities.* Retrieved January 25, 2007 from www.aoa.gov/PRESS/publications/Older-Adults-and-Mental-Health-2001.pdf.

U.S. Department of Health and Human Services, Office of Minority Health. (2001c). *National Standards for Culturally and Linguistically Appropriate Services in Health Care final report, March 1, 2001.* Washington, DC: U.S. Department of Health and Human Services, OPHS, Office of Minority Health.

U.S. Department of Health and Human Services. (2003). *Executive summary: Low income home energy assistance report to congress for FY 2003.* Retrieved December 28, 2006 from http://acf/hhs.gov/programs/liheap/data/execsum.htm.

U.S. Department of Health and Human Services. (2006). *Over 38 million people with Medicare now receiving prescription drug coverage. News release, June 14, 2006.* Retrieved January 28, 2007 from http://hhs.gov/news/press/2006pres/20060614.html.

U.S. Department of Health, Education and Welfare. (1964). Foster care. *Aging, 16,* 1–3.

U.S. Department of Health, Education and Welfare. (1979). *Healthy people: The surgeon general's report on health promotion and disease prevention* (PHS Pub. No. 79–55071). Washington, DC: Government Printing Office.

U.S. Department of Housing and Urban Development. (2001). *Housing choice voucher program fact sheet.* Retrieved January 25, 2002, from www.hud.gov/section8.cfm.

U.S. Department of Housing and Urban Development. (2002). *Home equity conversion mortgage program.* Retrieved January 2, 2007, from www.hud.gov/offices/hsg/sfh/hecm/hecm—df.cfm.

U.S. Department of Labor, Bureau of Labor Statistics. (1990). Thirty-eight million persons do volunteer work. Press Release 90–154, March 29. Washington, DC: U.S. Department of Labor, Bureau of Labor Statistics.

U.S. Department of Labor. (2000a). *Annual current population survey (Table 22).* Retrieved January 20, 2002 from www.bls.gov/cps/cpsaat22.pdf.

U.S. Department of Labor. (2000b). *Report of the working group on phased retirement.* Retrieved January 26, 2007 from www.dol.gov/ebsa/publications/phasedr1.htm.

U.S. Department of Labor. (2006a). *Persons not in the labor force by desire and availability for work, age, and sex.* Retrieved January 25, 2007, from http://www.findarticles.com/p/articles/mi_m2553/is_1_53/ai_n16107929.

U.S. Department of Labor. (2006b). *Senior Community Service Employment Program (SCSEP).* Retrieved January 15, 2007, from www.doleta.gov/seniors.

U.S. Department of Labor. (2006c). *Women and retirement savings.* Retrieved January 12, 2007 from www.dol.gov/ebsa/publications/women.html.

U.S. Department of Labor. (2007). *Volunteering in the United States, 2006.* Retrieved January 20, 2007, from www.bls.gov/news.release/volun.t04.htm.

U.S. Department of Transportation. (1980). *Elderly market for urban mass transit.* Washington, DC: Government Printing Office.

U.S. Department of Transportation. (1997). *Improving transportation for a maturing society. DOT-P10-97-01.* Retrieved June 14, 2001, from http://ntl.bts.gov/data/final-b2.pdf.

U.S. Department of Transportation. (2005a). *FTA authorization fact sheet other than urbanized area formula programs.* Retrieved November 16, 2007 from www.fta.dot.gov/documents/FTA_Rural_Program_Fact_Sheet_Sept05.pdf.

U.S. Department of Transportation. (2005b). *FTA authorization fact sheet. Elderly persons and persons with disabilities programs.* Retrieved November 16, 2007 from www.fta.dot.gov/documents/FTA_Elderly_and_Indiv_with_Disab_Fact_Sheet_Sept05.pdf.

U.S. Department of Transportation. (2005c). *FTA authorization fact sheet. New Freedom Program.* Retrieved November 16, 2007 from www.fta.dot.gov/documents/FTA_New_Freedom_Fact_Sheet_Sept05.pdf.

U.S. Equal Employment Opportunity Commission. (2006). *Age Discrimination in Employment Act (ADEA) Charges FY 1992-FY 2005.* Washington, DC. Retrieved December 12, 2006 from www.eeoc.gov/stats/adea.html.

U.S. General Accounting Office. (1991a). *Longstanding transportation problems need more federal attention* (Pub. No. HRD-91-117). Washington, DC: Government Printing Office.

U.S. General Accounting Office. (1991b). *Older Americans Act: Promising practice in information and referral services* (GAO Pub. No. PEMD 91-31). Washington, DC: Government Printing Office.

U.S. General Accounting Office. (1992). *Elderly Americans health, housing, and nutrition gaps between the poor and nonpoor: Report to the Chairman, Select Committee on Aging, House of Representatives* (Rep. No. GAO/PEMD-92-29; B—249013). Washington, DC: U.S. General Accounting Office.

U.S. General Accounting Office. (1993). *Long-term care case management: State experiences and implication for federal policy.* Washington, DC: Author.

U.S. General Accounting Office. (1995). *Supplemental Security Income: Growth and changes in recipient population call for re-examining program* (GAO Pub. No. HEHS-95-137). Washington, DC: Government Printing Office.

U.S. General Accounting Office. (2005). *Elderly housing: Federal housing programs that offer assistance for the elderly.* Retrieved January 2, 2007 from www.gao.gov/new.items/d05174.pdf.

U.S. Senate Special Committee on Aging. (1990). *Developments in aging: 1989, Vol. 1.* Washington, DC: Government Printing Office.

U.S. Senate Special Committee on Aging. (1991a). *Developments in aging: 1990, Vol. 1.* Washington, DC: Government Printing Office.

U.S. Senate Special Committee on Aging. (1991b). *Lifelong learning for an aging society* (No. 102-J). Washington, DC: U.S. Senate Special Committee on Aging.

U.S. Senate Special Committee on Aging. (1992). *Developments in aging: 1991, Vol. 1.* Washington, DC: Government Printing Office.

U.S. Senate Special Committee on Aging. (1993). *Developments in aging: 1992, Vol. 1.* Washington, DC: Government Printing Office.

U.S. Senate Special Committee on Aging. (2000). *Developments in aging: 1997 and 1998, Vol. 1* (Report 106-229). Retrieved June 2, 2001 from www.gpo.gov/congress/senate/senate221p106.html.

U.S. Small Business Administration. (1995). *SCORE: Service Corps of Retired Executives.* Retrieved May 4, 2001 from www.score.org.

Verbrugge, L. M., Gruber-Baldini, A. L., & Fozard, J. L. (1996). Age differences and age changes in activities: Baltimore Longitudinal Study of Aging. *Journal of Gerontology: Psychological Sciences and Social Sciences, 51*(1), S30–S41.

Wachs, M. (1979). *Transportation for the elderly.* Berkeley, CA: University of California Press.

Wacker, R. R. (1985). *Long term care admission agreements in Colorado: A review.* Denver, CO: Advocacy Assistance Program.

Wacker, R. R. (1992). *What do you think? An evaluation of the Weld County senior nutrition program.* Greeley, CO: University of Northern Colorado.

Wacker, R. R. (1996). *Improving quality of care for nursing home residents: An innovative community program to enhance certified nurse aide training: Final report to the Retirement Research Foundation.* Greeley, CO: University of Northern Colorado.

Wacker, R. R., & Blanding, C. (1994). *Comprehensive leisure and aging study: Final report.* Washington, DC: National Recreation and Park Association.

Waggoner, G. (1996). Adopt an elder: Linking youth and the elderly. *Activities, Adaptation, and Aging, 20,* 41–52.

Wagner, D. L. (1995a). Senior center research in America: An overview of what we know. In D. Shollenberger (Ed.), *Senior centers in America: A blueprint for the future: Outcomes of a national meeting convened to develop recommendations for programs, policies, and funding of senior center programs of the future.* Washington, DC: National Council on the Aging.

Wagner, D. L. (1995b). Senior centers and the "new" elderly cohorts of tomorrow. In D. Shollenberger (Ed.), *Senior centers in America: A blueprint for the future: Outcomes of a national meeting convened to develop recommendations for programs, policies, and funding of senior center programs of the future.* Washington, DC: National Council on the Aging.

Wagner, D. L. (2003). *Workplace programs for family caregivers: Good business and good practice.* Retrieved January 12, 2007 from www.caregiver.org/caregiver/jsp/content/pdfs/op_2003_workplace_programs.pdf.

Wagner, E. H., Grothaus, L. C., Hecht, J. A., & LaCroix, A. Z. (1991). Factors associated with participation in a senior health promotion program. *The Gerontologist, 31,* 598–602.

Wagnild, G., & Grupp, K. (1991). Major stressors among elderly home care clients. *Home Healthcare Nurse, 9,* 15–21.

Wake Forest University School of Medicine. (2002). *National study of adult day services.* Retrieved January 2, 2007 from www.rwjf.org/newsroom/featureDetail.jsp?featureID = 183&type = 2.

Waldman, S. (1985). A legislative history of nursing home care. In R. J. Vogel & H. C. Palmer (Eds.), *Long-term care: Perspectives from research and demonstrations* (pp. 507–535). Rockville, MD: Aspen.

Waldrop, J., & Stern, S. M. (2003). *Disability status: 2000—C2KBR-17, U.S. Census Bureau,* Washington, DC: Government Printing Office.

Walker, D., & Beauchene, R. E. (1991). The relationship of loneliness, social isolation, and physical health to dietary adequacy of independently living elderly. *Journal of the American Dietetic Association, 91,* 300–305.

Walker, D. A., & Clarke, M. (2001). Cognitive behavioural psychotherapy: A comparison between younger and older adults in two inner city mental health teams. *Aging & Mental Health, 5,* 197–199.

Walker, J., Bisbee, C., Porter, R., & Flanders, J. (2004). Increasing practitioners' knowledge of participation among elderly adults in senior center activities. *Educational Gerontology, 30,* 353–366.

Walker, S. N. (1889). Health promotion for older adults: Directions for research. *American Journal of Health Promotion, 3,* 47–52.

Walster, E., Berscheid, E., & Walster, G. W. (1973). New directions in equity research. *Journal of Personality and Social Psychology, 25,* 176–184.

Ward, C. (1997). Evaluation of intergenerational programs. In S. Newman, C. Ward, T. Smith, J. Wilson, & J. McCrea (Eds.), *Intergenerational programs: Past, present, and future* (pp. 117–126). Bristol, PA: Taylor & Francis.

Warrick, L., Netting, E., Christianson, J., & Williams, F. (1992). Hospital-based case management: Results from a demonstration. *The Gerontologist, 32,* 781–788.

Warshaw, G. (1988). *Health promotion and aging: Preventive health services.* Surgeon general's workshop: Health promotion and aging. Washington, DC: Government Printing Office.

Webber, P. A., Fox, P., & Burnette, D. (1994). Living alone with Alzheimer's disease: Effects on health and social service utilization patterns. *The Gerontologist, 34,* 8–14.

Weinstock, R. (1978). *The graying of the campus.* New York: Educational Facilities Laboratory.

Weissert, W. (1977). Adult day care programs in the United States: Current research projects and a survey of ten centers. *Public Health Reports, 92,* 49–56.

Wellman, N. S., Rosenzweig, L. Y., & Lloyd, J. L. (2002). Thirty years of the older Americans nutrition program. *The American Dietetic Association, 102*(3), 348–350.

Wellman, B., & Wortley, S. (1989). Brothers' keepers: Situating kinship relations in broader networks of social support. *Sociological Perspectives, 32,* 273–306.

Wellman, N. S. (1994). The nutrition screening initiative. *Nutrition Reviews, 52*(8), S44–S47.

Wells, J. (2002). *Setting the PACE: Alternative senior care programs keep up with the needs of the nation's elderly, providing participants with a sense of community and independence.* Retrieved January 22, 2007 from www.onlok.org/html/newsroom/press.asp?id = 240000151&catid = 240000339&scatid = 240000245&t = newsdetail.

West, G. E., Delisle, M.A., Simard, C., & Drouin, D. (1996). Leisure activities and service knowledge and use among the rural elderly. *Journal of Aging and Health, 8,* 254–279.

Whaley, J. S., & Hutchinson, A. B. (1993a). *National standards for Older Americans Act information and referral services.* Washington, DC: National Information and Referral Support Center.

Whaley, J. S., & Hutchinson, A. B. (1993b). *Implementation guide for Older Americans Act information and referral services.* Washington, DC: National Information and Referral Support Center.

White, J. V., Ham, R. J., & Lipschitz, D. A. (1991). *Report of nutritional screening: Vol. 1. Toward a common view.* Washington, DC: Nutrition Screening Initiative.

White, M., Gundrum, G., Shearer, S., & Simmons, J. (1994). A role for case managers in the physician office. *Journal of Case Management, 3,* 62–68.

White House Conference on Aging. (1995). *The road to an aging policy for the 21st century: Final report of the 1995 White House Conference on Aging.* Washington, DC: White House Conference on Aging.

White House Conference on Aging. (2006). *The booming dynamics of aging: From awareness to action. Final report of the 2005 White House Conference on Aging.* Retrieved September 20, 2006 from www.whcoa.gov/about/about.asp#report.

Whittaker, J. M. (2005). *Issues in aging: Unemployment and older workers.* Retrieved January 26, 2007 from http://www.opencrs.com/rpts/RL32757_20050131.pdf.

Wiencek, T. (1991). How the Older Workers' Benefit Protection Act affects employers. *Practice Lawyer, 37,* 69–76.

Wiener, J. M. (2003). An assessment of strategies for improving quality of care in nursing homes. *The Gerontologist, 43, Special Issue II,* 19–27.

Wiener, J. M., Sullivan, C. M., & Skaggs, J. (1996). *Spending down to Medicaid: New data on the role of Medicaid in paying from nursing home care.* AARP Public Policy Institute Report No. 9607. Washington, DC: American Association of Retired Persons.

Wilke, H., & Lazette, J. T. (1970). The obligation to help: The effects of amount of prior help on subsequent helping behavior. *Journal of Experimental Social Psychology, 6,* 488–493.

Williams, A. L., Haber, D., Weaver, G. D., & Freeman, J. L. (1998). Altruistic activity: Does it make a difference in the senior center? *Activities, Adaptation & Aging, 22*(4), 31–39.

Williamson, J. B. (1974). The stigma of public dependency: A comparison of alternative forms of public aid to the poor. *Social Problems, 22,* 213–238.

Wilson, L., & Simson, S. (1993). Senior volunteerism policies at the local level: Adaptation and leadership in the 21st century. *Journal of Volunteer Administration, 11*(4), 15–23.

Wingard, D. L., Jones, D. W., & Kaplan, R. M. (1987). Institutional care utilization by the elderly: A critical review. *The Gerontologist, 27,* 156–163.

Wolf, R. S. (1996). Understanding elder abuse and neglect. *Aging, 367,* 4–9.

Wolfe, W. S., Olson, C. M., Kendall, A., & Frongillo, E. A. (1998). Hunger and food insecurity in the elderly. *Journal of Aging and Health, 10*(3), 327–350.

Woolcock, M. (2001). The place of social capital in understanding social and economic outcomes. *Canadian Journal of Policy Research, 2*(1), 11–17.

Wright, B. (2004). *Assisted living in the United States. AARP Public Policy Institute.* Retrieved December 28, 2006 from http://assets.aarp.org/rgcenter/post-import/fs62r_assisted.pdf.

Wu, K. B. (2006) *Sources of income for older persons in 2004. AARP Public Policy Institute.* Retrieved January 12, 2007 from http://assets.aarp.org/rgcenter/econ/dd148_income.pdf.

Wurtman, J. J., Lieberman, H., Tsay, R., Nader, T., & Chew, B. (1988). Calorie and nutrient intakes of elderly and young subjects measured under identical conditions. *Journal of Gerontology, 79,* 117–131.

Yamada, Y. (2002). Profile of home care aides, nursing home aides, and hospital aides: Historical changes and data recommendations. *The Gerontologist, 42,* 199–206.

Yankelovich, D. (2005). *Ferment and change: Higher education in 2015. Chronicle of Higher Education, November.* Retrieved January 13, 2007 from www.chronicle.com/weekly/v52/i14/14b00601.htm.

Yee, J. L., & Schulz, R. (2000). Gender differences in psychiatric morbidity among family caregivers: A review and analysis. *The Gerontologist, 40,* 147–164.

Yeo, G. (1993). Ethnicity and nursing homes: Factors affecting use and successful components for culturally sensitive care. In C. M. Barresi & D. E. Stull (Eds.), *Ethnic elderly and long term care* (pp. 161–177). New York: Springer.

Yin, T., Zhou, Q., & Bashford, C. (2002). Burden on family members caring for frail elderly: a meta-analysis of interventions. *Nursing Research, 51,* 199–208.

Young, K. (1992). LIR program and organizational models. In R. Fischer, M. Blazey, & H. Lipman (Eds.), *Students of the third age* (pp. 25–37). New York: Macmillan.

Zarit, S. (1996). Interventions with family caregivers. In S. Zarit & B. Knight (Eds.), *A guide to psychotherapy and aging* (pp. 139–162). Washington, DC: American Psychological Association.

Zarit, S. H., Stephens, M. A. P., Townsend, A., & Greene, R. (1998). Stress reduction for family caregivers: Effects of adult day care use. *Journal of Gerontology, 53B,* S267–S277.

Zarit, S., & Zarit, J. (1998). *Mental disorders in older adults: Fundamentals of assessment and treatment.* New York: Guilford.

Zbylot, S., Job, C., McCormick, E., Boulter, C., & Moore, A. (1995). A case-mix classification system for long-term care facilities. *Nursing Management, 26*(4), 49–54.

Zedlewski, S., Barnes, R., Burt, M., McBride, T., & Meyer, J. (1990). *The needs of the elderly in the 21st century* (Urban Institute Rep. No. 90–5). Washington, DC: Urban Institute.

Zedlewski, S. R., & Schaner, S. G. (2006). *Older adults engaged as volunteers.* Retrieved January 3, 2007 from www.urban.org/publications/311325.html.

Zhan, L., Cloutterbuck, J., Keshian, J., & Lombardi, L. (1998). Promoting health: Perspectives from ethnic elderly women. *Journal of Community Health Nursing, 15*(1), 31–44.

Index

About the Authors

Robbyn R. Wacker, Ph.D., is Assistant Vice President for Research, Dean of the Graduate School and International Admissions, and Professor of Gerontology at the University of Northern Colorado in Greeley, Colorado. Her research interests include international aging social policy and psychosocial predictors of community service use among older adults. Prior to obtaining her doctorate, she provided legal assistance to older adults through the Title III Legal Services program. Along with her administrative duties, She continues to be an active researcher in the field of gerontology. She has published over 60 referred presentations, scholarly articles, books, and conference proceedings. She has earned numerous university and professional awards, including UNC's Academic Leadership Excellence Award, Outstanding Achievement Award in Sponsored Programs, and the Mortar Board Excellence Award for Teaching, and was selected by the Harvard Graduate School of Education to attend its summer Management Development Program for leaders in higher education.

Karen A. Roberto, Ph.D., is the Director of the Center for Gerontology, Interim Director of the Institute of Society, Culture, and Environment, and Professor of Adult Development and Aging at Virginia Polytechnic Institute and State University and Adjunct Research Professor of Community Medicine and Geriatrics at the Edward Via College of Osteopathic Medicine in Blacksburg, Virginia. Her research examines psychosocial aspects of aging. Within this realm, her primary focus is on older women's adaptation to life with chronic illness (e.g., osteoporosis, pain). Other research interests include family relationships and caregiving, health care decision making, and elder mistreatment. She has published over 100 scholarly articles and book chapters and is the editor/author of six books. She is a fellow of the Gerontological Society of America, the Association for Gerontology in Higher Education, and the National Council on Family Relations. In 2004 she received the Gordon Streib Academic Gerontologist Award from the Southern Gerontological Society, and in 2006 Virginia Tech awarded her the University Alumni Award for Excellence in Research.